THE ESSENCE OF

Shaolin White Crane

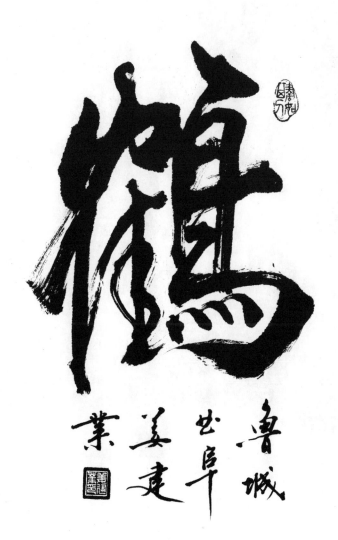

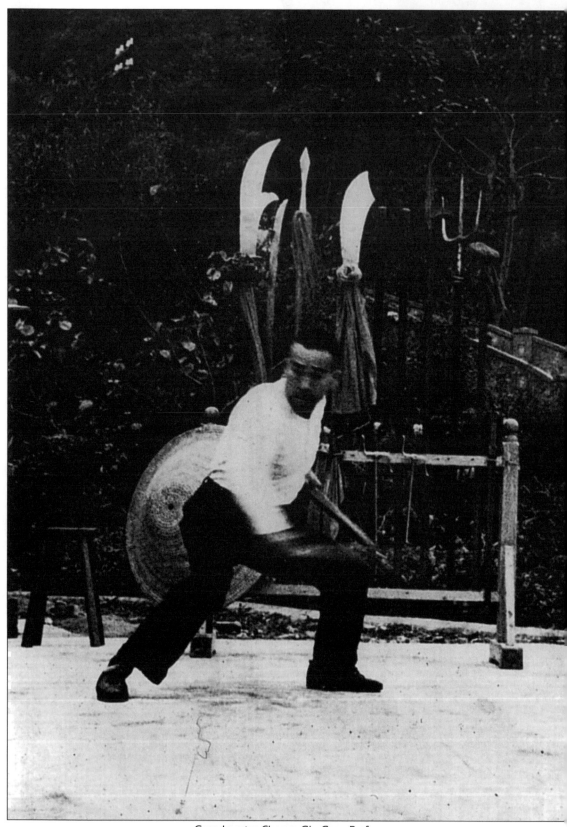

Grandmaster Cheng, Gin-Gsao Performs
Two-Short Rods (Shuang Jian), 1965

THE ESSENCE OF
Shaolin White Crane
MARTIAL POWER AND QIGONG

少林白鶴

Dr. Yang, Jwing-Ming

YMAA Publication Center
Jamaica Plain, Mass. USA

YMAA Publication Center
Main Office:
   4354 Washington Street
   Roslindale, Massachusetts, 02131
   617-323-7215 • ymaa@aol.com • www.ymaa.com

10   9

Publisher's Cataloging in Publication
(Prepared by Quality Books Inc.)

Yang, Jwing-Ming, 1946-
   The essence of Shaolin white crane : martial power and qigong / Yang
Jwing-Ming.
   p. cm.
   ISBN: 1-886969-35-3

   1. Martial arts—China. 2. Ch'i kung.   I. Title.

GV1100.7.A2Y36 1996   796.8'0951
                                          QBI96-20389

Printed in Canada.

Figure 8-14 modified from LifeArt by TechPool Studios Corp. USA, Copyright © 1994.

Disclaimer:
The author and publisher of this material are NOT RESPONSIBLE in any
manner whatsoever for any injury which may occur through reading or following the instructions in this manual.
The activities, physical or otherwise, described in this material may be too
strenuous or dangerous for some people, and the reader(s) should consult a
physician before engaging in them.

OTABIND

This book is bound
"Otabind" to lay
flat when opened.

THE ESSENCE OF
Shaolin White Crane
MARTIAL POWER AND QIGONG

少林白鶴

Dr. Yang, Jwing-Ming

YMAA Publication Center
Jamaica Plain, Mass. USA

YMAA Publication Center
Main Office:
4354 Washington Street
Roslindale, Massachusetts, 02131
617-323-7215 • ymaa@aol.com • www.ymaa.com

ISBN:1-886969-35-3

10   9

Publisher's Cataloging in Publication
(Prepared by Quality Books Inc.)

Yang, Jwing-Ming, 1946-
   The essence of Shaolin white crane : martial power and qigong / Yang
Jwing-Ming.
   p. cm.
   ISBN: 1-886969-35-3

   1. Martial arts—China. 2. Ch'i kung. I. Title.

GV1100.7.A2Y36 1996   796.8'0951
                                       QBI96-20389

Printed in Canada.

Figure 8-14 modified from LifeArt by TechPool Studios Corp. USA, Copyright © 1994.

Disclaimer:
The author and publisher of this material are NOT RESPONSIBLE in any
manner whatsoever for any injury which may occur through reading or following the instructions in this manual.
The activities, physical or otherwise, described in this material may be too
strenuous or dangerous for some people, and the reader(s) should consult a
physician before engaging in them.

This book is bound
"Otabind" to lay
flat when opened.

To My White Crane Master
Cheng, Gin-Gsao

謹奉獻給曾金灶師父

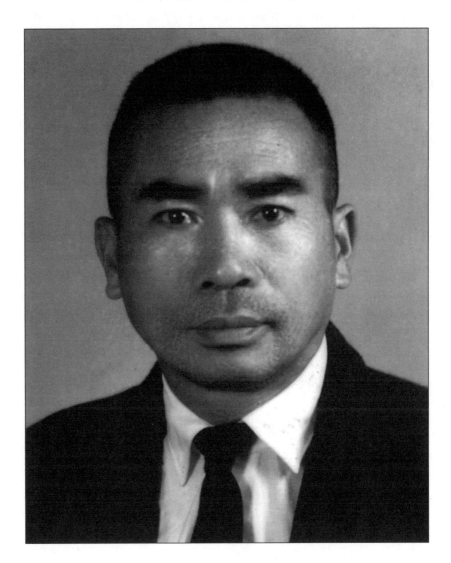

Proverbs:

"The Taller the Bamboo Grows, the Lower It Bows."

"The Truly Humble Always Know Others, and Do Not Care If Other People Know Them."

"Those Who Have to Criticize Others are Those Whose Minds are Void."

"The Yin Side of Dignity is False Pride and Self-Spite."

"Those Who Despise Themselves are Always Concerned With Their Dignity."

ACKNOWLEDGMENTS

Thanks to Tim Comrie for his photography, Jerry Leake for design and layout, and Deborah Clark for the cover design. Thanks also to Yang, Mei-Ling and Ramel Rones for general help, to Ray Ahles, Jeff Grace, Corlius Birkill, Marc Noblitt, Andrew Murray, Jeffrey Pratt, Doug Smith and many other YMAA members for proofing the manuscript and for contributing many valuable suggestions and discussions. Special thanks to James O'Leary for his editing, and a very special thanks to the artist Chow Chian-Chiu for his beautiful painting on the cover of this book.

ABOUT THE AUTHOR

Dr. Yang, Jwing-Ming, Ph.D.
楊俊敏

Dr. Yang, Jwing-Ming was born on August 11th, 1946, in *Xinzhu Xian* (新竹縣), Taiwan (台灣), Republic of China (中華民國). He started his *Wushu* (武術)(*Gongfu* or *Kung Fu*, 功夫) training at the age of fifteen under the *Shaolin White Crane* (*Bai He*, 少林白鶴) Master Cheng, Gin-Gsao (曾金灶). Master Cheng originally learned *Taizuquan* (太祖拳) from his grandfather when he was a child. When Master Cheng was fifteen years old, he started learning White Crane from Master Jin, Shao-Feng (金紹峰), and followed him for twenty-three years until Master Jin's death.

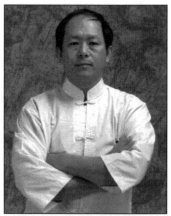

Dr. Yang, Jwing-Ming

In thirteen years of study (1961-1974 A.D.) under Master Cheng, Dr. Yang became an expert in the White Crane Style of Chinese martial arts, which includes both the use of barehands and of various weapons such as saber, staff, spear, trident, two short rods, and many other weapons. With the same master he also studied White Crane *Qigong* (氣功), *Qin Na* (or *Chin Na*, 擒拿), *Tui Na* (推拿) and *Dian Xue* massages (點穴按摩), and herbal treatment.

At the age of sixteen, Dr. Yang began the study of *Yang Style Taijiquan* (楊氏太極拳) under Master Kao Tao (高濤). After learning from Master Kao, Dr. Yang continued his study and research of *Taijiquan* with several masters and senior practitioners such as Master Li, Mao-Ching (李茂清) and Mr. Wilson Chen (陳威伸) in *Taipei* (台北). Master Li learned his *Taijiquan* from the well-known Master Han, Ching-Tang (韓慶堂), and Mr. Chen learned his *Taijiquan* from Master Chang, Xiang-San (張祥三). Dr. Yang has mastered the *Taiji* barehand sequence, pushing hands, the two-man fighting sequence, *Taiji* sword, *Taiji* saber, and *Taiji Qigong*.

When Dr. Yang was eighteen years old he entered *Tamkang College* (淡江學院) in *Taipei Xian* to study Physics. In college he began the study of traditional *Shaolin Long Fist* (*Changquan or Chang Chuan*, 少林長拳) with Master Li, Mao-Ching at the Tamkang College Guoshu Club (淡江國術社)(1964-1968 A.D.), and eventually became an assistant instructor under Master Li. In 1971 he completed his M.S. degree in Physics at the National Taiwan University (台灣大學), and then served in the Chinese Air Force from 1971 to 1972. In the service, Dr. Yang taught Physics at the Junior Academy of the Chinese Air Force (空軍幼校) while also teaching *Wushu*. After being honorably discharged in 1972, he returned to Tamkang College to teach Physics and resumed study under Master Li, Mao-Ching. From Master Li, Dr. Yang learned Northern Style *Wushu*, which includes both barehand (especially kicking) techniques and numerous weapons.

In 1974, Dr. Yang came to the United States to study Mechanical Engineering at Purdue University. At the request of a few students, Dr. Yang began to teach *Gongfu* (*Kung Fu*), which resulted in the foundation of the Purdue University Chinese Kung Fu Research Club in the spring of 1975. While at Purdue, Dr. Yang also taught college-credited courses in *Taijiquan*. In May of 1978 he was awarded a Ph.D. in Mechanical Engineering by Purdue.

In 1980, Dr. Yang moved to Houston to work for Texas Instruments. While in Houston he founded Yang's Shaolin Kung Fu Academy, which was eventually taken over by his disciple Mr. Jeffery Bolt after he moved to Boston in 1982. Dr. Yang founded Yang's Martial Arts Academy (YMAA) in Boston on October 1, 1982.

In January of 1984 he gave up his engineering career to devote more time to research, writing, and teaching. In March of 1986 he purchased property in the Jamaica Plain area of Boston to be used as the headquarters of the new organization, Yang's Martial Arts Association. The organization has continued to expand, and, as of July 1st 1989, YMAA has become just one division of Yang's Oriental Arts Association, Inc. (YOAA, Inc).

In summary, Dr. Yang has been involved in Chinese *Wushu* since 1961. During this time, he has spent thirteen years learning *Shaolin* White Crane (*Bai He*), *Shaolin* Long Fist (*Changquan*), and *Taijiquan*. Dr. Yang has more than twenty-eight years of instructional experience: seven years in Taiwan, five years at Purdue University, two years in Houston, Texas, and fourteen years in Boston, Massachusetts.

In addition, Dr. Yang has also been invited to offer seminars around the world to share his knowledge of Chinese martial arts and *Qigong*. The countries he has visited include Canada, Mexico, France, Italy, Poland, England, Ireland, Portugal, Switzerland, Germany, Hungary, Spain, Holland, Latvia, and Saudi Arabia.

Since 1986, YMAA has become an international organization, which currently includes 29 schools located in Poland, Portugal, France, Latvia, Italy, Holland, Hungary, South Africa, Saudi Arabia, Canada, and the United States. Many of Dr. Yang's books and videotapes have been translated into languages such as French, Italian, Spanish, Polish, Czech, Bulgarian, and Hungarian.

Dr. Yang has published twenty other volumes on the martial arts and Qigong:

1. ***Shaolin Chin Na***; Unique Publications, Inc., 1980.

2. ***Shaolin Long Fist Kung Fu***; Unique Publications, Inc., 1981.

3. ***Yang Style Tai Chi Chuan***; Unique Publications, Inc., 1981.

4. ***Introduction to Ancient Chinese Weapons***; Unique Publications, Inc., 1985.

5. ***Chi Kung — Health and Martial Arts***; YMAA Publication Center, 1985.

6. ***Northern Shaolin Sword***; YMAA Publication Center, 1985.

7. ***Tai Chi Theory & Martial Power*** (formerly *Advanced Yang Style Tai Chi Chuan, Vol.1, Tai Chi Theory and Tai Chi Jing*); YMAA Publication Center, 1996.

8. ***Tai Chi Chuan Martial Applications*** (formerly *Advanced Yang Style Tai Chi Chuan, Vol.2, Martial Applications*); YMAA Publication Center, 1996.

9. ***Analysis of Shaolin Chin Na***; YMAA Publication Center, 1987.

10. ***The Eight Pieces of Brocade***; YMAA Publication Center, 1988.

11. ***The Root of Chinese Chi Kung — The Secrets of Chi Kung Training***; YMAA Publication Center, 1989.

12. ***Muscle/Tendon Changing and Marrow/Brain Washing Chi Kung — The Secret of Youth***; YMAA Publication Center, 1989.

13. ***Hsing Yi Chuan — Theory and Applications***; YMAA Publication Center, 1990.

14. ***The Essence of Tai Chi Chi Kung — Health and Martial Arts***; YMAA Publication Center, 1990.

15. ***Arthritis — The Chinese Way of Healing and Prevention*** (formerly *Qigong for Arthritis*); YMAA Publication Center, 1996.

16. ***Chinese Qigong Massage — General Massage***; YMAA Publication Center, 1992.

17. ***How to Defend Yourself***; YMAA Publication Center, 1992.

18. ***Baguazhang — Emei Baguazhang***; YMAA Publication Center, 1994.

19. ***Comprehensive Applications of Shaolin Chin Na — The Practical Defense of Chinese Seizing Arts***; YMAA Publication Center, 1995.

20. ***Taiji Chin Na — The Seizing Art of Taijiquan***; YMAA Publication Center, 1995.

Dr. Yang has also published the following videotapes:

1. ***Yang Style Tai Chi Chuan and Its Applications***; YMAA Publication Center, 1984.

2. ***Shaolin Long Fist Kung Fu — Lien Bu Chuan and Its Applications***; YMAA Publication Center, 1985.

3. ***Shaolin Long Fist Kung Fu — Gung Li Chuan and Its Applications***; YMAA Publication Center, 1986.

4. ***Shaolin Chin Na***; YMAA Publication Center, 1987.

5. ***Wai Dan Chi Kung, Vol. 1 — The Eight Pieces of Brocade***; YMAA Publication Center, 1987.

6. ***Chi Kung for Tai Chi Chuan***; YMAA Publication Center, 1990.

7. ***Qigong for Arthritis***; YMAA Publication Center, 1991.

8. ***Qigong Massage — Self Massage***; YMAA Publication Center, 1992.

9. ***Qigong Massage — With a Partner***; YMAA Publication Center, 1992.

10. ***Defend Yourself 1 — Unarmed Attack***; YMAA Publication Center, 1992.

11. ***Defend Yourself 2 — Knife Attack***; YMAA Publication Center, 1992.

12. ***Comprehensive Applications of Shaolin Chin Na 1***; YMAA Publication Center, 1995.

13. ***Comprehensive Applications of Shaolin Chin Na 2***; YMAA Publication Center, 1995.

14. ***Shaolin Long Fist Kung Fu — Yi Lu Mai Fu & Er Lu Mai Fu***; YMAA Publication Center, 1995.

15. ***Shaolin Long Fist Kung Fu — Shi Zi Tang***; YMAA Publication Center, 1995.

16. ***Taiji Chin Na***; YMAA Publication Center, 1995.

17. ***Emei Baguazhang — 1; Basic Training, Qigong, Eight Palms, and Applications***; YMAA Publication Center, 1995.

18. ***Emei Baguazhang — 2; Swimming Body Baguazhang and Its Applications***; YMAA Publication Center, 1995.

19. ***Emei Baguazhang — 3; Bagua Deer Hook Sword and Its Applications***; YMAA Publication Center, 1995.

20. ***Xingyiquan —12 Animal Patterns and Their Applications***, YMAA Publication Center, 1995.

21. ***24 and 48 Simplified Taijiquan***; YMAA Publication Center, 1995.

FOREWORD

Master Liang, Shou-Yu

梁守渝

White Crane martial skills and *Gongfu* training have been popularly recognized as one of the most effective southern martial styles in China. It is a beautiful and brilliant flower of great renown, grown in the garden of Chinese *Wushu* (i.e., martial arts society). White Crane martial arts emphasize **the training of the *Yi*** (i.e., wisdom mind) **and the *Qi* internally**, demanding use of the *Yi* to lead the *Qi* (以意引氣), and **as the *Yi* arrives, the *Qi* also arrives** (意到氣到). When the *Qi* is manifested, awe is inspired (吐氣生威). The style includes a great variety of hand techniques, and trains "**moving the hands soft and reaching the target hard**" (運手柔，著手剛). It specializes in emitting the elastic-shaking *Jin* (trembling *Jin*)(彈抖勁), the stepping is light, agile, and firm.

Dr. Yang has practiced White Crane *Gongfu* since he was a youth. He has conducted profound study and research of the Ancestral Crane style (Jumping Crane)(宗鶴、縱鶴). When he practices his sequences, the manifestations of his shaking *Jin* and bumping *Jin* are very powerful. It is impossible to reach this stage if one has not practiced many years of refined *Gong* (i.e., hard refined study).

This book, ***The Essence of Shaolin White Crane*** is the foundation of White Crane *Gongfu*. It contains the most important and fundamental essence of the style. It is said: "**training fist without training *Gong*** (i.e., *Qigong*), **when old, all emptiness**" (練拳不練功，到老一場空).

In this book, other than introducing a general theory of *Qigong* and *Jin,* Master Yang introduces two complete sets of White Crane Hard *Qigong* and one complete set of White Crane Soft *Qigong.* These *Qigong* practices are seldom revealed to Western martial society. In addition, he profoundly discusses how to use torso, waist, and chest movements to manifest Shaking *Jin.* This is very helpful and useful for those martial artists who are interested in *Jin* manifestation. The reason for this is that it does not matter which style of martial arts a person has learned, the essential keys of using the torso, waist, and the chest to manifest the *Jin* remain the same. This is especially useful in applications during sparring and combat.

White Crane *Qigong* is useful not only for *Jin* manifestation. Because it emphasizes spine and chest movement, it is also very effective for improving health. Many illnesses arise out of the poor condition of the torso. White Crane Soft *Qigong* has proven to be one of the most effective means of strengthening and regaining health in the torso.

I deeply believe that this book is yet another valuable contribution from Dr. Yang to Western martial arts society.

Liang, Shou-Yu
September 7, 1995

PREFACE

It is commonly accepted that Okinawan *Karate* was heavily influenced by the Chinese White Crane style. In the last ten years, many readers — especially Okinawan *Karate* practitioners — have asked me to write a book about White Crane Martial Arts. However, I have been hesitant to do so. The reason for this is that it is very difficult to express the feeling of this art through words. I have been training this art for more than thirty years, and deeply realize that this art is like a piece of profound classical music or painting, the essence of which cannot be described correctly and easily in words. This is especially true if this book is to be used for instruction. It is not easy to teach through a book if a person is to write a piece of profound classical music or paint with the correct feeling.

White Crane style is very different from most other martial styles. The sequences within it are constructed from many moving patterns which manifest the *Jin* (martial power) of the style instead of the techniques themselves. From each *Jin* movement or pattern, many techniques can then be derived. The quality, depth, and number of techniques which can be derived from each pattern depends on how profoundly you have understood and felt the essence of each *Jin's* manifestation. If you do not catch this root, the art you derive will be shallow and often meaningless.

After having pondered for many years, I believe that the best way to pass this art down by word is first to emphasize White Crane *Qigong,* which will help the reader to build the root and foundation of the style. Only after a reader has practiced this *Qigong* for a long time and has understood the **feeling** and the essence of each *Qigong* pattern, both **internally** and **externally**, does it make sense that he or she may begin to apply this *Qigong* movement into the *Jin* patterns.

This is like learning how to paint. First, you must learn how to use a brush and then you apply this basic skill into the painting of an object. Only after long practice will you be able to create and place your own feeling into the art and make it alive.

I spent thirteen years learning White Crane from Master Cheng, Gin-Gsao (曾金灶), and did not even complete half of his training. Master Cheng learned his first martial art, *Taizuquan* (太祖拳), from his grandfather, and then White Crane from Grand Master Jin, Shao-Feng (金紹峰). In fact, most of his arts were obtained during twenty-three years of learning from Grandmaster Jin. After his master's death, he and three of his classmates stayed to protect their master's tomb for three years, then they separated. He then took up residence on *Gu Qi Feng* mountain (古奇峰) in my hometown, living like a hermit. Although Master Cheng could not read or write, his martial morality and talent reached one of the highest levels possible. Even though I spent thirteen years learning from him, I believe that, compared to him, what I know is still very shallow.

I left Taiwan and Master Cheng for the United States in 1974 to pursue my doctoral degree at Purdue University. Two years later, and unknown to me at the time, Master Cheng died of a stroke. After my graduation, I had my first vacation home in 1979. I went back to Taiwan to show my respect at his grave. In front of his tomb, I swore that I would not let the arts he taught me die; the knowledge he had passed down would not be buried under the ground. Since then, I have written many books and have become involved in converting Chinese culture into Western forms. For example, 60 to 70% of the techniques which I have documented in my *Qin Na* books originated with Master Cheng. In addition, due to my understanding of White Crane style I have a unique understanding of the essence of my *Taijiquan.* It was from this understanding that my *Taijiquan* books were written. The reason for this is that **White Crane is classified as a Soft-Hard style**. The soft side of its theory and essence remains the same in *Taijiquan.*

White Crane has a history which stretches back a thousand years, and throughout which many styles have been derived. Nevertheless, the theory of each style remains fundamentally the same. It is impossible for any individual, even a master, to understand and experience all of White Crane's variations. Therefore, you should remain humble and keep your eyes and mind open. You should treat this book only as a reference, which hopefully will guide you to the entrance of the style.

In the first part of this book, the general concepts of Chinese martial arts will be reviewed. Next, a basic summary of Chinese *Qigong* theory will be provided. The history and training theory of Southern White Crane martial styles will then be surveyed and discussed. In the second part of this book, the theory of Martial Arts *Qigong* will be introduced. From this theoretical foundation, the hard side and the soft side of White Crane Martial *Qigong* and its training methods will be introduced discussed. From this second part, you should obtain a strong foundation and a basic understanding of how martial arts power, called *Jin,* is manifested. Finally, in the third part of this book, *Jin* theory will be reviewed, followed by the introduction of various *Jin* practices in Southern White Crane styles.

This book proposes to be an authority on neither Chinese Martial Arts Qigong nor Southern White Crane martial arts training. Rather, it exists to offer you a reference to the author's personal knowledge and understanding. The main purpose of this book is to agitate and encourage other traditional Chinese martial artists to open their minds and share their knowledge with the general public. In addition, this book seeks to reveal the long hidden potential connection between Chinese White Crane styles and Japanese *Karate* styles.

Dr. Yang, Jwing-Ming
Dublin, Ireland
March 10, 1995

C O N T E N T S

Part I. General Concepts
基本概念

Chapter 1. About Chinese Martial Arts 中國武功介紹

Chapter 2. About Chinese Qigong 中國氣功介紹

Chapter 3. About White Crane Martial Arts 白鶴拳介紹

Part II. White Crane Qigong
白鶴氣功

Chapter 4. Theory 理論

Part III. White Crane Jin
白鶴勁

Part I

General Concepts

基本概念

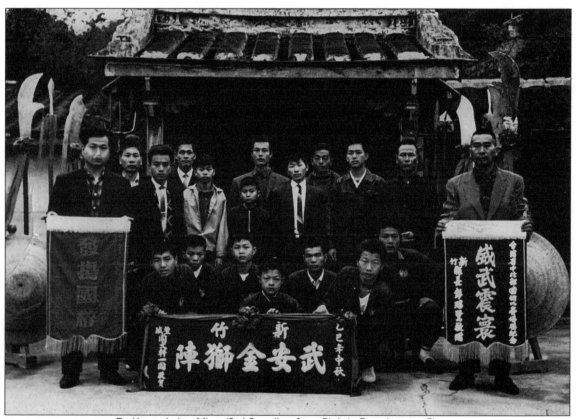

Dr. Yang, Jwing-Ming (3rd Standing from Right), Grandmaster Cheng,
Gin-Gsao (1st Standing from Right), and Dr. Yang's Classmates, 1965

Chapter 1

About Chinese Martial Arts

中國武功介紹

1-1. Introduction

The word for "martial" in Chinese is *"Wu"* (武). This word is constructed from two Chinese words *"Zhi"* (止) and *"Ge"* (戈). *"Zhi"* means "to stop," "to cease," or "to end" and *"Ge"* means "spear," "lance," or "javelin," and implies "general weapons." From this you can see that the original meaning of martial arts in China is **to stop or to end the usage of weapons** (止戈為武). *"Wushu"* (武術) means "martial techniques"; this implies the techniques which can be used to stop a fight. This means that Chinese martial arts were created to stop fighting instead of starting it. It is defensive instead of offensive. This concept was very different from that which was obtained by Western society in the 1960's. At that time, Chinese martial arts were commonly lumped together under the term *"Kung Fu"* (功夫) and were considered solely as fighting skills. In fact, the Chinese meaning of *"Kung"* (Gong, 功) means "energy" and *"Fu"* (夫) means "time." If you are learning or doing something which takes a great deal of time and effort to accomplish, then it is called *Gongfu* (Kung Fu). This can be learning how to play the piano, to paint, to learn martial arts, or to complete a difficult task which takes time and patience.

Even though Chinese martial arts were imported into Western society more than thirty years ago, many questions still remain. The most common and confusing questions today are: Where does the style I am learning come from? What are its theoretical roots and foundation? How good are the styles which I am practicing? What are the differences between the internal styles and the external styles? What are the differences between the southern styles and northern styles? How do we define hard, soft-hard, and soft styles? How is Japanese *Karate* different from Korean *Tae Kwon Do,* and how are these styles different from Chinese martial arts? How do these styles relate to each other? What is Martial Arts *Qigong?* How different is this *Qigong* from other schools of *Qigong,* such as Medical *Qigong,* Scholar *Qigong,* and Religious *Qigong?*

In order to answer these questions, you must first study and understand the history of Chinese martial arts. Furthermore, you should search and comprehend its theoretical roots and cultural background. **Knowledge of past history and an understanding of its roots will enable you to appreciate the consequences which exist today.**

Therefore, this chapter will first survey Chinese martial arts history and its cultural relationship with neighboring countries in the past. From this survey, you will obtain a general concept of how this art developed. Then, we will trace back how this art was developed and became popular today in the West. From this you will be able to analyze the style you are learning.

Next, we will summarize some of the important concepts in Chinese martial society, such as the differences between internal styles and external styles, how the southern styles developed differently from the northern styles, the definition of the hard, soft-hard, and soft styles, the four fighting categories of Chinese martial arts, and the *Dao* of Chinese martial arts.

Finally, I would like to remind the reader that embodying the martial moralities is more important than learning martial arts skills themselves. Learning martial arts is only a process of self-discipline which can promote your morality and spiritual level to a higher stage. Therefore, in the fourth section of this chapter, some of the martial moralities will be reviewed and discussed.

1-2. A Brief History of Chinese Martial Arts - East and West

It is impossible to survey the history of all the existing Chinese martial arts in a single book. There are two reasons for this.

A. Since ancient times, there have probably been more than five thousand martial styles created in China. After long periods of testing and experimenting in martial arts society or in battle, the arts of quality continued to survive, while those which were ineffective slowly became disregarded and died out. According to recent reports out of China, there could be more than one thousand martial styles which still exist and are practiced there, each with its own history. It is not easy to collect all of this history for every style.

B. Since most martial artists in ancient times were illiterate, the history of each style was often passed down orally. After a few generations, the history would become like a story. In fact, there are only a few existing famous styles, such as *Taijiquan, Shaolin Quan,* and some military martial styles, in which the history was documented in writing. Moreover, the documentation for these styles was extremely scarce and its accuracy often questioned.

Therefore, in this section, I would first like to briefly summarize a portion of the known history of the East. Then, based on my personal observations of the evolution of Chinese martial arts in the West for the past 22 years, I will offer my opinion and conclusion on Chinese martial arts in Western society.

1. Historical Survey of Chinese Martial Arts

Chinese martial arts probably started long before recorded history. Martial techniques were discovered or created during the long epoch of continuous conflict between humans and animals, or between different tribes of humans themselves. From these battles, experiences were accumulated and techniques discovered which were passed down from generation to generation.

Later, with the invention of weapons — whether sticks, stones, or animal bones — different types and shapes of weapons were invented, until eventually metal was discovered. At the beginning, metal weapons were made from copper, tin and/or bronze, and after thousands of years of metallurgical development, the weapons became stronger and sharper. Following the advancement of weapon fabrication, new fighting techniques were created. Different schools and styles originated and tested one another.

Many of these schools or styles created their forms by imitating different types of fighting

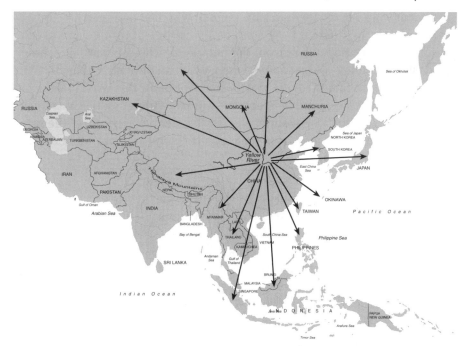

Figure 1-1. China and Her Neighboring Countries

techniques from animals (e.g., tiger, panther, monkey, bear or snake), birds (e.g., eagle, crane, or chicken), or insects (e.g., praying mantis). The reason for imitating the fighting techniques of animals came from the belief that animals possessed natural talents and skills for fighting in order to survive in the harsh natural environment. The best way to learn effective fighting techniques was by studying and imitating these animals. For examples, the sharp spirit of the eagle was adopted, the pouncing/fighting of the tiger and eagle's strong claws was imitated, and the attacking motions of the crane's beak and wings were copied.

Since the martial techniques first developed in very ancient times, they gradually became part of Chinese culture. The philosophy of these fighting arts and culture has in turn been influenced by other elements of Chinese culture. Therefore, the *Yin/Yang Taiji* theory was adopted into techniques, and the *Bagua* (Eight Trigrams) concept was blended into fighting strategy and skills.

Chinese culture initially developed along the banks of the Yellow River (黃河)(Figure 1-1). After many thousands of years, this culture spread out. It eventually spread so wide that it reached every corner of Asia. China is called *"Zhong Guo"* (中國), which means "Central Kingdom," by its neighboring countries. The reason for this was because China possessed a much longer developmental history in artistic, spiritual, religious, and scholastic fields, as well as many others; Chinese history stretches back more than seven thousand years. To the neighboring countries, China was an advanced cultural center from which they could learn and absorb cultural forms. Over thousands of years, the Chinese people themselves have immigrated to every corner of Asia, carrying with them their arts and customs. From this prolonged exchange, Chinese culture became the cultural foundation of many other Asian countries. Naturally, Chinese martial arts, which were considered a means of defense and fighting in battle, have also significantly influenced other Asian societies.

However, since the martial arts techniques and the methods of training could decide victory or defeat in battle, almost all Chinese martial arts were considered highly secret between countries, and even between different stylists. In ancient times, it was so important to protect the secret of a style that usually a master would kill a student who had betrayed him, in order to keep the techniques secret. It is no different from a modern government protecting its technology for purposes of national security. For this reason, the number of Chinese martial techniques which were revealed to outside countries was limited. Often, when an outlander came to China to learn martial arts, he first had to obtain the trust of a master. Normally, this would take more than ten years of testing from the teacher in order to achieve mutual understanding. Moreover, the techniques exported were still limited to the surface level. **The deeper essence of the arts, especially the internal cultivation of *Qi* and how to apply it to the martial techniques, normally remained a deep secret.**

For example, it is well known in China that in order to compete and survive in a battle against other martial styles, each martial style must contain four basic categories of fighting techniques. They are: **hand striking, kicking, wrestling,** and ***Qin Na*** (seizing and controlling techniques). When these techniques were exported to Japan, they splintered over time to become many styles. For example, punching and kicking became *Karate,* wrestling became *Judo,* and *Qin Na* became *Jujitsu.* Actually, the essence and secret of Chinese martial arts developed in Buddhist and Daoist monasteries was not completely revealed to Chinese lay society until the Qing Dynasty (1644-1912 A.D.). These secrets have been revealed to Western countries only in the last three decades.

There was an extreme scarcity of documentation before 500 A.D. with regard to martial arts organization and techniques. The most complete documents which exist today concern the *Shaolin* Temple. However, since *Shaolin* martial arts significantly influence the overwhelming majority of Chinese martial arts society today, we should be able to obtain a fairly accurate concept from studying *Shaolin* history. The following is a brief summary of *Shaolin* history according to recent publications by the *Shaolin* Temple itself.

The Shaolin Temple

Buddhism traveled to China from India during the Eastern Han Ming emperor period (東漢明帝)(58-76 A.D.)(Chinese emperors are given special names upon their coronation; it is customary to address them by this name, followed by the title "emperor"). Several hundred years after this, as several emperors became sincere Buddhists, Buddhism became very respected and popular in China. It is estimated that by 500 A.D., there probably existed more than ten thousand Buddhist temples. In order to absorb more Buddhist philosophy during these five hundred years, some monks were sent to India to study Buddhism and bring back Buddhist classics. Naturally, some Indian monks were also invited to China for preaching.

According to one of the oldest books, **Deng Feng County Recording** (*Deng Feng Xian Zhi,* 登封縣志), a Buddhist monk name Batuo (跋陀) came to China for Buddhist preaching in 464 A.D.[1.] Deng Feng was the county in Henan Province where the *Shaolin* Temple was eventually located.

Thirty-one years later, the *Shaolin* Temple was built in 495 A.D., by the order of Wei Xiao Wen emperor (魏孝文帝)(471-500 A.D.) for Batuo's preaching. Therefore, Batuo can be considered the first chief monk of the *Shaolin* Temple. However, there is no record regarding how and what Batuo passed down by way of religious *Qigong* practice. There is also no record of how or when Batuo died.

However, the most influential person in this area was the Indian monk Da Mo (達摩). Da Mo, whose last name was Sardili (沙地利) and who was also known as Bodhidharma, was once the prince of a small tribe in southern India. He was of the *Mahayana* school of Buddhism, and was considered by many to have been a *bodhisattva,* or an enlightened being who had renounced nirvana in order to save others. From the fragments of historical records, it is believed that he was born about 483 A.D.

Da Mo was invited to China to preach by the Liang Wu emperor (梁武帝). He arrived in Canton, China in 527 A.D. during the reign of the Wei Xiao Ming emperor (魏孝明帝)(516-528 A.D.) or the Liang Wu emperor(梁武帝)(502-557 A.D.). When the emperor decided he did not like Da Mo's Buddhist theory, the monk withdrew to the *Shaolin* Temple. When Da Mo arrived, he saw that the priests were weak and sickly, so he shut himself away to ponder the problem. When he emerged after nine years of seclusion, he wrote two classics: *Yi Jin Jing* (*Muscle/Tendon Changing Classic*, 易筋經) and *Xi Sui Jing* (*Marrow/Brain Washing Classic*, 洗髓經).

The *Yi Jin Jing* taught the priests how to build their *Qi* to an abundant level and use it to improve health and change their physical bodies from weak to strong. After the priests practiced the *Yi Jin Jing* exercises, they found that not only did they improve their health, but they also greatly increased their strength. When this training was integrated into the martial arts forms, it increased the effectiveness of their martial techniques. This change marked one more step in the growth of the Chinese martial arts: Martial Arts *Qigong*.

The *Xi Sui Jing* taught the priests how to use *Qi* to clean their bone marrow and strengthen their immune systems, as well as how to nourish and energize the brain, helping them to attain Buddhahood. Because the *Xi Sui Jing* was hard to understand and practice, the training methods were passed down secretly to only a very few disciples in each generation. Da Mo died in the *Shaolin* Temple in 536 A.D. and was buried on *Xiong Er* mountain (熊耳山). If you are interested in knowing more about *Yi Jin Jing* and *Xi Sui Jing,* please refer to the book, "***Muscle/Tendon Changing and Marrow/Brain Washing Chi Kung***" by YMAA.

During the revolutionary period between the Sui Dynasty (隋) and the Tang Dynasty (唐), in the 4th year of Tang Gao Zu Wu De (621 A.D., 唐高祖武德四年), Qin King Li, Shi-Ming (秦王李世民) had a serious battle with Zheng King Wang, Shi-Chong (鄭帝王世充). When the situation was urgent for The Qin King, 13 *Shaolin* monks assisted him against Zheng. Later, Li, Shi-Ming became the first emperor of the Tang Dynasty (618-907 A.D.), and he rewarded the *Shaolin* Temple with 40 Qing (about 600 acres) of land donated to the temple. He also permitted the Temple to own and train its own soldiers. At that time, in order to protect the wealthy property of the *Shaolin* Temple from bandits, martial arts training was a necessity for the monks. The priest martial artists in the temple were called "monk soldiers" (*Seng Bing,* 僧兵). Their responsibility, other than studying Buddhism, was training martial arts to protect the property of the *Shaolin* Temple.

For nearly three hundred years, the *Shaolin* Temple legally owned its own martial arts training organization, and continued to absorb martial skill from outside the temple into its training system.

During the Song Dynasty (960-1278 A.D.) *Shaolin* continued to gather more martial skills from outside of the Temple. They blended these arts into the *Shaolin* training. During this period, one of the most famous *Shaolin* martial monks, Jueyuan (覺遠) traveled around the country in order to learn and absorb high levels of martial skill into *Shaolin.* He went to Lan Zhou (蘭州) to meet one of the most famous martial artists, Li Sou (李叟). From Li Sou, he met Li Sou's friend, Bai, Yu-Feng (白玉峰) and his son. Later all four returned to the *Shaolin* Temple and studied together. After ten years of mutual study and research, Li Sou left Shaolin; Bai, Yu-Feng and his son decided to stay in *Shaolin* and became monks. Bai, Yu-Feng's monk name was Qiu Yue Chan Shi (秋月禪師). Qiu Yue Chan Shi is known for his barehand fighting and narrow blade sword techniques. According to the book ***Shaolin Temple Record*** (少林寺志), he developed the then existing Eighteen Buddha Hands techniques into One Hundred Seventy Three Techniques. Not only that, he compiled the existing techniques contained within *Shaolin* and wrote the book, ***The***

Essence of the Five Fist (五拳精要). This book included and discussed the practice methods and applications of the Five Fist (Animal) Patterns. The five animals included: **Dragon, Tiger, Snake, Panther,** and **Crane**. This record confirms that the Five Animal Patterns martial skills already existed for some time in the *Shaolin* Temple.

From the same source, it is recorded that in the Yuan Dynasty (元代), in the year 1312 A.D., the monk Da Zhi (大智和尚) came to the *Shaolin* Temple from Japan. After he studied *Shaolin* martial arts (barehands and staff) for nearly 13 years (1324 A.D.), he returned to Japan and spread *Shaolin Gongfu* to Japanese martial arts society. Later, in 1335 A.D. another Buddhist monk named Shao Yuan (邵元和尚) came to *Shaolin* from Japan. He mastered calligraphy, painting, *Chan* theory (i.e., Ren), and *Shaolin Gongfu* during his stay. He returned to Japan in 1347 A.D., and was considered and regarded a *"Guohuen"* (Country Spirit 國魂) by the Japanese people. This confirms that *Shaolin* martial techniques were imported into Japan for at least seven hundred years.

Later, when the Manchus took over China and established the Qing Dynasty, in order to prevent the Han race (pre-Manchurian) Chinese from rebelling against the government, martial arts training was forbidden from 1644 to 1911 A.D. In order to preserve the arts, *Shaolin* martial techniques spread to laymen society. All martial arts training in the *Shaolin* Temple was carried out secretly during this time. Moreover, the *Shaolin* monk soldiers had decreased in number from thousands to only a few hundred. According to the *Shaolin* Historical Record, the *Shaolin* Temple was burned three times from the time it was built until the end of the Qing Dynasty (1911 A.D.). Because the *Shaolin* Temple owned such a large amount of land and had such a long history, it became one of the richest temples in China. It was also because of this that *Shaolin* had been attacked many times by bandits. In ancient China, bandit groups could number more than ten thousand; robbing and killing in Chinese history was very common.

During Qing's ruling period, the most significant influence on the Chinese people occurred during the year 1839-1840 A.D. (Qing Dao Guang 20th year, 清道光二十年). This was the year that the Opium War between Britain and China broke out. After the loss of the War, China started to realize that relying on traditional fighting methods, using traditional weapons and barehands could not defeat guns. The values of the long, traditional Chinese culture were questioned. The traditional dignity and pride of the Chinese people started to quaver, and doubt that China was the center of the world started to arise. Their confidence and trust in self-cultivation started to break. This situation continued to worsen. In 1900 A.D. (Qing Guangxu 20th year, 清光緒二十年), when the joint forces of the eight powerful countries (Britain, France, The United States, Japan, Germany, Austria, Italy, and Russia) occupied Beijing in the wake of the Boxer Rebellion, Chinese dignity was brought to its lowest point. Many Chinese started to despise their own culture, which had been built and developed on principles of spiritual cultivation and humanistic morality. They believed that these traditional cultural foundations could not save their country. In order to save the nation, they needed to learn from the West. Chinese minds started to open and guns and cannons became more popular.

After 1911, the Qing Dynasty fell in a revolution led by Dr. Sun, Yat-Sen (孫中山). Due to the mind expanding influence of their earlier occupation, the value of traditional Chinese martial arts was re-evaluated, and the secrets of Chinese martial arts were gradually revealed to the public. From the 1920's to the 1930's, many martial arts books were published. However, this was also the Chinese Civil War period, during which Chiang, Kai-Shek (蔣介石) tried to unify the country. Unfortunately, in 1928, there was a battle in the area of the *Shaolin* Temple. The Temple was burned for the last time by Warlord Shi, You-San's (石友三) military. The fire lasted for more than 40 days, and all the major buildings were destroyed. The most priceless books and records on martial arts were also burned and lost.

It was also during this period that, in order to preserve Chinese martial arts, President Chiang, Kai-Shek ordered the establishment of the Nanking Central *Guoshu* Institute (南京中央國術館) at Nanking in 1928. For this institute, many famous masters and practitioners were recruited. The traditional name *"Wushu"* (martial techniques, 武術) was renamed *"Zhong Guo Wushu"* (Chinese martial techniques, 中國武術) or simply *"Guoshu"* (country techniques, 國術). This was the first time in Chinese history that under the government's power, all the different styles of Chinese martial arts sat down and shared their knowledge together. Unfortunately, after only three generations, World War II started in 1937 A.D., and all training was discontinued.

After the second World War in 1945, mainland China was taken over by communists. Under communist rule, all religions were forbidden. Naturally, all *Shaolin* training was also prohibited. Later, under the communist party, *Wushu* training was established at the National Athletics Institute (國家體育學院). In this organization, portions of the martial training and applications were purposely deleted by the communist party in order to discourage possible unification of martial artists against the government. From Chinese history, it is well known that almost all revolutions which succeeded did so due to the unification of Chinese martial artists. Sadly, only the aesthetic and acrobatic parts of the arts were preserved and developed. Eventually, it became known that the athletes trained during this period did not know how to fight or defend themselves. Performance was the goal of this preservation. This situation was not changed until the late 1980's. After the communist government realized that the essence of the arts — martial training and applications — started to die out following the death of many traditional masters, the traditional training was once again encouraged. Unfortunately, many masters had already been killed during the so-called "Cultural Revolution," and many others had lost their trust of the communist party, and were not willing to share their knowledge.

In order to bring Chinese *Wushu* into Olympic competition, China had expended a great deal of effort to promote *Wushu*. With this motivation, the *Shaolin* Temple again received attention from the government. New buildings were constructed and a grand hotel was built. The *Shaolin* Temple became an important tourist location! In addition, many training activities and programs were created for interested martial artists around the world. Moreover, in order to preserve the dying martial arts, a team called the "Martial Arts Investigation Team" (武術挖掘小組) was organized by the government. The mission of this team is to search for surviving old traditional masters and to put their knowledge in book or videotape form.

This situation was very different in Taiwan. When Chiang, Kai-Shek retreated from mainland China to Taiwan, he brought with him many well known masters, who passed down the Chinese martial arts there. Traditional methods of training were maintained and the arts were preserved in the traditional way. Unfortunately, due to modern new life styles, not too many youngsters were willing to dedicate the necessary time and patience for the training. The level of the arts has therefore reached the lowest level in Chinese martial history. Many secrets of the arts which were the accumulation of thousand years of human experience have rapidly died out. In order to preserve the arts, the remaining secrets began to be revealed to the general public, and even to Western society. It is good that books and videotapes have been widely used both in mainland China and Taiwan to preserve the arts.

Many of the Chinese martial arts were also preserved in Hong Kong, Indo-China, Malaysia, The Philippines, Indonesia, Japan, and Korea. It is widely recognized that now, in order to preserve the arts, all interested Chinese martial artists should be united and share their knowledge openly.

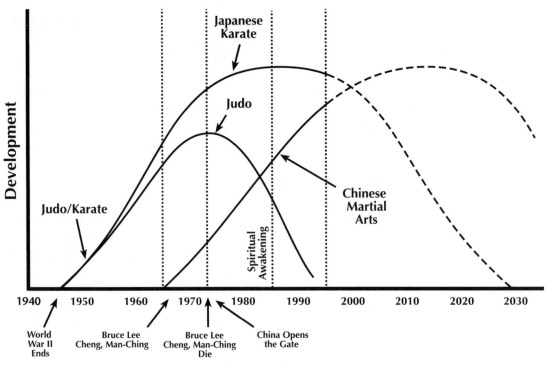

Figure 1-2. History of Oriental Martial Arts Development in Western Society

If we calm down and look backward at the martial arts history in China, we can see that in the early 1900's, the Chinese martial arts still carried the traditional ways of training. The level of the arts remained high. From then until World War II, the level of arts degenerated very rapidly. From the War until now, in my opinion, the arts have not even reached one-half of their traditional levels.

All of us should understand that martial arts training today is no longer useful for war. The chances for using it in self-defense have also been reduced to minimum compared to that of ancient times. This is an art whose knowledge has taken the Chinese thousands of years to accumulate. What remains for us to learn is the spirit of the arts. **From learning these arts, we will be able to discipline ourselves and promote our understanding of life to a higher spiritual level.** From learning the arts, we will be able to maintain healthy conditions in our physical and mental bodies.

2. A History of Chinese Martial Arts in the West

If we trace back the history of Chinese martial arts in Western society, we can see that even before the 1960's, *Karate* and *Judo* had already been imported into Western society and had been popular for nearly twenty years (Figure 1-2). Most Chinese culture was still isolated and conservatively hidden in communist China. Later, when Bruce Lee's (李小龍) motion pictures were introduced to the public, they presented a general concept of Chinese *Kung Fu (Gongfu)*, which stimulated and excited Western oriental martial arts society to a great level. This significantly influenced the young baby-boomer generation in America. During the period of unrest in America during the war in Viet Nam, these films provided both a heroic figure for young Americans to admire, as well as a positive Asian personality with whom they could easily relate. Many troubled youngsters started to abuse drugs during this time in an attempt either to escape from the reality and truth of the cruel world, or to prove to themselves that they had courage and bravery. Under these conditions, Bruce Lee's movies brought to the young generation both excitement and challenge. Since then, Chinese *Kung Fu* has become popularly known in Western society.

At that time the term *"Kung Fu"* was widely misinterpreted to mean "fighting," and very few people actually knew that the meaning of *"Kung Fu"* is "**Hard Work**"; an endeavor which normally requires a person to take a great deal of time and energy to accomplish. It was even more amazing that, after the young generation saw these movies, they started to mix the concepts from what they had learned from movies with the background they had learned from *Karate, Judo, Aikido,* and their own imagination. Since then, a new generation of American Styles of Chinese *Kung Fu* originated, and hundreds of new *Kung Fu* styles have been created. These practitioners did not know that the movies they had watched were a modified version of Chinese martial arts derived from Bruce Lee's Chinese martial art, *Wing Chun (Yongchun)* style. For cinematic purposes, they had been mixed with the concepts of *Karate,* Western Boxing, and some kicking techniques developed by Bruce Lee himself. At that time, there were only a very few traditional Chinese martial arts instructors residing in the West, and even fewer were teaching.

During this period Cheng, Man-Ching (鄭曼清) brought the concept of one of the Chinese internal martial arts, *Taijiquan,* to the West. Through his teaching and publications, a limited portion of the public finally grasped the correct concepts of a small branch of Chinese martial arts. This again brought to Western society a new paradigm for pursuing Chinese martial arts. *Taijiquan* gradually became popular. However, the American Style of Chinese *Kung Fu* still occupied the major market of the Chinese martial arts society in America. The Viet Nam War finally ended. When President Nixon levered open the tightly closed gate to mainland China in 1972, the Western public finally had a better chance to understand Chinese culture. From the more frequent communications, acupuncture techniques for medical purposes, used in China for more than four thousand years, were exported to the West. In addition, Chinese martial arts also slowly migrated westward. The period from the 1970's to the early 1980's can be regarded as an educational time for this cultural exchange. While the Americans' highly developed material sciences entered China, Chinese traditional medical and spiritual sciences (*Qigong*) started to influence American society.

During this period, many Western doctors went to China to study traditional Chinese medicine, while many Chinese students and professors came to America to study material sciences. In addition to this, many American Chinese martial artists started to awaken and re-evaluate the art they had learned during the 1960's. Many of the young generation went to China to explore and learn directly from Chinese authorities. It was a new and exciting period in the late 1970's and early 1980's. Because of the large market and new demand, many Chinese martial artists poured into America from China, Taiwan, Hong Kong, and Indo-China. However, this generated a great force which opposed the American Styles of Chinese *Kung Fu* created during the 1960's. The Chinese martial arts society was then divided more or less against each other. Not only that, martial artists who came from different areas of Asia also grouped themselves in camps against each other. Coordination and mutual support in Chinese martial arts for tournaments or demonstration was almost nonexistent.

Then, in the late 1980's, many American Chinese martial artists trained in China started to become aware of some important facts. They discovered that what they had learned emphasized only the beauty of the arts, and that martial purposes, which are the essence and root of the arts, were missing. They started to realize that what they had learned were arts which had been modified by the Chinese communist party in the 1950's. The actual combative Chinese martial arts were still hidden from lay society, and were passed down conservatively in traditional ways. Many of these artists were disappointed and started to modify what they had learned to transform their techniques into more martial forms, while many others started to learn from martial artists from Taiwan, Hong Kong, and Indo-China.

When mainland China finally realized this in the late 1980's, they decided to bring the martial purpose once again into the martial arts. Unfortunately, the roots of the beautiful martial arts which had been developed for nearly forty years were already firm and very hard to change. As mentioned earlier, the situation was especially bad when it was realized that many of the older generation of martial artists had either been killed by the Red Guard during the "Cultural Revolution," or had simply passed away. Those who controlled the martial/political power and could change the wrong path into the correct one had built successful lives in the beauty arts. The government therefore established the Martial Arts Investigating Team (武術挖掘小組) to find those surviving members of the old generation in order to preserve the arts through videotapes or books while still possible. They also started to bring sparring into national tournaments in hopes that through this effort, the real essence of the martial arts could be rediscovered. Therefore, *San Shou* (i.e., sparring, 散手) was brought back to the tournament circuit in the early 1990's. In *San Shou* training, certain effective fighting techniques were chosen for their special training, and each successfully delivered technique was allocated a point value. It was much like many other sports. However, the strange fact is that many *Wushu* athletes in China today do not know how to fight, and many *San Shou* fighters do not train *Wushu* at all. In my opinion, *Wushu* is *San Shou* and *San Shou* is *Wushu*. They cannot and should not be separated.

In Europe, Bruce Lee's movies also started a fashion of learning *Kung Fu*. People there were only one step behind America. Unfortunately, from 1960 to 1980, there were very few traditional Chinese martial artists immigrating to Europe. Few traditional masters taught in Europe, and they dominated the entire market. Later, in the early 1980's, many European martial artists went to mainland China, Taiwan, and Hong Kong to train for short periods of time in order to learn *Kung Fu*. Unfortunately, after years of training, they realized that it is very difficult to comprehend the deep essence of an art simply by studying a few months here and there. The situation was especially sad for martial artists who went to mainland China at that time. At the beginning of the 1990's, China significantly changed its training from gymnastic *Wushu* to more traditional styles. The worst thing that happened was, after many years of effort to bring *Wushu* into the Olympic games, China failed in its bid to host the summer games. China has since paid less attention to the development of *Wushu*. Even the young generation in China now treats *Wushu* as an old fashioned pursuit, and pays more attention to Western material satisfaction and political reform. The spirit of training has now been reduced significantly.

In America, since 1985 Mr. Jeffery Bolt and many other Chinese martial arts practitioners, such as Nick Gracenin, Pat Rice, Sam Masich, etc. have tried to unify the Chinese martial arts community in the hope of bringing together the great martial artists from China, Taiwan, Hong Kong, and Indo-China through tournaments and friendship demonstrations. Their ultimate goal is that these masters would become friends and finally promote Chinese martial arts to a higher quality. After ten years of effort, the organization, the United States of America Wushu-Kung Fu Federation (U.S.A.W.K.F.) was established. Although there are still many opposing forces and obstacles to this unification, I believe that the future is bright, and can foresee the continued success of this enterprise in the future.

1-3. Common Knowledge of Chinese Martial Arts

In order to clarify the confusion regarding some important Chinese martial arts concepts which commonly exist in Western martial arts society, this section will explain some essential

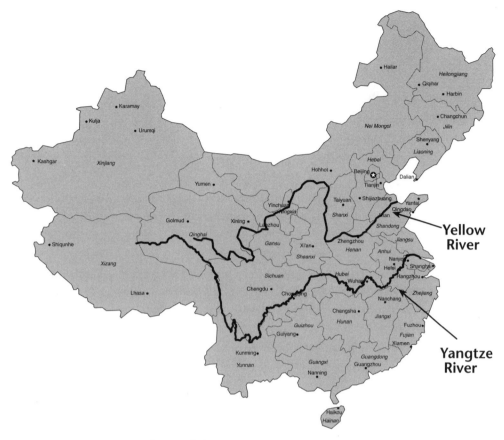

Figure 1–3. The Yangtze and Yellow Rivers in China

points, such as the differences between Northern Styles and Southern Styles, Internal Styles and External Styles. Hopefully, through study of this section, you will gain a better understanding of Chinese martial arts.

1. Northern Styles and Southern Styles

Chinese martial arts can be categorized into northern styles and southern styles. The geographic line making this distinction is the Yangtze River (*Chang Jiang,* 長江, which means Long River) (Figure 1-3). The Yangtze River runs across southern China from the west to the east.

Generally speaking, the northern region of the Yangtze River is bordered by large fields, highlands, and desert. For this reason, horse riding was common, like Texas in the United States. People in the north are more open minded compared to those of the south. The common foods are wheat, soybeans, barley and sorghum, which can be grown in the dry highlands.

In the southern region, there are more plains, mountains, and rivers. Rain is common in the south. Population density is much higher than that in the north. The common food is rice. Other than horses, the most common means of transportation is by boat. There is a common saying: "southern boats and northern horses" (南船北馬). This implies that the southern people use boats, while the northern people use horses for communications.

Because of a long history of development shaped by the above distinctions, the northern Chinese are generally taller than southern Chinese. It is believed that this is from the difference in diet. Moreover, northern Chinese are used to living in a wide open environment. After thousands of years of martial arts development, northern people perfected long range fighting, and therefore they preferred to use their legs more. This is not the case in southern China, which is more crowded and where the people, generally speaking, are shorter than those of the north. Moreover, because boats are so common, many martial techniques were actually developed to fight on boats. Since you must be steady on a boat, the techniques developed therefore emphasize hand techniques with a firm root. High kicks are limited.

From the above factors, we can conclude:

1. Northern Chinese are generally taller, and therefore prefer long or middle range fighting, while southern Chinese are shorter, so middle and the short range fighting are emphasized.

2. Northern styles emphasize more kicking techniques for long range fighting, while southern stylists specialize in more hand techniques and a limited number of low kicks. This is why it is commonly said: "southern fist and northern leg" (南拳北腿) in Chinese martial arts society.

3. Southern stylists focus on training a firm root, while northern stylists like to move and jump around. Moreover, northern martial stylists have more expertise in horse riding, and martial techniques from horse back, while southern martial styles specialize more in fighting on boats and on the ground.

4. Because southern styles generally emphasize more hand techniques, grabbing techniques such as *Qin Na* have developed more.

Many styles were created near the Yellow river which carried within them the characteristics of both northern and southern styles. For example, the *Shaolin* Temple is located in Henan Province (河南省), which is located just to the south of the Yellow river. The *Shaolin* Temple has trained both northern and southern styles for most of its history.

2. Internal Styles and External Styles

Before we go into the differences between internal and external styles, you should first recognize one important point: **all Chinese styles, both internal and external, come from the same root**. If a style does not share this root, then it is not a Chinese martial style. This root is the Chinese culture. Throughout the world, various civilizations have created many different arts, each one of them based on that civilization's cultural background. Therefore, it does not matter which style you are discussing; as long as it was created in China, it must contain the essence of Chinese art, the spirit of traditional Chinese virtues, and the knowledge of traditional fighting techniques which have been passed down for thousands of years.

Martial artists of old looked at their experiences and realized that in a fight there are three factors which generally decide victory. These three factors are **speed**, **power**, and **techniques**. Among these, speed is the most important. This is because, if you are fast, you can get to the opponent's vital areas more easily, and get out again before he can get you. Even if your power is weak and you only know a limited number of techniques, you still have a good chance of inflicting a serious injury on the opponent. The reason for this is there are many vital areas such as the eyes, groin, and throat, where you do not need too much power to make an attack effective.

If you already have speed, then what you need is power. Even if you have good speed and techniques, if you don't have power, your attacks and defense will not be as effective as possible. You may have met people with great muscular strength but no martial arts training who were able to defeat skilled martial artists whose power was weak. Finally, once you have good speed and power, if you can develop good techniques and a sound strategy, then there will be no doubt that victory will be yours. Therefore, in Chinese martial arts, increasing speed, improving power and studying the techniques, are the most important subjects. In fact, speed and power training are considered the foundation of effectiveness in all Chinese martial arts styles.

Moreover, it does not matter what techniques a style creates, they all must follow certain basic principles and rules. For example, all offensive and defensive techniques must effectively protect vital areas such as the eyes, throat, and groin. Whenever you attack, you must be able to access your opponent's vital areas without exposing your own.

The same applies to speed and power training. Although each style has tried to keep their methods secret, they all follow the same general rules. For example, developing muscle power should not be detrimental to your speed, and developing speed should not decrease your muscular power. Both must be of equal concern. Finally, the training methods you use or develop should be appropriate to the techniques which characterize your style. For example, in Eagle and Crane styles, the speed and power of grabbing are extremely important, and should be emphasized.

In Chinese martial arts society, it is also said: "**First, bravery; second, power; and third, Gongfu.**"[2] When the situation occurs, among the factors necessary for winning, the first and most crucial is how brave you are. If you are scared and nervous, then even if you have fast speed, strong power, and good techniques, you will not be able to manifest all of these into the action. From this proverb, you can see that compared to all other winning factors, bravery is the most important.

As mentioned earlier, it is generally understood in Chinese martial arts society that, before the Liang Dynasty (502-555 A.D.), martial artists did not study the use of *Qi* to increase speed and power. After the Liang Dynasty martial artists realized the value of *Qi* training in developing speed and power. It quickly became one of the major concerns in almost all styles. Because of this two part historical development, we should discuss this subject by dividing it into two eras. The dividing point should be the Liang dynasty, when Da Mo was preaching in China (527-536 A.D.).

It is generally believed that before Da Mo, although *Qi* theory and principles had been studied and widely applied in Chinese medicine, they were not used in the martial arts. Speed and power, on the other hand, were normally developed through continued training. Even though this training emphasized a concentrated mind, it did not provide the next step and link this to developing *Qi*. Instead, these martial artists concentrated solely on muscular power. This is why styles originating from this period are classified as external styles.

As mentioned earlier, Da Mo passed down two classics — the ***Yi Jin Jing*** (*Muscle/Tendon Changing Classic*) and the ***Xi Sui Jing*** (*Marrow/Brain Washing Classic*). The ***Yi Jin Jing*** was not originally intended to be used for fighting. Nevertheless, the martial *Qigong* based on it was able to significantly increase power, and it became a mandatory course of training in the *Shaolin* Temple. This had a revolutionary effect on Chinese martial arts, leading to the establishment of an internal foundation, based on *Qi* training.

As time passed, several martial styles were created which emphasized a soft body, instead *of* the stiff muscular body developed by the *Shaolin* priests. These newer styles were based on the belief that, since *Qi* (internal energy) is the root and foundation of physical strength, a martial artist should first build up this internal root. This theory holds that when *Qi* is abundant and full, it can energize the physical body to a higher level, so that power can be manifested more effectively and efficiently. In order to build up *Qi* and circulate it smoothly, the body must be relaxed and the mind must be concentrated. We recognize at least two internal styles as having been created during this time (550-600 A.D.): *Hou Tian Fa* (後天法) (Post-Heaven Techniques) and *Xiao Jiu Tian* (小九天) (Small Nine Heavens). According to some documents, these two styles were the original sources of *Taijiquan,* the creation of which is credited to Chang, San-Feng of the late Song Dynasty (around 1200 A.D.).[3]

In summary: The various martial arts are divided into external and internal styles. While the external styles emphasize training techniques and building up the physical body through some martial *Qigong* training, the internal styles emphasize the build up of *Qi* in the body. In fact, all styles, **both internal and external, have martial *Qigong* training**. The external styles train the physical body and Hard *Qigong* first, and gradually become soft and train Soft *Qigong,* while the internal styles train Soft *Qigong* first, and later apply the built up *Qi* to the physical techniques. It is said: **"Externally, train tendons, bones, and skin; and internally train one mouthful of *Qi.*"**[4] This means that it does not matter whether you are studying an external or an internal style, if you want to manifest the maximum amount of power, you have to train both externally and internally. Externally means the physical body, and internally means the *Qi* circulation and level of *Qi* storage in the body, which is related to the breathing.

It is said that: **"The external styles are from hard to soft and the internal styles are from soft to hard, the ways are different but the final goal is the same."**[5] It is also said: **"External styles are from external to internal, while internal styles are from internal to external. Although the approaches are different, the final goal is the same."**[6] Again, it is said: **"External styles first *Li* (muscular strength) and then *Qi,* while internal styles first *Qi* and later *Li.*"**[7] The preceding discussion should have given you a general idea of how to distinguish external and internal styles. Frequently, internal and external styles are also judged by how the *Jin* is manifested. *Jin* is defined as *"Li* and *Qi,"* (*Li* means muscular strength). It is how the muscles are energized by the *Qi* and how this manifests externally as power. It is said: "The internal styles are as soft as a whip, the Soft-Hard styles (half external and half internal) are like rattan, and the external styles are like a staff." If you are interested in this rather substantial subject, please refer to Dr. Yang's books ***Tai Chi Theory & Martial Power*** (formerly *Advanced Yang Style Tai Chi Chuan, Vol. 1*).

3. Martial Power — Jin

Jin training is a very important part of the Chinese martial arts, but there is very little written on the subject in English. Theoretically, *Jin* can be defined as **"using the concentrated mind to lead the *Qi* to energize the muscles and thus manifest the power to its maximum level."** From this, you can see that *Jin* is related to the training of the mind and *Qi.* That means *Qigong.*

Traditionally, many masters have viewed the higher levels of *Jin* as a secret which should only be passed down to a few trusted students. Almost all Oriental martial styles train *Jin.* The differences lie in the depth to which *Jin* is understood, in the different kinds of *Jin* trained, and in the range and characteristics of the emphasized *Jins.* For example, Tiger Claw style emphasizes hard and strong *Jin,* imitating the tiger's muscular strength; muscles predominate in most of the techniques. White Crane, Dragon, and Snake are softer styles, and the muscles are used relatively less. In *Taijiquan* and *Liu He Ba Fa,* the softest styles, Soft *Jin* is especially emphasized and muscle usage is cut down to a minimum.

The application of *Jin* brings us to a major difference between the Oriental martial arts and those of the West. Oriental martial arts traditionally emphasize the training of *Jin,* whereas this concept and training approach is relatively unknown in other parts of the world. In China, martial styles and martial artists are judged by their *Jin.* How deeply is *Jin* understood and how well is it applied? How strong and effective is it, and how is it coordinated with martial technique? When a martial artist performs his art without *Jin* it is called "Flower fist and brocade leg"

(花拳繡腿). This is to scoff at the martial artist without Jin who is weak like a flower and soft like brocade. Like dancing, his art is beautiful but not useful. It is also said "Train *Quan* and not *Gong,* when you get old, all emptiness."[8] This means that if a martial artist emphasizes only the beauty and smoothness of his forms and doesn't train his *Gong,* then when he gets old, he will have nothing. The *"Gong"* here means *"Qigong,"* (氣功) and refers to the cultivation of *Qi* and its coordination with *Jin* to develop the latter to its maximum, and to make the techniques effective and alive. Therefore, if a martial artist learns his art without training his *"Qigong"* and *"Jin Gong"* (勁功), once he gets old the techniques he has learned will be useless, because he will have lost his muscular strength.

Often *Jin* has been considered a secret transmission in Chinese martial arts society. This is so not only because it was not revealed to most students, but also because it cannot be passed down with words alone. *Jin* must be experienced. It is said that the master "passes down *Jin.*" Once you feel *Jin* done by your master, you know what is meant and are able to work on it by yourself. Without an experienced master it is more difficult, but not impossible, to learn about *Jin.* There are general principles and training methods which an experienced martial artist can use to grasp the keys of this practice. If you read Chapter 7 and Chapter 8 of this book carefully and practice patiently and perseveringly, and remember to remain humble, to question and ponder, you will no doubt be able to learn *Jin* and become a real master.

4. Hard Styles, Soft-Hard Styles, and Soft Styles

Chinese martial styles can also be distinguished from the ways they manifest *Jin* (martial power); they can thus be categorized into Hard, Soft-Hard, and Soft Styles. Generally speaking, the Hard Styles use more muscular power. In these styles, the *Qi* is led to the muscles or generated in the local area, then the muscles are tensed up to trap the *Qi* there in order to energize muscular power to its maximum efficiency. In order to reach this goal, once the *Qi* is led to the muscles, commonly the breath is held temporarily to trap the *Qi* in the muscles. Then, this muscular power is used for attack or defense. This kind of *Jin* manifestation is like using a staff to strike. It is easy for a beginner to manifest Hard *Jin.* When this power is used upon an opponent's body, external injury can be inflicted immediately. A typical Hard Style is Tiger Claw (虎爪), which imitates the tiger's use of strong muscular power for fighting. **With Hard *Jin*, because the muscles and tendons are more tensed in order to protect the ligaments of the joints, few injuries are caused from power manifestation.** This kind of *Jin* can be achieved more easily by beginners. Generally speaking, external styles are more likely to be Hard Styles.

The second category is Soft-Hard Styles. In these styles, the muscles and tendons remain relaxed, and the movements are soft to allow the *Qi* to move freely from the Lower *Dan Tian* to the limbs. Just before the attack reaches the opponent's body, suddenly the muscles and tendons are tensed. This kind of power is first soft and then hard. According to past experience, this kind of power is like the strike of rattan. When this Soft-Hard power is applied to the opponent's body, both external and internal injuries can be inflicted. The reason for softness at the beginning is to allow the *Qi* to move freely from the Lower *Dan Tian* to the limbs, and the reason for the hardening through tensing the muscles and tendons is to protect against pulling and damaging of the ligaments in the joints. It also offers the attacker strong physical support for the power, which can be bounced back from the opponent's body. Typical Soft-Hard Styles are White Crane (白鶴) or Snake (蛇).

Finally, the third category is Soft Styles. In these styles, the muscles and tendons are relaxed as much as possible to allow the *Qi* to circulate from the Lower *Dan Tian* to the limbs for striking. However, right before contact with the opponent's body, the physical body remains relaxed.

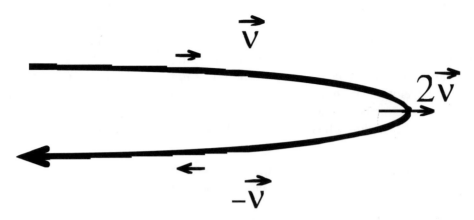

Figure 1–4. Whipping Speed

In order to protect the ligaments in the elbows and shoulders from being pulled and injured, right before the limbs reach their maximum extension, they are immediately pulled back. **From this pulling action, the muscles and tendons are tensed instantly to protect the ligaments, and then immediately relaxed again.** This action is just like a whip. Although the physical body is relaxed, the power generated is the most harmful and penetrating possible, and can reach to the deep places of the body. Therefore, internal injury or organ damage can occur. Naturally, this kind of *Jin* manifestation is dangerous for beginners. The reason for the penetration of the power is the whipping motion. Theoretically speaking, when you snap a whip forward with a speed V, and then pull back with another speed V, at the turning point between forward and backward, the speed at which the whip contacts the target is 2V (Figure 1-4). From here, you can see that speed in whipping is the key to power's penetration. This is like a surgical technology from the 1970's, in which water from a high pressure nozzle was used for cutting. Typical Soft Styles are *Taijiquan* (太極拳) and *Liu He Ba Fa* (六合八法).

At this point, we can superficially perceive the internal styles or Soft Styles and the external styles or Hard Styles. Consider Figure 1-5. The left line represents the amount of muscular power manifested, and the right line represents the *Qi* which is built up. From this figure, you can see that those styles which emphasize mostly muscular power or which use local *Qi* to energize the muscles are toward the left, while those styles which use less muscular power are toward the right hand side. Naturally, the more a style is toward the right, the softer and more relaxed the physical body should be, and greater concentration is needed to build up *Qi* and lead it to the limbs. We will discuss *Jin* in more detail in Chapter 7 of this book. The purpose of this section is only to offer you a simple idea of how *Jin* and different styles are related.

5. Four Categories of Fighting Skills

The name of Chinese martial arts has been changed from period to period. However, the most common name recognized is *"Wuyi"* (武藝). *Wuyi* means "martial arts," and includes all categories of martial arts which are related to battle. For example: archery, horse riding, dart throwing, the design and manufacture of weapons, armor, or even the study of battlefield tactics.

In actual combat, individual fighting techniques are called *"Wushu"* (武術), which means "martial techniques." After many thousands of years of knowledge accumulation and fighting experience, martial techniques can be divided into four major categories. These four categories are: kicking (*Ti,* 踢), hand striking (*Da,* 打), wrestling (*Shuai,* 摔), and *Qin Na* (*Chin Na*) (*Na,* 拿).

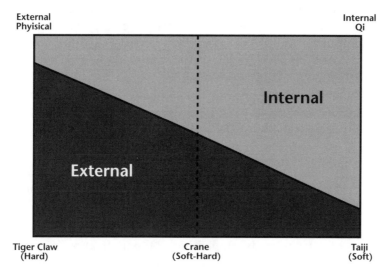

Figure 1–5. Hard Styles, Soft-Hard Styles, and Soft Styles

Kicking is using the legs to kick the opponent's vital areas, sweep the opponent's legs, or block the opponent's kicking. Hand striking is using the hands, forearms, elbows, or shoulders to block an attack or to strike the opponent. Wrestling is using grabbing, tripping, sweeping, bumping, etc. to make the opponent lose his balance, and then to take him down. Finally, *Qin Na* itself has four categories of techniques, including Sealing the Veins/Arteries, Sealing the Breath, Cavity Press, and Joint Locking.

Technically speaking, **wrestling techniques are designed against kicking and striking, *Qin Na* techniques are to be used in countering wrestling, while kicking and hand striking are used to conquer the techniques of *Qin Na* joint locking**. From this, you can see that all have special purposes and mutually support and can conquer each other. In order to make the techniques effective, all four categories of fighting techniques are required in any Chinese martial style.

As mentioned previously, when these techniques were imported into Japan, they were somehow divided into many different styles. For example, *Karate* specializes in hands striking and kicking, *Judo* excels in wrestling, and *Jujitsu* emphasizes joint locking skills. Finally, *Aikido* is a mixture of wrestling and *Qin Na*.

Truly speaking, in order to become a proficient martial artist, you must learn northern styles and also southern styles, allowing you to cover all ranges of fighting skills. You should also understand both internal and external styles. Although the basic theory of *Qi* cultivation for both styles is the same, the training methods are often quite different. Learning both internal and external styles will offer you various angles for viewing the same thing. Most importantly, in order to make your martial arts training complete, you should learn all four categories of fighting techniques. These four categories are often included in any Chinese martial arts style.

6. The Dao of Chinese Martial Arts

As mentioned at the beginning of this book, the most fundamental philosophy of Chinese martial arts is to stop the fight. The word "martial" (武) is constructed by the two Chinese words "stop" (止) and "weapons" (戈), and means to cease the battle. This concept is very important, especially in ancient times when there was even more violence and fighting between different races and nations than there is today. In order to protect yourself and your country, you needed to learn the martial arts. From this perspective, you can see that martial arts are defensive, and are a way of using fighting skills to stop actual fighting. If you examine Chinese history, you will see that even after China had become a huge country and its culture had reached one of the highest levels in the world, it never thought of invading or conquering other countries. On the contrary, throughout its history, China has tried to prevent invasion by the Mongols from the North, the Manchus from the North-East, and many small incursions from Korea and the tribes to its west. Even though China invented gun powder before even the Song Dynasty, except for a short period of time, it has never developed itself into a powerful killing weapon. If China had possessed the intention of conquering the world at that time, its military technologies were probably up to the task.

China's most basic human philosophies originated with Confucianism and Daoism. These philosophies emphasize peace, harmony, and the love of the human race. War is necessary only when it is needed for self-protection.

From this fundamental philosophy and cultural development, we can see that almost all the Chinese martial arts techniques were developed under the motivation for self-defense, and not for offense. However, there is one style called *"Xingyiquan"* (Shape-Mind Fist, 形意拳), which was created by Marshal Yue Fei (岳飛) during the Chinese Southern Song Dynasty (南宋) (1127-1278 A.D.), which emphasizes attack. If we consider the background of the creation of this style, we can understand why this style was created for offense. At that time, the Mongols had taken over the northern half of China and captured the Song emperor. For survival purposes, a new emperor was established and the empire moved to the South of China. At all times, the Chinese were preparing against an invasion by the Mongols. Martial arts training was one of the most important aspects of the country's affairs in order to survive. *Xingyiquan* was created as a military style, with which a person could reach a higher fighting capability in a short time. *Xingyiquan* trains forward movements instead of backward. Although the basic techniques are simple, they are powerful and effective. If you are interested in more information on *Xingyiquan,* please refer to the book **Hsing Yi Chuan- Theory and Applications**, by Master Liang, Shou-Yu and Dr. Yang, Jwing-Ming.

According to Chinese philosophy, in order to achieve harmony and peace with your enemy, when there is a conflict, you must not merely conquer his or her body. True power or capability for fighting is in showing your opponents that they do not have a chance of victory. Therefore, after a physical conflict, there should be spiritual harmony with your enemy. Only then can peace be reached. Killing and conquest can only produce more hate and killing in the future. In China, **the highest level of fighting is no fight**. If you are able to anticipate and avoid a fight, then you have won the war.

For example, there is a tavern near my studio. Occasionally, an inebriated person decides that he wants to come in and challenge the school. Often, this will agitate the students, and the younger ones want to fight. One time, a drunken Viet Nam veteran walked into the school and challenged them to fight. Again, some students were agitated and angry. I told them I would handle it this time. I politely and carefully approached him, asked his name and if there was anything that I could do to help him. He told me how strong and great he used to be, how brave he was in the war, and how well he was able to fight. I listened and nodded my head to show my acknowledgment of his past glory. After he saw that I was actually listening to his story, his manner became more gentle. Then, I asked him to sit down and told him I was busy with class right now; I would fight him after class if it was all the same to him. Next, I went to prepare some hot tea and gave it to him. I told him the tea would help him while he was waiting. Half an hour later, he woke up and sneaked out the door without being noticed. Since then, every time he passes the studio, he will smile and wave to me. Although we do not know each other deeply, at least we have become friends, and he has never bothered us again since then.

Another story was told to me by my Grandmother. A long time ago, there was a family that owned a small farm. The father worked very hard to make the farm successful, so that he would be able to leave it to his two sons when he died. The elder son, who was married, was named De-Xin (德信), while the younger son, who was not married, was named De-Yi (德義).

One day, the father became very sick, and he knew that he would soon die. He gathered his sons together and said to them, " I wish to give this farm to both of you. Share it equally, and help each other to make it successful. I hope that it makes you as happy as it has made me." With these words the father quietly passed away.

The sons divided the land equally, and set about the task of building their own farms. Even though they had divided the land, they still cooperated, helping each other with the more difficult chores. However, not long after the father died, De-Xin's wife decided that she and De-Xin had not received enough land. After all, De-Yi was single and didn't need as much land as they did. She began urging her husband to request more land from his brother.

Finally, after considerable provocation from his wife, De-Xin demanded more land from De-Yi. Because De-Xin was much bigger and stronger, the only thing De-Yi could do was to concede in angry silence, and let his brother occupy more land.

However, De-Xin's wife was still not satisfied. When she saw how easy it was to get more land from her brother-in-law, she again urged her husband to demand more land. Again, De-Yi could only consent to his brother's demands. Still, De-Xin's wife was not satisfied, and finally she demanded that De-Yi leave all the land to her and her husband.

De-Yi requested help from his relatives and friends, and begged them to mediate the conflict. No one would help. They knew it was unfair for De-Yi to be forced off his land, but they were afraid because they knew of De-Xin's violent temper.

Finally, De-Yi decided to take a stand for what he knew was right. He decided to stay, even though his brother wanted him to leave. For this defiance, De-Xin beat him very, very badly. De-Yi was finally forced to leave his home and become a traveling street beggar.

One day, while traveling in the Putian (浦田) region of Fujian Province (福建), he saw several *Shaolin* priests in town on an expedition to purchase food. He knew that the *Shaolin* monks were good in *Gongfu,* and he thought that if he could learn *Gongfu,* he could beat De-Xin and regain the land that was rightfully his. He decided to follow the monks, and when they reached the temple he would request that they accept him as a student of *Gongfu.*

When he arrived at the temple, he requested to see the Head Priest. The Head Priest welcomed him, and asked him why he had requested the meeting. De-Yi told the Head Priest his sad story, and asked to be taught *Gongfu* so that he could regain his land.

The Head Priest looked at him, pondered for a few minutes, and finally said, "De-Yi, if you are willing to endure the painfully hard training, then you are accepted as a student here." With deep appreciation, De-Yi knelt down and bowed to the Head Priest.

Early the next morning, De-Yi was summoned to the back yard of the temple. The Head Priest was standing in front of a young willow tree, holding a calf. He said to De-Yi, "Before you learn any *Gongfu,* you must first build up your strength. To do this you must hold this calf in your arms and jump over this willow tree fifty times in the morning and fifty times in the evening. De-Yi replied, "Yes, master. This is a simple task and I will do it every day."

From then on, De-Yi held the calf in his arms and jumped over the willow tree every morning and every evening. Days passed, weeks passed, months passed, years passed. The calf grew into a cow and the small willow tree grew into a big tree. Still, De-Yi held the cow in his arms and jumped over the tree.

One day, he requested to see the Head Priest. He asked, "Dear Master, I have held the cow and jumped over the willow tree for three years already. Do you think I am strong enough to train *Gongfu?*"

The Head Priest looked at him and the cow. He smiled and said: "De-Yi, you do not have to learn anymore. You have completed your *Gongfu* training. Your strength is enough to regain your lost land. You should take this cow home with you and use it to cultivate your land."

De-Yi looked at the Head Priest with surprise and asked: "If I have not learned any martial arts, what do I do if my brother comes to fight me again for my land?" The Head Priest laughed and said, "Do not worry, De-Yi. If your brother comes to fight you again, simply pick up the cow and run towards him. There will be no fight."

De-Yi half believed the Head Priest, but he also thought that perhaps the Head priest was joking with him. He took the cow and left the *Shaolin* Temple. When he arrived home, he started to cultivate his land.

De-Xin soon discovered his brother's return. He decided to beat up his young brother again and teach him an unforgettable lesson. After that, De-Yi would never dare to return. When De-Yi came to the rice field, he saw his brother running towards him, shouting in anger.

When De-Yi saw his brother running toward him, he remembered what the Head Priest had said and immediately picked up the cow and ran towards his brother. This surprised and shocked De-Xin. He just could not believe that his brother possessed such strength. He turned around and ran away, never to return again.

From this story, I learned two lessons. The first is that you need patience and endurance to succeed. Big success always comes from many little efforts. The second lesson is that the best way to win a fight is without fighting. Often you can win a fight with wisdom, and this is better than beating up someone.

I remember that my White Crane master told me something that affected my perspective of Chinese martial arts completely. He told me that the goal of a martial artist's learning was not fighting. It is neither for showing off nor for proving you are capable of conquering other people. He said **the final goal of learning is to discover the meaning of life. Therefore, what I was learning from him was not a martial art, but the way of life**. I could not accept this concept when I was young. However, now I am fifty. I can start to understand what he meant.

In the last twenty years, I have had many questions in my mind. Why are we here? What do we expect ourselves to accomplish in our lifetime? Do we come to this life as just an animal, without a deep meaning, or do we come to this life to comprehend and to experience the deep meaning of our lives?

In my opinion, there are many ways of understanding the meaning of life. You can learn piano with all of your effort (energy and time). From the learning process, you learn to know yourself and to discipline yourself. Finally, you achieve the capability to use your wisdom mind to control your emotional mind, and reach a high stage of spiritual understanding of your life. Often, whenever I listen to music composed by Beethoven, Mozart, or another great composer or musician, I am so touched and inspired. I always wonder how these people could create such a high spiritual level of music which influences the human race for hundreds of years. I deeply believe that in order for them to reach such a deep level of understanding, they must have gone through the same process of emotional and physical self-conquest. I believe that through music, these composers comprehended the meaning of their lives. Naturally, the meaning may well be beyond our understanding. However, their spirit has always inspired the following generations.

Naturally, you may also learn painting or any art which can cultivate your spirit to a higher level. However, it does not matter which way you choose — in order to reach to a high level of spiritual growth, you must face your biggest enemy. This enemy is yourself. **The only way to defeat this enemy is through self-discipline and an understanding of life.**

For example, have you ever thought about why the highest levels of Chinese martial arts were always created either in Buddhist or Daoist monasteries? Why has it been monks who have developed all these deadly martial arts? One of the main reasons, as explained earlier, was self-defense against the bandits. However, the other reason is that, through training martial arts, you learn how to use your wisdom mind to conquer or control your emotional mind. This is one of the most effective ways of reaching a high level of spiritual understanding of life.

I also remember a story told to me by my master about a very famous archer, Yang, You-Ji (養由基), who lived during the Chinese Spring and Autumn period (722-481 B.C.) (春秋). When Yang, You-Ji was a teenager, he was already well-known for his superior skill in archery. Because of this, he was very proud of himself. One day, he was in his study, when he heard the call of an oil seller just outside his house. Curious, he went out of his house and saw an old man selling cooking oil on the street. He saw the old man place the oil jar, which had a tiny hole the size of the coin, on the ground and then use the ladle to scoop a full measure of oil and pour it from chest height into the jar without losing a single drop, or even touching the sides of the hole. Yang, You-Ji was amazed at this old man's steady hand, and the accuracy with which he was able to pour the oil into the jar. He asked the old man: "Old man, how did you do that?" (To call an aged person old man in China is not impolite, but a sign of respect.) The old man looked at him, the well-known teenage archer of the village, and said: "Young man, would you like to see more?" The young man nodded his head.

The old man then asked him to go into the house and bring out a bench. The old man placed a Chinese coin, which had a very tiny hole in the center for threading purposes, on the hole in the jar. Then, the old man ladled a full scoop of oil and climbed onto a bench. Standing on the bench, he poured the oil all the way down from such a high place, through the hole in the coin and into the jar. This time, Yang, You-Ji kept his eyes wide open, and was shocked at the old man's amazing skill. He asked the old man: "How did you do that? I have never seen such an amazing thing before." The old man looked at him and smiled. He said: "There is nothing but practicing."

Suddenly, Yang, You-Ji understood that his archery was good because he practiced harder than others. There was nothing of which to be proud. Thereafter, he became very humble and practiced even harder. When he reached his thirties, he was considered the best archer in the entire country, and was honored to serve the emperor as a body guard. But in his late fifties, he disappeared from the palace, and nobody ever knew where he went.

Twenty years later, one of his friends heard that Yang, You-Ji was on Tian Mountain of Xinjiang Province (天山，新疆), and decided to find him. After months of traveling, he finally arrived at the mountain and located his friend. He stepped in Yang's house and they recognized each other. However, when Yang saw his friend's bow and arrow on his shoulder, he opened his eyes and said: "What are those funny things you are carrying on your back?" His friend looked at him and with mouth agape and said: "Wao! You must be the best archer existing today, since you have already gone through the entire experience of archery."

When I heard this story, I could not understand its actual meaning. Now, I begin to under-stand. **Everything we have experienced before is just one learning process in reaching the**

spirit of our life. Once this learning is completed, the process of learning is no longer necessary and ceases to exist. It is just like the Buddhists who believe that our physical body is only used to cultivate our spirit; once you have reached a high level of spirit, the physical body is no longer important.

Learning martial arts is the same. You are using the way of learning martial arts to understand the meaning of your life. The higher you have reached, the better you experience the spirit which is beyond other martial artists. One day, you will no longer be able to train or perform martial arts. However, your understanding and spirit will remain there, and you will retain your knowledge and spirit.

Next, you should understand that **the arts are alive and are creative**. To Chinese philosophy, if an art is not creative, then the art is dead. It is also because the art is creative that, after hundreds of years of development and creation, there can be many styles of the same art.

One afternoon, I went to visit my master and asked him why the same movement was applied differently by two of my classmates. He looked at me and asked: "Little Yang! How much is one plus one?" Without hesitation, I said: "Two." He smiled and shook his head, and said: "No! Little Yang, it is not two." I was confused and thought he was joking. He continued: "Your father and your mother together are two. After their marriage, they have five children. Now, it is not two but seven. You can see one plus one is not two but seven. The arts are alive and creative. If you treat them as dead, it is two. But if you make them alive, they can be many. This is the philosophy of developing Chinese martial arts. Now, I am forty-two; when you reach forty-two, if your understanding about the martial arts is the same as mine today, then I will have failed you, and also you will have failed me."

This also reminds me of a story I heard from Master Liang, Shou-Yu a few years ago. He said he knew a story of how Master Chang, San-Feng taught the *Taiji* Sword techniques to one of his students. He said, after a student completed his three years of *Taiji* Sword learning from Master Chang, he was so happy and could perform every movement in exactly the same way and feeling as Master Chang had taught him.

Then, Master Chang asked him to leave and practice for three years, and then come to see him. The student left. After three years of hard practice, the student came to see Master Chang. However, he was sad and ashamed to meet Master Chang. He bowed his head down and felt so sorry. He said to Master Chang: "Master Chang, after three years of practice, I am now very sad. The more I have practiced, the more I have lost the feeling I had three years ago. Now, I feel about a third of the forms are different from what you taught me originally."

Master Chang looked at him and said: "No good! No good! Go home and practice another three years and then come to see me." The student left in sorrow and sadness. He practiced harder and harder for the next three years. Then, he came to see Master Chang again. However, he felt even worse than the first time he came back. He looked at Master Chang very disappointedly. He said: "Master Chang! I don't know why. The more I have practiced, the worse it has become. Now, two thirds of the forms feel different from what you taught me."

Master Chang again looked at him and said: "No good! No good! Go home again and practice another three years and then come to see me." The student left very very sadly. This time, he practiced even harder than before. He put all his mind into understanding and feeling every movement of the forms he learned. After three years, again he returned to see Master Chang. This time, his face turned pale and he dared not look at Master Chang's face directly. He said: "Master Chang! I am sorry. I am a failure. I have failed you and myself. I feel now not even one form has the same feeling as you taught me."

When Master heard of this, he laughed loudly and very happily. He looked at the student and said: "Great! You have done well. Now, the techniques you have learned are yours and not mine anymore."

From this story, you can see that **the mentality of the arts is creative**. If the great musician Beethoven, after he learned all the techniques from his teacher never learned to create, then he would not have become so great. It is the same with the great painter Picasso. If he did not know how to be creative, then after he learned all the painting techniques from his teacher, he would never have become such a genius. Therefore, you can see that arts are alive and not dead. However, if you do not learn enough techniques and have not reached a deep level of understanding, then when you start to create, you will have lost the correct path and the arts will be flawed. It is said in Chinese martial arts society that: ""*Sifu* leads you into the door, cultivation depends on oneself."[9]

Furthermore, when you learn any art, you should understand **the mentality of learning is to feel and to gain the essence of the art**. Only if your heart can teach the essence of the arts, then will you have gained the root. With this root, you will be able to grow and become creative.

My master told me a story. Once upon a time a boy came to see an old man and asked him: "Honorable old man, I have heard that you are able to change a piece of rock into gold. Is that true?" "Yes, young man. Like others, do you want a piece of gold? Let me change one for you." The boy replied. "Oh no! I do not want a piece of gold. What I would like is to learn the trick you use to change rocks into gold."

What do you think about this short story? When you learn anything, if you do not gain the essence of the learning, you will remain on the surface, just holding the branches and flowers. However, if you are able to feel the arts deeply, then you will be able to create. **Feeling deeply enables you to ponder and finally to understand the situation.** Without this deep feeling, what you see will be only on the surface.

Once there was a wise king in Korea who had a fifteen year old son. This son had grown up comfortably in the palace, with all of the servants' attention. This made the king very worried, and he believed that his son would never be a good king whose concern was for his people. Therefore, he summoned a well known wise old man living in the deep woods.

In response to this call, the old man came to the palace. After he promised to teach the prince to be a wise, good king, he took the prince to the deep woods. After they arrived in the deep woods, the old man taught the young prince how to find food, how to cook, and how to survive in the jungle. Then he left the prince alone in the woods. However, he promised that he would come back a year later.

A year later, when the old man came back, he asked the prince what he thought about the woods. The prince replied: "I am sick of them. I need a servant. I hate it here. Take me home." However, the old man merely said: "Very good. That is good progress, but not enough. Please wait here for another year, and I will be back to see you again." Then, he left again.

A year again passed, and the old man came back to the woods, asking the prince again the same question. This time the prince said: "I see birds, I see trees, I see flowers and animals." His mind had started to accept the surrounding environment, and he recognized his role in the jungle. The old man was satisfied and said: "This is great progress. However, it is not enough, and therefore you must stay here for another year." This time, the prince was not even upset and said: "No problem." Once again, the old man left.

Another year passed, and the old man came back again. This time, when the old man asked the prince what he thought, the prince said: "I feel birds, woods, fish, animals, and many things around me here." This time, the old man was very happy and said: "Now I can take you home. If you can feel the things happening around you, then you will be able to concern yourself with the people's feelings, and you will be a good king." Then, the old man took him home.

This story is only to tell you that, when you do anything, you must put your mind into it, feel it, taste it, and experience it. Only then may you say that you understand it. **Without this deep feeling and comprehension, the arts you create will be shallow and lose their essence.**

Finally, I would like to point out an important thing. Normally, after more than thirty years of learning, studying, pondering, and practicing, all masters have experienced most of the possible creations of their art, and their understanding of it has reached to a very deep level. It is common that the master will keep this personal secret to himself until he has found someone he can really trust. This is often called the secret of the art.

There is another story which was told to me by Master Liang, Shou-Yu. About fifty years ago, there was a very famous clay doll maker in Beijing. Because he was so famous, he had many students. However, it did not matter how, when people purchased a doll, they could always tell which ones were made by the master and which ones were made by the students. It also did not matter how the students tried and pondered, they could not catch the secret of their master. They continued to believe that their master's dolls were better because he had more years of experience.

One day, this master became very sick and was dying. After he realized that he would die soon, he decided to reveal his last secret to his most trustworthy student. He summoned his student to his bed, and said: "You are the student whom I can trust most. You have been loyal to me in the past. Here, I would like to tell you the last of my secrets. But remember, **if you keep this secret to yourself, you will always enjoy wealth and glory. However, if you reveal it to everyone else, then you will be as poor as others**." Then he asked this student to make a doll in front of him.

Not long after, this student had completed his doll. Although the doll was well made, it looked like a student's doll instead of the master's. Then, the master looked at the student and said: "The difference between your doll and my doll is the expression on the face. The expression of the face must be natural and delightful. This is the final trick for you to remember." Then, he placed his index finger under the chin of the wet clay doll, and gently pushed the chin slightly upward. Immediately, the facial expression of the doll changed and became very natural. Now, the doll looked like the master's.

From this, you can see that normally, a secret is hidden in the obvious place. A practitioner can realize this secret suddenly when time passes by through continued pondering and practice. It is said in Chinese martial arts society that: "The great *Dao* is no more than two or three sentences. Once spoken, it is worth less than three pennies."[10]

From the above stories, you may have understood that **the creation of an in-depth art comes from continued learning, pondering, and practice**. Only then will the spirit of the art be high, and the art created be profound.

Conclusions:

1. Chinese martial arts were created mainly for defense, and not for offense.
2. The best fight is "the fight of no fight."
3. The reason for learning arts is to find and to understand yourself. From this understanding, you can promote the meaning of your life to a higher spiritual level.

4. The arts are creative. It is the same in Chinese martial arts. After you have learned and practiced for a long time, then you should blend what you have learned with your own ideas to make the arts even greater.

5. A deeply touching art is created from deep spiritual feelings. It is not an outward form. Forms are only the manifestation of the internal feeling.

6. The greatest secret is hidden in the most obvious place, and can only be obtained from continued pondering and practice.

1-4. Martial Moralities

Martial morality has always been a required discipline in Chinese martial arts society. Before you learn any martial techniques, you should first understand this subject.

In Chinese martial arts society, it is well known that a student's success is not determined by his external appearance, nor by how strong or weak he is, but rather by the student's way of thinking and his morality. Chinese martial artists have a saying: "A student will spend three years looking for a good teacher, and a teacher will test a student for three years." A wise student realizes that it is better to spend several years looking for a good teacher than to spend the time learning from a mediocre one. **A good teacher will lead you to the right path, and will help you to build a strong foundation for your future training**. A teacher who is not qualified, however, will not help you build a strong foundation, and may even teach you many bad habits. In addition, **good teachers will always set a good example for their students with their spiritual and moral virtue**. Good martial arts teachers do not teach only martial techniques, they also teach a way of life.

From a teacher's perspective, it is very hard to find good students. When people have just begun their studies, they are usually enthusiastic and sincere, and they are willing to accept discipline and observe proper manners. However, as time passes, you gradually get to see what they are really like, and sometimes it's quite different from how they acted in the beginning. Because of this, teachers quite frequently spend at least three years watching and testing students before they decide whether they can trust them and pass on to them the secrets of their style. This was especially so in ancient times when martial arts were used in wars, and fighting techniques were kept secret.

Martial Morality is called *"Wude"* (武德). Teachers have long considered *Wude* to be the most important criterion for judging students, and they have made it the most important part of the training in the traditional Chinese martial arts. *Wude* includes two aspects: the morality of deed and the morality of mind. Morality of deed includes: **Humility, Respect, Righteousness, Trust, and Loyalty**. Morality of mind consists of: **Will, Endurance, Perseverance, Patience,** and **Courage**. Traditionally, only those students who had cultivated these standards of morality were considered to be worthy of teaching. Of the two aspects of morality, the morality of deed is more important. The reason for this is very simple. Morality of deed concerns the student's relationship with master and classmates, other martial artists, and the general public. Students who are not moral in their actions are not worthy of being taught, since they cannot be trusted or even respected. Furthermore, without morality of deed, they may abuse the art and use their fighting ability to harm innocent people. Therefore, masters will normally watch their students carefully for a long time until they are sure that the students have matched their standards of morality of deed before letting them start serious training.

Morality of mind is for the self-cultivation which is required to reach the final goal. The Chinese consider that we have two minds, an "Emotional mind" (*Xin,* 心) and a "Wisdom mind" (*Yi,* 意). Usually, when a person fails in something it is because the emotional mind has dominated their thinking. The five elements in the morality of mind are the keys to training, and they lead the student to the stage where the wisdom mind can dominate. This self-cultivation and discipline should be the goal of any martial arts training philosophy.

Next, we will discuss these requirements of morality.

Martial Morality

(Wude, 武德)

Morality of Deed:

1. Humility (*Qian Xu;* 謙虛)

Humility comes from controlling your feelings of pride. In China it is said: "Satisfaction (i.e., pride) loses, humility earns benefits."[11] When you are satisfied with yourself, you will not think deeply, and you will not be willing to learn. However, if you remain humble, you will always be looking for ways to better yourself, and you will keep on learning. Remember, there is no limit to knowledge. It does not matter how deep you have reached, there is always a deeper level. Confucius said, "If three people walk by, there must be one of them who can be my teacher."[12] There is always someone who is more talented or more knowledgeable than you in some field. The Chinese say: "There is always a man beyond the man, there is a sky above the sky."[13] Since this is so, how can you be proud of yourself?

I remember a story that my White Crane master told me when I was seventeen years old. Once there was a bamboo that had just popped up out of the ground. It looked at the sky and smiled, and said to itself, "Someone told me that the sky is so high that it cannot be reached. I don't believe that's true." The sprout was young and felt strong. It believed that if it kept growing, one day it could reach the sky. So it kept growing and growing. Ten years passed, twenty years passed. Again it looked at the sky. The sky was still very high, and it was still far beyond its reach. Finally, it realized something, and started to bow down. The more it grew the lower it bowed. My teacher asked me to always remember that "The taller the bamboo grows, the lower it bows" (竹高愈躬).

There was another story a friend told me. Once upon a time, a student came to see a Zen master. He said, "Honorable Master, I have studied for many years, and I have learned so much of the martial arts and Zen theory already that I have reached a very high level. I heard that you are a great master, and I have therefore come to see if you can teach me anything more."

The master didn't reply. Instead, he picked up a teacup and placed it in front of the student. He then picked up the teapot and poured until the tea reached the rim of the cup, and then he kept on pouring until the tea overflowed onto the table. The student stared at the master in total confusion and said, "No, No, Master! The cup is overflowing!"

The master stopped pouring, looked at him and smiled. He said, "Young man, this is you. I am sorry that I cannot accept you as a student. Like this cup, your mind is filled up and I cannot teach you any more. If you want to learn, you must first empty your cup."

In order to be humble, you must first rid yourself of false dignity. This is especially true in front of a master. A person who is really wise knows when and how to bend, and always keeps his cup empty.

There is a story told to me by one of my students. There was once a Samurai swordsman who came to visit an old Zen master. The warrior said: "Respectable master! I have been a Samurai swordsman for many, many years. However, I have heard that you are a very knowledgeable master, so I come to ask you a very serious question and hopefully you may give me the answer. Will you teach me about heaven and hell?" The old master snapped his head up in disgust and said, "Teach you about heaven and hell? I doubt that you could even learn to keep your own sword from rusting, you ignorant fool. How dare you suppose that you could understand anything I might have to say?"

The old man went on and on, becoming even more insulting, while the young swordsman's surprise turned first to confusion, then to hot anger, rising by the minute. Master or no master, who can insult a Samurai and live?

As last, with teeth clenched and blood nearly boiling with fury, the warrior blindly drew his sword and prepared to end the old man's sharp tongue and life all in one moment. The master looked straight into his eyes and said gently, "That's hell."

At the peak of his rage, the Samurai realized that this was indeed his teaching; the master had bounded him into a living hell, driven by uncontrolled anger and ego. The young man, profoundly humbled, sheathed his sword and bowed to this great spiritual teacher. Looking up into the wise man's aged, beaming face, he felt more love and compassion than he had ever felt in his life, at which point the master raised his index finger, as would a schoolteacher and said, "And that's heaven."

From the above story, you can see that if you remain humble, you can see things clearly, since your mind is opened to accept criticism. If you are satisfied and proud, then you have closed your mind and remain in the circle of self-satisfaction. Naturally, no progress can be made.

2. **Respect** (*Zun Jing;* 尊敬)

Respect is the foundation of your relationship with your parents, teachers, your fellow students, other martial artists, and all other people in society. Respect makes a harmonious relationship possible. However, the most important type of respect is self-respect. If you can't respect yourself, how can you respect others or expect them to respect you? Respect must be earned, you cannot request or demand it.

In China, it is said: "Those who respect themselves and others will also be respected."[14] For example, if you despise yourself and become a villain in this society, then you have lost your self-respect. Since you have abused your personality and humility as a human, why should other people respect you? Only when you have demonstrated that you are deserving of respect will respect come to you automatically and naturally.

I remember my grandmother told me a story. A long time ago a girl named Li-Li got married, and went to live with her husband and mother-in-law. In a very short time Li-Li found that she couldn't get along with her mother-in-law at all. Their personalities were very different, and Li-Li was infuriated by many of her mother-in-law's habits, the worst of which was constant criticism.

Days passed days, weeks passed weeks, but Li-Li and her mother-in-law never stopped arguing and fighting. What made the situation even worse was that, according to ancient Chinese tradition, Li-Li had to bow to her mother-in-law and obey her every wish. All the anger and unhappiness in the house caused everyone great distress.

Finally, Li-Li could not stand her mother-in-law's bad temper and dictatorship any longer, so she decided to do something about it. Li-Li went to see her father's good friend Mr. Huang, who sold herbs. She told him the problem, and asked if he would give her some poison so that she could solve the problem once and for all.

Mr. Huang thought for a while, and finally he said, "Li-Li, I will help you to solve your problem, but you must listen to me and obey what I tell you." Li-Li said, "Yes, Mr. Huang, I will do whatever you tell me to do." Mr. Huang went into the back room, and returned in a few minutes with a package of herbs. He told Li-Li, "You can't use a quick-acting poison to get rid of your mother-in-law, because that would cause people to become suspicious. Therefore, I have given you a number of herbs that will slowly build up poison in her body. Every other day prepare some pork or chicken, and put a little of these herbs in her serving. Now, in order to make sure that nobody suspects you when she dies, you must be very careful to act very friendly toward her. Don't argue with her, obey her every wish, and treat her like a queen."

Li-Li was so happy. She thanked Mr. Huang, and hurried home to start her plot of murdering her mother-in-law. Weeks went by, and months went by, and every other day Li-Li served the specially treated food to her mother-in-law. She remembered what Mr. Huang had said about avoiding suspicion, so she controlled her temper, obeyed her mother-in-law, and treated her like her own mother.

After six months had passed, the whole household had changed. Li-Li had practiced controlling her temper so much that she found that she almost never got mad or upset. She hadn't had an argument in six months with her mother-in-law, who now seemed much kinder and easier to get along with. The mother-in-law's attitude toward Li-Li had changed, and she began to love Li-Li like her own daughter. She kept telling friends and relatives that Li-Li was the best daughter-in-law one could ever find. Li-Li and her mother-in-law were now treating each other just like a real mother and daughter.

One day Li-Li came to see Mr. Huang and again asked for his help. She said, "Dear Mr. Huang, please help me to keep the poison from killing my mother-in-law! She's changed into such a nice woman, and I love her like my own mother. I do not want her to die because of the poison I gave to her."

Mr. Huang smiled and nodded his head. "Li-Li," he said, "There's nothing to worry about. I never gave you any poison. All of the herbs I gave you were simply to improve her health. The only poison was in your mind and your attitude toward her, but that has been all washed away by the love which you gave to her."

From this story you can see that before anyone can respect you, you must first respect others. Remember, "The person who loves others will also be loved."

There was also another story my grandmother told me. In China, there was once a family made up of a father, a mother, a ten year old son, and a grandmother. Every mealtime they sat together around the table. The grandmother was quite old. Her hands had begun to shake all the time, and she had difficulty holding things. Whenever she ate, she couldn't hold the rice bowl steady and spilled rice all over the table.

The daughter-in-law was very upset by this. One day she complained to her husband, "My dear husband, every time your mother eats she spills her food all over the table. This makes me so sick I can't eat my own food!" The husband didn't say anything. He knew that he couldn't keep his mother's hands from shaking.

In a few days, when the husband had done nothing to solve the problem, his wife spoke to him again. "Are you going to do something about your mother or not? I cannot stand it any more." After arguing for a while, the husband sadly gave in to his wife's suggestion, and agreed that his mother should sit at a separate table, away from the rest of the family. When dinner time came, the grandmother found herself sitting alone at a separate table. And to make things worse, she had to eat from a cheap, chipped bowl because she had dropped and broken several others.

The grandmother was very sad, but she knew she couldn't do anything about it. She began to think of the past, and how much time and love she had given her son as he was growing up. She had never complained, but had always been there when he was sick or when he needed anything. Now she felt deserted by her family, and her heart was broken.

Several days passed. The grandmother was still very sad, and the smile began to disappear from her face. Her ten year old grandson had been watching everything, and he came to her and said, "Grandma, I know you are very unhappy about how my parents are treating you, but don't worry. I think I know how to get them to invite you back to the table, but I'll need your help."

Hope began to grow in the grandmother's heart. "But what do you want me to do?" she asked. The boy smiled and said, "Tonight at dinner time, break your rice bowl, but make it look like an accident." Grandmother's eyes opened wide in wonder. "But why?" she asked. "Don't worry," he said, "Leave it to me."

Dinner time came. She was curious about what her grandson was going to do, so she decided to do as he had asked. When her son and daughter-in-law were not looking, she picked up the old and chipped rice bowl that she had to eat out of, then dropped it on the floor and broke it. Immediately her daughter-in-law stood up, ready to complain. However, before she could say anything, the grandson stood up and said, "Grandma, why did you break that bowl? I wanted to save it for my mother when she gets old!"

When the mother heard this her face turned pale. She suddenly realized that everything she did was an example to her son. The way she was treating her mother-in-law was teaching her son how to devalue her when she got old. She suddenly felt very ashamed. From that day on, the whole family ate together around the same table.

From this, you can see that how we love, value and respect teachers and elders is exactly how we deserve to be treated when we are old. Real love is something that cannot be purchased. Respect your parents and love them always. Only then will you deserve the respect and love of your own children.

3. Righteousness (*Zheng Yi;* 正義)

Righteousness is a way of life. Righteousness means that if there is something you should do, you don't hesitate to take care of it, and if there is something that you should not do, you don't get involved with it. Your wisdom mind should be the leader, not your emotional mind. If you can do this, then you will feel clear spiritually, and avoid being plagued by feelings of guilt. If you can demonstrate this kind of personality you will be able to avoid evil influences, and you will earn the trust of others.

In the period of the Warring States (戰國, 475-222 B.C.), the two neighboring states of Zhao (趙) and Qin (秦) were often fighting against each other. In Zhao's court, there were two capable and talented officers — a military commander named Lian Po (廉頗), and a civilian official named Lin, Xiang-Ru (藺相如). Because of these two men, the state of Qin dared not launch a full-scale invasion against Zhao.

Originally, Lin, Xiang-Ru's position was far lower than that of General Lian Po. But later on, when Lin, Xiang-Ru was assigned as an ambassador to Qin, he won a diplomatic victory for the Zhao. This led the Zhao king to assign him to more important positions, and before too long his rank climbed higher than Lian Po's. Lian Po was very unhappy, and unwilling to accept this. He kept telling his subordinates that he would find an opportunity to humiliate Lin, Xiang-Ru.

When Lin, Xiang-Ru heard of this, he avoided meeting Lian Po face to face at any occasion. One day, some of Lin, Xiang-Ru's officers came to see him and said, "General Lian Po has only talked about what he intends to do, yet you have already become so afraid. We feel very humiliated and would like to resign."

Lin, Xiang-Ru then asked them, "If you were to compare General Lian Po and the Qin's King, who would be more prestigious?" "Of course General Lian Po cannot compare with the King of Qin!" they replied.

"Right!" he exclaimed. "And when I was an ambassador to Qin I had the courage to denounce the King of Qin right to his face. Thus, I have no fear of General Lian Po! The State of Qin dares not attack Zhao because of General Lian Po, and myself. If the two of us are at odds with each other, Qin will take advantage of this opportunity to invade us. The interests of this country come first with me, and I am not going to haggle with Lian Po because of personal hostilities!"

Later, when Lian Po heard of this, he felt extremely ashamed. He tore off his shirt, and with a birch rod tied to his back, he went to Lin, Xiang-Ru's home to request retribution for his own false dignity. Lin, Xiang-Ru modestly helped Lian Po up from the ground and held his hand firmly. From that time on, Lian Po and Lin, Xiang-Ru became close friends and served their country with the same heart.

There is another tale of events that happened during the Chinese Spring and Autumn Period (春秋, 722-481 B.C.). In the state of Jin (晉), there was a high-ranking official named Qi Xi (祁奚). When he was old and ready to retire, Duke Dao of Jin (晉悼公) asked him to recommend a candidate to replace himself. Qi Xi said, "Xie Hu (解狐) is an excellent man who is most suitable to replace me."

Duke Dao was very curious and said, "Isn't Xie Hu your political enemy? Why do you recommend him?" "You asked me who I thought was most suitable and most trustworthy for the job. Therefore, I recommended who I thought was best for this position. You did not ask me who was my enemy," Qi Xi replied.

Unfortunately, before Duke Dao could assign Xie Hu the new position, Xie Hu died. Duke Dao could only ask Qi Xi to recommend another person. Qi Xi said, "Now that Xie Hu is dead, the only person who can take my place is Qi Wu (祁午)."

Duke Dao was again very curious and said, "Isn't Qi Wu your son? Aren't you afraid that there may be gossip?" "You asked me only who was the most suitable for the position, and did not ask if Qi Wu was my son. I only replied with who was the best choice as a replacement."

As Qi Xi predicted, his son Qi Wu was able to contribute greatly. People believed that only a virtuous man like Qi Xi could recommend a really talented man. He would not praise an enemy to flatter him, and he would not promote his own son out of selfishness.

4. Trust (*Xin Yong;* 信用)

Trust includes being trustworthy, and also trusting yourself. You must develop a personality which other people can trust. For example, you should not make promises lightly, but if you have made a promise, you should fulfill it. **Trust is the key to friendship, and the best way of earning respect**. The trust of a friend is hard to gain, but easy to lose. Self-trust is the root of confidence. You must learn to build up your confidence and demonstrate it externally. Only then can you earn the trust and respect of others.

There is an ancient Chinese story about Emperor You of Zhou (周幽王, 781-771 B.C.). When Emperor You attacked the kingdom of Bao (褒), he won a beautiful lady named Bao Shi (褒姒). However, although she was beautiful, Bao Shi never smiled. In order to make her smile, the Emperor gave her precious pearls and jewels to wear, and delicious things to eat. He tried a thousand things but still Bao Shi wouldn't smile. The Emperor was the monarch of the country and yet he couldn't win a smile from the beautiful lady. It made him very unhappy.

At that time, the country of Zhou had platforms for signal fires around its borders. If an enemy attacked the capital, the fires were lit to signal the feudal lords that their emperor was in danger, and they would immediately send out troops to help. The fires were not to be lit unless the situation was critical. However, the emperor thought of a way to use them to please Bao Shi. He ordered the signal fires lit. The feudal lords thought that the capital city was in great danger, so a vast and mighty army of soldiers soon came running.

When Bao Shi saw all the troops rushing crazily about in a nervous frenzy, she unconsciously let out a great laugh. Emperor You was so happy that he smiled and smiled, and completely forgot about the lords, standing there staring blankly. After a while the Emperor said, "It's nothing. Everyone go home."

Emperor You completely forgot about the importance of the signal fires, and went so far as to light them several times in order to win Bao Shi's smile. The lords all knew that they had been made fools of, and were furious.

Later, Emperor You dismissed his empress, Lady Shen (申后), in favor of his concubine Bao Shi. Lady Shen's father was greatly angered, and united with a foreign tribe called the Quan Rong (犬戎) to attack Emperor You. When Emperor You's situation grew urgent, he ordered the signal fires lit, summoning the feudal lords to save him and the capital. Even as he died, the Emperor never understood that, because of the games he had played with the signal fires, not even one lord would come to save him.

It is a truth that it may take more than ten years of effort to earn the trust of a person, but that it can take only one night to destroy this trust. Once this trust is broken, it can take twenty years to regain it, if one ever regains it at all.

5. Loyalty (*Zhong Cheng*; 忠誠)

Loyalty is the root of trust. You should be loyal to your teacher and to your friends, and they should also be loyal to you. Loyalty lets mutual trust grow. In the Chinese martial arts, it is especially crucial that there be loyalty between you and your master. This loyalty is built upon a foundation of obedience to your master. Obedience is the prerequisite for learning. If you sincerely desire to learn, you should rid yourself of false dignity. You must bow to your teacher both mentally and spiritually. Only this will open the gates of trust. A teacher will not teach someone who is always concerned about his own dignity. Remember, in front of your teacher, you do not have dignity.

There was a story told to me when I was a child. A long time ago in Asia there was a king. Nobody had ever seen the king's real face, because whenever he met with his ministers and officials, and whenever he appeared in public, he always wore a mask. The face on the mask had a very stern and solemn expression. Because nobody could see the real expression on his face, all the officials and people respected him, obeyed him, and feared him. This made it possible for him to rule the country efficiently and well.

One day his wife said to him, "If you have to wear the mask in order to rule the country well, then what the people respect and show loyalty to is the mask and not you." The king wanted to prove to his wife that it was he who really ruled the country, and not the mask, so he decided to take the mask off and let the officials see his real face.

Without the mask, the officials were able to see the expression on his face and figure out what he was thinking. It wasn't long before the officials weren't afraid of him anymore.

A few months passed, and the situation got steadily worse. He had lost the solemn dignity which made people fear him, and even worse, the officials had started to lose respect for him. Not only did they argue with each other in front of him, they even began to argue with him about his decisions.

He soon realized that the unity and cooperation among his officials had disintegrated. His ability to lead the country had gradually disappeared, and the country was falling into disorder. The king realized that, in order to regain the respect of the people and his ability to rule the country, he had to do something. He therefore gave the order to behead all of the officials who had seen his face, and he then appointed new ones. He then put the mask back on his face. Soon afterward, the country was again united and under his control.

Do you have a mask on your face? Is it the mask that people are loyal to? Is what you show people on your face what you really think? Do we have to put a mask on in this masked society? How heavy and how thick is your mask? Have you ever taken your mask off and taken a good look at the real you in the mirror? If you can do this it will make you humble. Then, even if you have a mask on your face, your life will not be ruled by your mask.

Morality of Mind:

1. Will (*Yi Zhi;* 意志)

It usually takes a while to demonstrate a strong will. This is because of the struggle between the emotional mind and the wisdom mind. If your wisdom mind governs your entire being you will be able to suppress the disturbances that come from the emotional mind, and your will can last. A strong will depends upon the sincerity with which you commit yourself to your goal. This has to come from deep within you, and can't be just a casual, vague desire. Oftentimes, the students who show the greatest eagerness to learn in the beginning, quit the soonest, while those who hide their eagerness deep inside their hearts stay the longest.

There is a Chinese story from ancient times about a ninety year old man who lived together with his sons, daughters-in-law, and grandsons near the mountain Bei (北山). In front of his house were two mountains, *Taixing* (太行) and *Wangwu* (王屋), which blocked the road to the county seat and made travel very inconvenient. One day he decided to remove these two mountains to the coast nearby and dump the dirt into the sea. His neighbors laughed at him when they heard of this. However, he replied, "Why is this so impossible? I will die soon, but I have sons and my sons will have grandsons without end. However, the mountain remains the same. Why can't I move it?" Isn't it true that where there is a will, there is a way?

There is another story about the famous poet Li Bai (李白). When Li Bai was young he studied at a school far away from his home. He lacked a strong will, so before the end of his studies he gave up and decided to go home. While crossing over a mountain on the way home he passed an old lady sitting in front of her house. In her hands she held a metal pestle which she was grinding on the top of a rock. Li Bai was very curious and asked her what she was doing. She said, "I want to grind this pestle into a needle." When Li Bai heard of this he was very ashamed, and decided to return to school and finish his studies. He later became one of the greatest poets in China.

There is another well-known story which tells of a famous archer named Hou Yi (后羿). When Hou Yi heard that there was a famous archery master in the North, he decided to ask the master to take him as a student. After three months of travel, Hou Yi finally arrived in the cold northern territory. Before long, he found the home of the famous master. He knocked on the door, and when the old master came out, Hou Yi knelt down and said, "Honorable master, would you please accept me as your disciple?" The old master replied, "Young man, I can't accept any students. I am not as good as you think, and besides, I am already old." But Hou Yi would not accept no for an answer. "Honorable master," he said, "I have made up my mind: I swear I will not get up until you promise to take me as your student."

The master closed the door without a word, leaving Hou Yi outside. Before long it got dark and started to snow, but Hou Yi remained in his kneeling position without moving. One whole day passed, but the master never appeared again. Hou Yi continued to kneel on the ground in front of the door. A second day passed, and a third day. Finally, the master opened the door and said, "Young man, if you really want to learn my archery techniques, you must first pass a few tests." "Of course, master," Hou Yi replied with great happiness.

"The first is a test of your patience and perseverance. You must go back home and every morning and evening watch three sticks of incense burn out. Do this for three years and then come back to see me."

Hou Yi went home and started to watch the incense each morning and evening. At first, he got bored and impatient very quickly. However, he was determined to keep his promise, so he continued to watch the incense. Six months later, watching the incense burn had become a habit. He started to realize that he had become patient, and even began to enjoy his morning and evening routine. He began to concentrate his mind, focusing on the head of the incense as it burned down the stick. From practicing concentration and calming his mind, he learned to distinguish between the real and the false. After the three years were up, he found that every time he concentrated and focused his eyes on something, that object would be enlarged in his mind, and all other surrounding objects would disappear. He did not realize that he had learned the most important factor in becoming a good archer — **a concentrated and calm mind**. After he finished this test, he was very happy and traveled to the North to see his master.

The master told him, "You have passed the first test, now you must pass a second. You must go back and day and night watch your wife weave at her loom, following the shuttle with your eyes as it moves incessantly to and fro. You must do this for three years and then come back to see me."

Hou Yi was very disappointed, because he had thought that his master would teach him now that he had completed his three years of patience training. However, because his heart was set on learning from this famous master, he left and went home. He sat by his wife's loom and focused his eyes on the shuttle as it moved to and fro. As with the incense, he didn't enjoy himself at first, but after one year passed he began to get used to the fast shuttle motion. After another two years, he found that when he concentrated on the shuttle, it would move more slowly. Without realizing it, he had learned the next important part of an archer's training — **concentrating on a moving object**. He returned to his master and told his master what he had found. Instead of beginning his instruction, he was asked to return home and make 10 rice baskets a day for the next three years. Chinese rice baskets were made out of rattan, and one needed to have very strong wrists and arms to make them. Even a very good basket maker could hardly make five a day, and Hou Yi was being asked to make ten a day!

Although disappointed, Hou Yi returned home to do as he was told. In the beginning he hardly slept, spending almost every hour of the day in making baskets. His hands were numb and bleeding, his shoulders were sore, and he was always tired, but he persisted in working to finish ten baskets a day. After six months he found that his hands and shoulders were no longer in pain, and he could make ten baskets a day easily. By the end of three years, he could make twenty a day. He surely had achieved the last requirement of a good archer — **strong and steady arms and shoulders**. Hou Yi finally realized that all his efforts for the last nine years had actually been the training for how to become a good archer. He was now able to shoot very well with his concentrated mind and strong arms.

Proud and happy, he returned to his master, who said, "You have studied hard and learned well. I can't teach you any more than what you already know." With this the master turned his head and walked away.

Hou Yi was thinking that all his master had taught him in the last nine years was expressed in only three sentences. He couldn't believe that this was all there was to learn. He decided to put his master, who by now was two hundred yards away, to a test. He pulled an arrow from his quiver, aimed at the tassel on his master's hat, and released. His master instantly sensed the arrow coming his way, pulled and notched an arrow, and shot it back to meet the coming arrow in the air. Both arrows dropped to the ground. Hou Yi saw this and without stopping shot a second arrow, and this second arrow suffered the same fate. He couldn't believe that his master could shoot and meet his arrows in mid-air three times in a row, so he loosed a third arrow. He suddenly realized that his master had run out of arrows. While he was wondering what his master was going to do, his master plucked a branch from a nearby willow tree and used this branch as an arrow. Again it met Hou Yi's arrow in mid-air. This time, Hou Yi ran toward his master, knelt before him, and said, "Most respected master, now I realize one thing. The thing that I cannot learn from you is experience, which can only come from practicing by myself."

Of course, part of the story is exaggerated. However, masters in China often used this story to encourage the students to strengthen their will, to think, and to research. What the master can give you is a key to the door. To enter the door and find things inside is your own responsibility. The more experience you have, the better you will be.

2. Endurance, Perseverance, and Patience

(*Ren Nai, Yi Li, Heng Xin;* 忍耐，毅力，恒心)

Endurance, perseverance, and patience are the manifestations of a strong will. People who are successful are not always the smartest ones, but they are always the ones who are patient and who persevere. **People who are really wise do not use wisdom only to guide their thinking, they also use it to govern their personalities**. Through cultivating these three elements you will gradually build up a profound mind, which is the key to the deepest essence of learning. If you know how to use your mind to ponder as you train, it can lead you to a deeper stage of understanding. If you can manifest this understanding in your actions you will be able to surpass others.

Of all the stories that my master told me, my favorite one is about the boy who carved the Buddha. Once upon a time, there was a twelve year old boy whose parents had been killed during a war. He came to the *Shaolin* Temple and asked to see the Head Priest. When he was led to the Head Priest, the boy knelt down and said, "Honorable Master, would you please accept me as your *Gongfu* student? I will respect, obey, and serve you well, and I won't disappoint you."

As the Head Priest looked at the boy, he felt that he had to give him a test before he could accept him as a student. He said, "Boy, I would like to teach you *Gongfu,* but I have to leave the temple for one year to preach. Could you do me a favor while I am gone?" The boy was glad to have a chance to prove that he could be a good student, and so he said, "Certainly, honorable Master! What do you want me to do?"

The Head Priest led the boy out of the temple and pointed to a big tree. He said, "I have always wanted a good carving of the Buddha. See that tree? Could you chop it down and make a Buddha for me?" The boy replied enthusiastically, "Yes, Master! When you return, I will have finished the Buddha for you." The next morning the Head Priest departed, leaving the boy to live with the monks. A few days later the boy chopped down the tree, and got ready to make the Buddha. The boy wanted to carve a beautiful Buddha and make the Head Priest happy. He worked night and day, patiently carving as carefully as he could.

A year later the Head Priest came back from his preaching. The boy was very anxious and excited. He showed the Head Priest his Buddha, which was five feet tall. He hoped to earn the Head Priest's trust, and he eagerly waited to be praised. But the Head Priest looked at the Buddha, and he knew that the boy had sincerely done his best. However, he decided to give the boy a further test. He said, "Boy, it is well done. But it seems it is too big for me. It is not the size which I was expecting. Since I have to leave the temple again to preach for another year, could you use this time to make this Buddha smaller?"

The boy was very disappointed and unhappy. He had thought that when the Head Priest saw the Buddha, he would be accepted as a student and he could start his *Gongfu* training. However, in order to make the Head Priest happy he said, "Yes, Master. I will make it smaller." Even though the boy had agreed, the Head Priest could see from the boy's face that this time he did not agree willingly, from his heart. However, he knew that this time the test would be a real one.

The next morning the Head Priest left, and again the boy stayed with the monks to fulfill this promise. The boy started carving the Buddha, trying to make it smaller, but he was disappointed and very unhappy. However, he forced himself to work. After six months had gone by, he found that he had carved an ugly, unhappy Buddha.

The boy was very depressed. He found that he couldn't work on the Buddha when he was so unhappy, so he stopped working. Days passed days, weeks passed weeks. The date of the Head Priest's return was getting closer. His chances of becoming a student of the Head Priest were getting slimmer and slimmer, and his unhappiness was growing deeper and deeper.

One morning, he suddenly realized an important thing. He said to himself, "If completing the Buddha is the only way I can learn *Gongfu,* why don't I make it good and enjoy it?" After that, his attitude changed. Not only was he happy again, he also regained his patience and his will was stronger. Day and night he worked. The more he worked, the happier he was, and the more he enjoyed his work. Before the boy noticed it, the year was up and he had almost completed his happy and refined Buddha.

When the Head Priest came back, the boy came to see him with his new Buddha. This carving was two feet tall, and smiling. When the priest saw the Buddha, he was very pleased. He knew that the boy had accomplished one of the hardest challenges that a person can face: conquering himself. However, he decided to give the boy one final test. He said, "Boy, you have done well. But it seems it is still too big for me. In a few days I have to leave the temple again for another year of preaching. During this time, could you make this Buddha even smaller?" Surprisingly, this time the boy showed no sign of being disappointed. Instead, he said, "No problem, Master. I will make it smaller." The boy had learned how to enjoy his work.

The Head Priest left again. This time, the boy enjoyed his work. Every minute he could find he spent at his task, carefully making the carving more lifelike and refined. His sincerity, his patience, and his growing maturity became expressed in the Buddha's face.

One year later, the Head Priest returned. The boy handed him a Buddha which was only two inches tall, and which had the best artwork one could ever find. The Head Priest now believed that this boy would be a successful martial artist. The boy had passed the test. He went on to become one of the best students in the *Shaolin* Temple.

As mentioned earlier, we have two kinds of minds. One comes from our emotions, and the other is generated from our wisdom and clear judgment. Do you remember times when you knew you should do a certain thing, but at the same time you didn't want to do it? It was your wisdom mind telling you to do it, and your lazy emotional mind saying no. Which side won? Once you can follow your wisdom mind, you will have conquered yourself and you will surely be successful.

3. Courage (*Yong Gan;* 勇敢)

Courage is often confused with bravery. Courage originates with the understanding that comes from the wisdom mind. Bravery is the external manifestation of courage, and can be considered to be the child of the wisdom and the emotional minds. For example, if you have the courage to accept a challenge, that means your mind has understood the situation and made a decision. Next, you must be brave enough to face the challenge. Without courage, the bravery cannot last long. Without the profound comprehension of courage, bravery can be blind and stupid.

Daring to face a challenge that you think needs to be faced is courage. But successfully manifesting courage requires more than just a decision from your wisdom mind. You also need a certain amount of psychological preparation so that you can be emotionally balanced; this will give your bravery a firm root so that it can endure. Frequently you do not have enough time to think and make a decision. A wise person always prepares, considering the possible situations that might arise, so that when something happens he will be ready and can demonstrate bravery.

There is a story from China's Spring and Autumn period (春秋, 722-481 B.C.). At that time, there were many feudal lords who each controlled a part of the land, and who frequently attacked one another.

When an army from the nation of Jin attacked the nation of Zheng (鄭), the Zheng ruler sent a delegation to the Jin (晉) army to discuss conditions for their withdrawal. Duke Wen of Jin (晉文公) (636-627 B.C.) made two demands: first, that the young Duke Lan (蘭) be set up as heir apparent; second, that the high official Shu Zhan (叔詹), who opposed Lan's being made heir apparent, be handed over to the Jin. The Zheng ruler refused to assent to the second condition.

Shu Zhan said, "Jin has specified that it wants me. If I do not go, the Jin armies that now surround us will certainly not withdraw. Wouldn't I then be showing myself to be afraid of death and insufficiently loyal?" "If you go," said the Zheng ruler, "You will certainly die. Thus I cannot bear to let you go."

"What is so bad about letting a minister go to save the people and secure the nation?" asked Shu Zhan. The ruler of Zheng then, with tears in his eyes, sent some men to escort Shu Zhan to the Jin encampment.

When Duke Wen of Jin saw Shu Zhan, he was furious and immediately ordered that a large tripod be prepared to cook him to death. Shu Zhan, however, was not the least bit afraid. "I hope that I can finish speaking before you kill me," he said. Duke Wen told him to speak quickly.

Relaxed, Shu Zhan said, "Before, while you were in Zheng, I often praised your virtue and wisdom in front of others, and I thought that after you returned to Jin you would definitely become the most powerful among the feudal lords. After the alliance negotiations at Wen, I also advised my lord to follow Jin. Unfortunately, he did not accept my suggestion. Now you think that I am guilty, but my lord knows that I am innocent and stubbornly refused to deliver me to you. I was the one who asked to come and save Zheng from danger. I am this kind of person; accurately forecasting events is called wisdom, loving one's country with all one's heart is called loyalty, not fleeing in the face of danger is called courage, and being willing to die to save one's country is called benevolence. I find it hard to believe that a benevolent, wise, loyal, and courageous minister can be killed in Jin!" Then, leaning against the tripod, he cried, "From now on, those who would serve their rulers should remember what happens to me!"

Duke Wen's expression changed greatly after hearing this speech. He ordered that Shu Zhan be spared and had him escorted back to Zheng.

There is another story about a famous minister, Si, Ma-Guang (司馬光), and his childhood during the Song Dynasty (宋, 1019-1086 A.D.). When he was a child, he was playing with a few of his playmates in a garden where there was a giant cistern full of water next to a tree.

One of the children was very curious about what was in the giant cistern. Since the cistern was much taller than the child, he climbed up the tree to see inside. Unfortunately, he slipped and fell into the cistern and started to drown.

When this happened, all of the children were so scared and they did not know what to do. Some of them were so afraid that they immediately ran away. Si, Ma-Guang, however, without hesitation picked up a big rock and threw it at the cistern and broke it. The water inside flowed out immediately, and the child inside was saved.

This story teaches that when a crisis occurs, in addition to wisdom and a calm mind, you must also be brave enough to execute your decision.

References

1. 登封縣志．少林武術大全，德虔編著。北京體育出版社

2. 一膽，二力，三功夫

3. ***Compilation of the Yang's Taijiquan, Saber, Sword, and Fighting Set,*** by Chen, Yan-Lin, 1943.
楊氏太極拳，刀，劍，桿，散手合編。陳炎林著。

4. 外練筋骨皮，內練一口氣。

5. 外家由硬而軟，內家由軟而硬，其法雖異，其的則同。

6. 外家由外而內，內家由內而外，其途雖異，其終的則一致。

7. 外家先力爾氣，內家先氣後力。

8. 練拳不練功，到老一場空。

9. 師父領進門，修行在自身。

10. 大道不過三兩句，說破不值三文錢。

11. 滿招損，謙受益。

12. 子曰："三人行，必有我師。"

13. 人外有人，天外有天。

14. 自敬敬人者，人恆敬之。

Chapter 2

About Chinese Qigong

中國氣功介紹

2-1. Introduction

From the last chapter, you can see that *Qigong* has always been an important part of Chinese martial arts training. Without *Qigong* training, a martial artist will have lost the origin of martial power, and what he or she uses will only be muscular power. This will make Chinese martial arts no different from the western fighting arts. The most unique elements of Chinese martial arts are in the *Qigong* training, and the buildup of internal energy (i.e., *Qi*). Moreover, through mental concentration, *Qi* can be led throughout the physical body to boost its functioning to a higher level. However, the most important aspect of *Qigong* training is to learn to feel yourself, to understand yourself and to deal with your own mind. This is the path of self-discipline and spiritual cultivation. From this training, you will begin to understand the way of your life more deeply. From this, you can see that **the way of Chinese martial arts is a way of life, and your life can be built upon an understanding of Chinese martial arts**. This bridge between these two mountains is the practice of the *Qigong*.

Qigong has been studied and developed in China for more than four thousand years. It is not easy for any person to achieve a deep, profound understanding and feeling for such arts in a short time. To help you grasp the concepts of martial *Qigong* training, you must first build the foundation of knowledge and understanding. This will provide you with a baseline reference for all your further study and evaluation.

This chapter will provide you with a simple *Qigong* practice "road-map" which can guide you to the garden of *Qigong* practice. You should study it carefully. If you are able to understand this chapter, you will soon grasp the rationale of every training method in this book. In the next section, first I will define the terminology of *Qi, Qigong* and their relationship to humanity. Having this definition, we will not treat *Qi* as mysterious. Then, in order to help you understand the historical background of *Qigong,* different categories of *Qigong* will be briefly summarized in section 2-3. Next, in section 2-4, the theoretical foundations of *Qigong* will be discussed. From comprehension of this section, you will have less doubt in your *Qigong* practice. Then, the relationships among *Qi,* Health, and Martial Arts will be explained in section 2-5. Finally, general *Qigong* training procedures will be reviewed in section 2-6. If you wish to learn more about *Qigong,* please refer to books: ***The Root of Chinese Chi Kung and Muscle/Tendon Changing and Marrow/Brain Washing Chi Kung***, by YMAA.

2-2. Qi, Qigong, and Human Beings

Before we discuss the relationship of *Qi* with the human body, we should first define *Qi* and *Qigong*. We will first discuss the general concept of *Qi*, including both the traditional understanding and the possible modern scientific paradigms, which allows us to use modern concepts to explain *Qigong*. If you would like to investigate these subjects in more detail, please refer to the YMAA book *The Root of Chinese Chi Kung.*

A General Definition of Qi

Qi is the energy or natural force which fills the universe. The Chinese have traditionally believed that there are three major powers in the universe. These Three Powers (*San Cai,* 三才) are Heaven (*Tian,* 天), Earth (*Di,* 地), and Man (*Ren,* 人). Heaven (the sky or universe) has Heaven *Qi* (*Tian Qi*), the most important of the three, which is made up of the forces which the heavenly bodies exert on the earth, such as sunshine, moonlight, the moon's gravity, and the energy from the stars. In ancient times, the Chinese believed that weather, climate, and natural disasters were governed by Heaven *Qi*. Chinese people still refer to the weather as Heaven *Qi* (*Tian Qi,* 天氣). Every energy field strives to stay in balance, so whenever the Heaven *Qi* loses its balance, it tries to rebalance itself. Then the wind must blow, rain must fall, even tornadoes or hurricanes must happen in order for the Heaven *Qi* to reach a new energy balance.

Under Heaven *Qi*, is Earth *Qi*. It is influenced and controlled by Heaven *Qi*. For example, too much rain will force a river to flood or change its path. Without rain, the plants will die. The Chinese believe that Earth *Qi* is made up of lines and patterns of energy, as well as the earth's magnetic field and the heat concealed underground. These energies must also balance, otherwise disasters such as earthquakes will occur. When the *Qi* of the earth is balanced, plants will grow and animals thrive.

Finally, within the Earth *Qi*, each individual person, animal, and plant has its own *Qi* field, which always seeks to be balanced. When any individual thing loses its *Qi* balance, it will sicken, die, and decompose. All natural things, including mankind and our Human *Qi*, grow within and are influenced by the natural cycles of Heaven *Qi* and Earth *Qi*. Throughout the history of *Qigong*, people have been most interested in Human *Qi* and its relationship with Heaven *Qi* and Earth *Qi*.

In China, Qi is defined as any type of energy which is able to demonstrate power and strength. This energy can be electricity, magnetism, heat, or light. For examples, electric power is called "electric *Qi*" (*Dian Qi,* 電氣), and heat is called "heat *Qi*" (*Re Qi,* 熱氣). When a person is alive, his body's energy is called "human *Qi*" (*Ren Qi,* 人氣).

Qi is also commonly used to express the energy state of something, especially living things. As mentioned before, the weather is called "Heaven *Qi*" (*Tian Qi,* 天氣) because it indicates the energy state of the heavens. When something is alive it has "vital *Qi*" (*Huo Qi,* 活氣), and when it is dead it has "dead *Qi*" (*Si Qi,* 死氣) or "ghost *Qi*" (*Gui Qi,* 鬼氣). When a person is righteous and has the spiritual strength to do good, he is said to have "Normal *Qi* or Righteous *Qi*" (*Zheng Qi,* 正氣). The spiritual state or morale of an army is called "energy state" (*Qi Shi,* 氣勢).

You can see that the word *Qi* has a wider and more general definition than most people think. It does not refer only to the energy circulating in the human body. Furthermore, the word *"Qi"* can represent the energy itself, and it can even be used to express the manner or state of the energy. It is important to understand this when you practice *Qigong*, so that your mind is not channeled into a narrow understanding of *Qi*, which would limit your future understanding and development.

A Narrow Definition of Qi

Now that you understand the general definition of *Qi,* let us look at how *Qi* is defined in *Qigong* society today. As mentioned before, among the Three Powers, the Chinese have been most concerned with the *Qi* which is related to our health and longevity. Therefore, after four thousand years of emphasizing Human *Qi,* when people mention *Qi* they usually mean the *Qi* circulating in our bodies.

If we look at the Chinese medical and *Qigong* documents that were written about two thousand years ago, the word *"Qi"* was written " 炁 ." This character is constructed of two words, " 无 " on the top, which means "nothing;" and " 灬 " on the bottom, which means "fire." This means that the word *Qi* was actually written as "no fire" in ancient times. If we go back through Chinese medical and *Qigong* history, it is not hard to understand this expression.

In ancient times, **the Chinese physicians or *Qigong* practitioners were actually looking for the *Yin-Yang* balance of the *Qi* which was circulating in the body. When this goal was reached, there was "no fire" in the internal organs**. This concept is very simple. According to Chinese medicine, each of our internal organs needs to receive a specific amount of *Qi* to function properly. If an organ receives an improper amount of *Qi* (usually too much, i.e., too *Yang*), it will start to malfunction, and, in time, physical damage will occur. Therefore, the goal of the medical or *Qigong* practitioner was to attain a state of "no fire," which eventually became the word *Qi.*

However, in more recent publications, the *Qi* of "no fire" has been replaced by the word " 氣 ," which is again constructed of two words, " 气 " which means "air," and " 米 " which means "rice." This shows that later practitioners realized that the *Qi* circulating in our bodies is produced mainly by the inhalation of air and the consumption of food (rice). Air is called *Kong Qi* (空氣), which means literally "space energy."

For a long time, people were confused about just what type of energy was circulating in our bodies. Many people believed that it was heat, others considered it to be electricity, and many others assumed that it was a mixture of heat, electricity, and light.

This confusion lasted until the early 1980's, when the concept of *Qi* gradually became clear. If we think carefully about what we know from science, we can see that (except possibly for gravity) there is actually only one type of energy in this universe, and that is electromagnetic energy. This means that light (electromagnetic waves) and heat (infrared waves) are also part of electromagnetic energy. This makes it very clear that the *Qi* circulating in our bodies is actually "bioelectricity," and that our body is a "living electromagnetic field."[1] This field is affected by our thoughts, feelings, activities, the food we eat, the quality of the air we breathe, our lifestyle, the natural energy that surrounds us, and also the unnatural energy which modern science inflicts upon us.

Next, let us define *Qigong.* Once you understand what *Qigong* is, you will be able to better understand the role that Chinese martial *Qigong* plays in Chinese martial arts and *Qigong* societies.

A General Definition of Qigong

We have explained that *Qi* is energy, and that it is found in the heavens, in the earth, and in every living thing. As mentioned in the first chapter that, in China, the word *"Gong"* (功) is often used instead of *"Gongfu"* (or *Kung Fu,* 功夫), which means energy and time. Any study or training which requires a lot of energy and time to learn or to accomplish is called *Gongfu.* The term can be applied to any special skill or study as long as it requires time, energy, and patience. Therefore, **the correct definition of *Qigong* is any training or study dealing with *Qi* which**

takes a long time and a lot of effort. You can see from this definition that *Qigong* is a science which studies the energy in nature. The main difference between this energy science and Western energy science is that *Qigong* focuses on the inner energy of human beings, while Western energy science pays more attention to the energy outside of the human body. When you study *Qigong*, it is worthwhile to also consider the modern, scientific point of view, and not restrict yourself to only the traditional beliefs.

The Chinese have studied *Qi* for thousands of years. Some of the information on the patterns and cycles of nature has been recorded in books, one of which is the **Yi Jing** (易經) (**Book of Changes**; 1122 B.C.). When the **Yi Jing** was written, the Chinese people, as mentioned earlier, believed that natural power included Heaven (*Tian*, 天), Earth (*Di*, 地), and Man (*Ren*, 人). These are called "The Three Powers" (*San Cai*, 三才) and are manifested by the three *Qi's*: Heaven *Qi*, Earth *Qi*, and Human *Qi*. These three facets of nature have their definite rules and cycles. The rules never change, and the cycles repeat regularly. The Chinese people used an understanding of these natural principles and the **Yi Jing** to calculate the changes of natural *Qi*. This calculation is called "The Eight Trigrams" (*Bagua*, 八卦). From the Eight Trigrams are derived the 64 hexagrams. Therefore, the **Yi Jing** was probably the first book which taught the Chinese people about *Qi* and its variations in nature and man. The relationship of the Three Natural Powers and their *Qi* variations were later discussed extensively in the book **Theory of Qi's Variation** (*Qi Hua Lun*, 氣化論).

Understanding Heaven *Qi* is very difficult, and it was especially so in ancient times when the science was just developing. But since nature is always repeating itself, the experiences accumulated over the years have made it possible to trace the natural patterns. Understanding the rules and cycles of "heavenly timing" (*Tian Shi*, 天時) will help you to understand natural changes of the seasons, climate, weather, rain, snow, drought, and all other natural occurrences. If you observe carefully, you will be able to see many of these routine patterns and cycles caused by the rebalancing of the *Qi* fields. Among the natural cycles are those which repeat every day, month, or year, as well as cycles of twelve years and sixty years.

Earth *Qi* is a part of Heaven *Qi*. If you can understand the rules and the structure of the earth, you will be able to understand how mountains and rivers are formed, how plants grow, how rivers move, what part of the country is best for someone, where to build a house and which direction it should face so that it is a healthy place to live, and many other things related to the earth. In China today there are people, called "geomancy teachers" (*Di Li Shi*, 地理師) or "wind water teachers" (*Feng Shui Shi*, 風水師), who make their living this way. The term "wind water" (*Feng Shui*) is commonly used because the location and character of the wind and water in a landscape are the most important factors in evaluating a location. These experts use the accumulated body of geomantic knowledge and the **Yi Jing** to help people make important decisions such as where and how to build a house, where to bury their dead, and how to rearrange or redecorate homes and offices so that they are better places to live and work in. Many people even believe that setting up a store or business according to the guidance of *Feng Shui* can make it more prosperous.

Among the three *Qi's*, Human *Qi* is probably the one studied most thoroughly. The study of Human *Qi* covers a large number of different subjects. The Chinese people believe that Human *Qi* is affected and controlled by Heaven *Qi* and Earth *Qi*, and that they in fact determine your destiny. Therefore, if you understand the relationship between nature and people, in addition to understanding "human relations" (*Ren Shi*, 人事), you will be able to predict wars, the destiny of a country, a person's desires and temperament, and even their future. The people who practice this profession are called "calculate life teachers" (*Suan Ming Shi*, 算命師).

However, the greatest achievement in the study of Human *Qi* is in regard to health and longevity. Since *Qi* is the source of life, if you understand how *Qi* functions and know how to regulate it correctly, you should be able to live a long and healthy life. Remember that you are part of nature, and you are channeled into the cycles of nature. If you go against this natural cycle, you may become sick, so it is in your best interest to follow the way of nature. This is the meaning of *"Dao,"* which can be translated as **"The Natural Way."**

Many different aspects of Human *Qi* have been researched, including acupuncture, acupressure, massage, herbal treatment, meditation, and *Qigong* exercises. The use of acupuncture, acupressure, and herbal treatment to adjust Human *Qi* flow has become the root of Chinese medical science. Meditation and Moving *Qigong* exercises are used widely by the Chinese people to improve their health or even to cure certain illnesses. In addition, Daoists and Buddhists use meditation and *Qigong* exercises in their pursuit of enlightenment.

In conclusion, **the study of any of the aspects of *Qi* including Heaven *Qi*, Earth *Qi*, and Human *Qi* should be called *Qigong*.** However, since the term is usually used today only in reference to the cultivation of Human *Qi* through meditation and exercises, we will only use it in this narrower sense to avoid confusion.

A Narrow Definition of Qigong

As mentioned earlier, the narrow definition of *Qi* is "the energy circulating in the human body." Therefore, **the narrow definition of *Qigong* is "the study of the *Qi* circulating in the human body."** Because our bodies are part of nature, the narrow definition of *Qigong* should also include the study of how our bodies relate to Heaven *Qi* and Earth *Qi*. Chinese *Qigong* consists today of several different fields: acupuncture, herbs for regulating human *Qi*, martial arts *Qigong*, *Qigong* massage, *Qigong* exercises, *Qigong* healing, and religious enlightenment *Qigong*. Naturally, these fields are mutually related, and in many cases cannot be separated.

The Chinese have discovered that the human body has twelve major channels (*Shi Er Jing*, 十二經) and eight vessels (*Ba Mai*, 八脈) through which the *Qi* circulates. The twelve channels are like **rivers** which distribute *Qi* throughout the body, and also connect the extremities (fingers and toes) to the internal organs. Here you should understand that the "internal organs" of Chinese medicine do not necessarily correspond to the physical organs as understood in the West, but rather to a set of clinical functions similar to each other, and related to the organ system. The eight vessels, which are often referred to as the extraordinary vessels, function like **reservoirs** and regulate the distribution and circulation of *Qi* in your body.

When the *Qi* in the eight reservoirs is full and strong, the *Qi* in the rivers is strong and will be regulated efficiently. When there is stagnation in any of these twelve channels or rivers, the *Qi* which flows to the body's extremities and to the internal organs will be abnormal, and illness may develop. You should understand that every channel has its particular *Qi* flow strength, and every channel is different. All of these different levels of *Qi* strength are affected by your mind, the weather, the time of day, the food you have eaten, and even your mood. For example, when the weather is dry the *Qi* in the lungs will tend to be more positive than when it is moist. When you are angry, the *Qi* flow in your liver channel will be abnormal. The *Qi* strength in the different channels varies throughout the day in a regular cycle, and at any particular time one channel is strongest. For example, between 11 AM and 1 PM the *Qi* flow in the Heart Channel is the strongest. Furthermore, the *Qi* level of the same organ can be different from one person to another.

Whenever the *Qi* flow in the twelve rivers or channels is not normal, the eight reservoirs will regulate the *Qi* flow and bring it back to normal. For example, when you experience a sudden shock, the *Qi* flow in the bladder immediately becomes deficient. Normally, the reservoir will immediately regulate the *Qi* in this channel so that you recover from the shock. However, if the reservoir *Qi* is also deficient, or if the effect of the shock is too great and there is not enough time to regulate the *Qi,* the bladder will suddenly contract, causing unavoidable urination.

When a person is sick, his *Qi* level tends to be either too positive (excessive, *Yang*) or too negative (deficient; *Yin*). A Chinese physician would either use a prescription of herbs to adjust the *Qi,* or else he would insert acupuncture needles at various spots on the channels to inhibit the flow in some channels and stimulate the flow in others, so that balance could be restored. However, there is another alternative, and that is to use certain physical and mental exercises to adjust the *Qi.* In other words, to use *Qigong.*

The above discussion is only to offer an idea of the narrow definition of *Qigong.* In fact, when people talk about *Qigong* today, most of the time they are referring to the mental and physical exercises that work with the *Qi.*

A Modern Definition of Qi

It is important that you know about the progress that has been made by modern science in the study of *Qi.* This will keep you from getting stuck in the ancient concepts and level of understanding.

In ancient China, people had very little knowledge of electricity. They only knew from acupuncture that when a needle was inserted into the acupuncture cavities, some kind of energy other than heat was produced which often caused a shock or a tickling sensation. It was not until the last few decades, when the Chinese people were more acquainted with electromagnetic science, that they began to recognize that this energy circulating in the body, which they called *Qi,* might be the same thing as what today's science calls "bioelectricity."

It is understood now that the human body is constructed of many different electrically conductive materials, and that it forms a living electromagnetic field and circuit. Electromagnetic energy is continuously being generated in the human body through the biochemical reaction in food and air assimilation, and circulated by the electromotive forces (EMF) generated within the body.

In addition, you are constantly being affected by external electromagnetic fields such as that of the earth, or the electrical fields generated by clouds. When you practice Chinese medicine or *Qigong,* you need to be aware of these outside factors and take them into account.

Countless experiments have been conducted in China, Japan, and other countries to study how external magnetic or electrical fields can affect and adjust the body's *Qi* field. Many acupuncturists use magnets and electricity in their treatments. They attach a magnet to the skin over a cavity and leave it there for a period of time. The magnetic field gradually affects the *Qi* circulation in that channel. Alternatively, they insert needles into cavities and then run an electric current through the needle to reach the *Qi* channels directly. Although many researchers have claimed a degree of success in their experiments, none has been able to publish any detailed and convincing proof of the results, or give a good explanation of the theory behind the experiment. As with many other attempts to explain the How and Why of acupuncture, conclusive proof is elusive, and many unanswered questions remain. Of course, this theory is quite new, and it will take more study and research before it is verified and completely understood. At present, there are many conservative acupuncturists who are skeptical.

To untie this knot, we must look at what modern Western science has discovered about bioelectromagnetic energy. Many bioelectricity-related reports have been published, and frequently the results are closely related to what is experienced in Chinese *Qigong* training and medical sci-

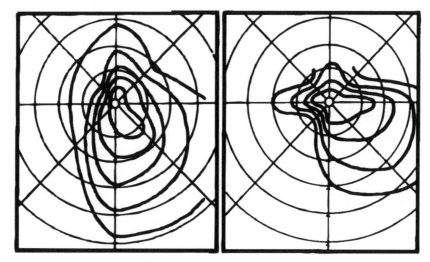

Figure 2–1. Electrical Conductivity Maps of the Skin Surface over Acupuncture Points

ence. For example, during the electrophysiological research of the 1960's, several investigators discovered that bones are piezoelectric; that is, when they are stressed, mechanical energy is converted to electrical energy in the form of electric current.[1] This might explain one of the practices of Marrow Washing *Qigong* in which the stress on the bones and muscles is increased in certain ways to increase the *Qi* circulation.

Dr. Robert O. Becker has done important work in this field. His book ***The Body Electric***[2] reports on much of the research concerning the body's electric field. It is presently believed that food and air are the fuels which generate the electricity in the body through biochemical reaction. This electricity, which is circulated throughout the entire body by means of electrically conductive tissue, is one of the main energy sources which keep the cells of the physical body alive.

Whenever you have an injury or are sick, your body's electrical circulation is affected. If this circulation of electricity stops, you die. But bioelectric energy not only maintains life, it is also responsible for repairing physical damage. Many researchers have sought ways of using external electrical or magnetic fields to speed up the body's recovery from physical injury. Richard Leviton reports: "Researchers at Loma Linda University's School of medicine in California have found, following studies in sixteen countries with over 1,000 patients, that low-frequency, low-intensity magnetic energy has been successful in treating chronic pain related to tissue ischemia, and has also worked in clearing up slow-healing ulcers, and in 90 percent of patients tested, raised blood flow significantly."[3]

Mr. Leviton also reports that every cell of the body functions like an electric battery and is able to store electric charges. He reports that: "Other biomagnetic investigators take an even closer look to find out what is happening, right down to the level of the blood, the organs, and the individual cell, which they regard as 'a small electric battery'."[3] This has convinced me that our entire body is essentially a big battery which is assembled from millions of small batteries. All of these batteries together form the human electromagnetic field.

Furthermore, much of the research on the body's electrical field relates to acupuncture. For example, Dr. Becker reports that the conductivity of the skin is much higher at acupuncture cavities, and that it is now possible to locate them precisely by measuring the skin's conductivity (Figure 2-1).[2] Many of these reports prove that the acupuncture which has been done in China for thousands of years is reasonable and scientific.

Some researchers use the theory of the body's electricity to explain many of the ancient "miracles" which have been attributed to the practice of *Qigong*. A report by Albert L. Huebner states: "These demonstrations of body electricity in human beings may also offer a new explanation of an ancient healing practice. If weak external fields can produce powerful physiological effects, it may be that fields from human tissues in one person are capable of producing clinical improvements in another. In short, the method of healing known as the laying on of hands could be an especially subtle form of electrical stimulation."[1]

Another frequently reported phenomenon is that when a *Qigong* practitioner has reached a high level of development, a halo would appear behind and/or around his head during meditation. This is commonly seen in paintings of Jesus Christ, the Buddha, and various Oriental immortals. Frequently the light is pictured as surrounding the whole body. This phenomenon may again be explained by the Body Electric theory. When a person has cultivated their *Qi* (electricity) to a high level, the *Qi* may be led to accumulate in the head. This *Qi* may then interact with the oxygen molecules in the air, and ionize them, causing them to glow.

Although the link between the theory of The Body Electric and the Chinese theory of *Qi* is becoming more accepted and better proven, there are still many questions to be answered. For example, how can the mind lead *Qi* (electricity)? How actually does the mind generate an EMF (electromotive force) to circulate the electricity in the body? How is the human electromagnetic field affected by the multitude of other electric fields which surround us, such as radio wiring or electrical appliances? How can we readjust our electromagnetic fields and survive in outer space or on other planets where the magnetic field is completely different from the earth's? You can see that the future of *Qigong* and bioelectric science is a challenging and exciting one. It is about time that we started to use modern technology to understand the inner energy world which has been for the most part ignored by Western society.

A Modern Definition of Qigong

If you now accept that the inner energy (*Qi*) circulating in our bodies is bioelectricity, then we can now formulate a definition of *Qigong* based on electrical principles.

Let us assume that the circuit shown in Figure 2-2 is similar to the circuit in our bodies. Unfortunately, although we now have a certain degree of understanding of this circuit from acupuncture, we still do not know in detail exactly what the body's circuit looks like. We know that there are twelve primary *Qi* channels (*Qi* rivers) and eight vessels (*Qi* reservoirs) in our body. There are also thousands of small *Qi* channels (*Luo*, 絡) which allow the *Qi* to reach the skin and the bone marrow. In this circuit, the twelve internal organs are connected and mutually related through these channels.

If you look at the electrical circuit in the illustration, you will see that:

1. The *Qi* channels are like the wires which carry electric current.

2. The internal organs are like the electrical components such as resistors and solenoids.

3. The *Qi* vessels are like capacitors, which regulate the current in the circuit.

How do you keep this electrical circuit functioning most efficiently? Your first concern is the resistance of the wire which carries the current. In a machine, you want to use a wire which has a high level of conductivity and low resistance, otherwise the current may melt the wire. Therefore, the wire should be of a material like copper or perhaps even gold. In your body, you want to keep the current flowing smoothly. This means that your first task is to remove anything which interferes with the flow and causes stagnation. Fat has low conductivity, so you should use diet and exercise to remove excess fat from your body. You should also learn how to relax your

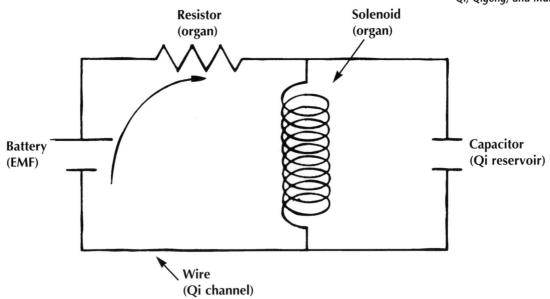

Resistor (organ)

Solenoid (organ)

Battery (EMF)

Capacitor (Qi reservoir)

Wire (Qi channel)

Figure 2–2. The Human Bioelectric Circuit is Similar to an Electric Circuit

physical body, because this opens all of the *Qi* channels. This is why relaxation is the first goal in *Taijiquan* and many *Qigong* exercises.

Your next concern in maintaining a healthy electrical circuit is the components - your internal organs. If you do not have the correct level of current in your organs, they will either burn out from too much current (*Yang*) or malfunction because of a deficient level of current (*Yin*). In order to avoid these problems in a machine, you use a capacitor to regulate the current. Whenever there is too much current, the capacitor absorbs and stores the excess, and whenever the current is weak, the capacitor supplies current to raise the level. The eight *Qi* vessels are your body's capacitors. *Qigong* is concerned with learning how to increase the level of *Qi* in these vessels so that they will be able to supply current when needed, and keep the internal organs functioning smoothly. This is especially important as you get older and your *Qi* level is generally lower.

Finally, in order to have a healthy circuit, you have to be concerned with the components themselves. If any of them are not strong and of good quality, the entire circuit will have problems. This means that the final concern in *Qigong* practice is how to maintain or even rebuild the health of your internal organs. Before we go any further, we should point out that there is an important difference between the circuit shown in the diagram and the *Qi* circuit in our bodies. This difference is that the human body is alive, and with the proper *Qi* nourishment, all of the cells can be regrown and the state of health improved. For example, if you are able to jog about three miles today, and if you keep jogging regularly and gradually increase the distance, eventually you will be able to easily jog five miles. This is because your body rebuilds and readjusts itself to fit the circumstances.

This means that, if we are able to increase the *Qi* flow through our internal organs, they can become stronger and healthier. Naturally, the increase in *Qi* must be slow and gradual so that the organs can adjust to it. In order to increase the *Qi* flow in your body, you need to work with the EMF (electromotive force) in your body. If you do not know what EMF is, imagine two containers filled with water and connected by a tube. If both containers have the same water level, then the water will not flow. However, if one side is higher than the other, the water will flow from that container to the other. In electricity, this potential difference is called electromotive force. Naturally, the higher the EMF is, the stronger the current will flow.

You can see from this discussion that the key to effective *Qigong* practice is, in addition to removing resistance from the *Qi* channels, learning how to increase the EMF in your body. Now let us see what the sources of EMF in the body are, so that we may use them to increase the flow of bioelectricity. Generally speaking, there are five major sources:

1. **Natural Energy.** Since your body is constructed of electrically conductive material, its electromagnetic field is always affected by the sun, the moon, clouds, the earth's magnetic field, and by the other energies around you. The major influences are the sun's radiation, the moon's gravity, and the earth's magnetic field. These affect your *Qi* circulation significantly, and are responsible for the pattern of your *Qi* circulation since you were formed. We are now also being greatly affected by the energy generated by modern technology, such as the electromagnetic waves generated by radio, TV, microwave ovens, computers, and many other things.

2. **Food and Air.** In order to maintain life, we take in food and air essence through our mouth and nose. These essences are then converted into *Qi* through biochemical reaction in the chest and digestive system (called the Triple Burner in Chinese medicine). When *Qi* is converted from the essence, an EMF is generated which circulates the *Qi* throughout the body. Consequently a major part of *Qigong* is devoted to getting the proper kinds of food and fresh air.

3. **Thinking.** The human mind is the most important and efficient source of bioelectric EMF. Any time you move to do something you must first generate an idea (*Yi*). This idea generates the EMF and leads the *Qi* to energize the appropriate muscles to carry out the desired motion. The more you can concentrate, the stronger the EMF you can generate, and the stronger the flow of *Qi* you can lead. Naturally, the stronger the flow of *Qi* you lead to the muscles, the more they will be energized. Because of this, the mind is considered the most important factor in *Qigong* training.

4. **Exercise.** Exercise converts the food essence (fat) stored in your body into *Qi,* and therefore builds up the EMF. Many *Qigong* styles have been created which utilize movement for this purpose.

5. **Converting Pre-Birth Essence into *Qi.*** The hormones produced by our endocrine glands are referred to as "Pre-Birth essence" in Chinese medicine. They can be converted into *Qi* to stimulate the functioning of our physical body, thereby increasing our vitality. Balancing hormone production when you are young and increasing its production when you are old are important subjects in Chinese *Qigong.*

From the foregoing, you can see that within the human body, there is a network of electrical circuitry. In order to maintain the circulation of bioelectricity, there must be a battery wherein to store a charge. Where then, is the battery in our body?

Chinese *Qigong* practitioners believe that there is a place which is able to store *Qi* (bioelectricity). This place is called the *Dan Tian* (i.e., elixir field). According to such practitioners, there are three *Dan Tians* in the human body. One is located at the abdominal area, one or two inches below the navel, called the *"Lower Dan Tian"* (*Xia Dan Tian,* 下丹田). The second is in the area of the lower sternum, and is called the *"Middle Dan Tian"* (*Zhong Dan Tian,* 中丹田). The third is the lower center of forehead (or the third eye), connected to the brain and is called the *"Upper Dan Tian"* (*Shang Dan Tian,* 上丹田).

The Lower *Dan Tian* is considered to be the residence of the Water *Qi*, or the *Qi* which is generated from the Original Essence (*Yuan Jing,* 元精). Therefore, *Qi* stored here is called Original *Qi* (*Yuan Qi,* 元氣). According to Chinese medicine, in this same area there is a cavity called *"Qihai"*

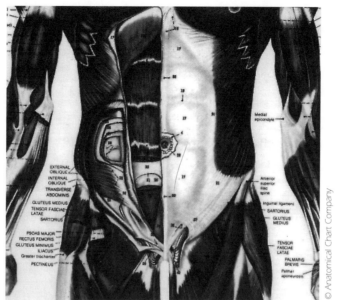

Figure 2–3. Anatomic Structure of the Abdominal Area

(Co-6)(氣海) which means *"Qi ocean."* This is consistent with the conclusions drawn by *Qigong* practitioners, who also call this area the "Lower *Dan Tian*" (lower elixir field). Both groups agree that this area is able to produce *Qi* or elixir like a field, and that here the *Qi* is abundant like an ocean.

In *Qigong* practice, it is commonly known that in order to build up the *Qi* to a higher level in the Lower *Dan Tian,* you must move your abdominal area (i.e., Lower *Dan Tian*) up and down through abdominal breathing. This kind of up and down abdominal breathing exercise is called *"Qi Huo"* (起火) and means "start the fire." It is also called "back to childhood breathing" (*Fan Tong Hu Xi,* 返童呼吸). Normally, after you have exercised the Lower *Dan Tian* for about ten minutes, you will have a feeling of warmth in the lower abdomen, which implies the accumulation of *Qi* or energy.

Theoretically and scientifically, what is happening when the abdominal area is moved up and down? If you look at the structure of the abdominal area, you will see that there are about six layers of muscle and fasciae sandwiching each other in this area (Figure 2-3). In fact, what you actually see is the sandwich of muscles and fat accumulated in the fasciae layers. When you move your abdomen up and down, you are actually using your mind to move the muscles, not the fat. Whenever there is a muscular contraction and relaxation, the fat slowly turns into bioelectricity. When this bioelectricity encounters resistance from the fasciae layers, it turns into heat. From this, you can see how simple the theory might be for the generation of *Qi.* Another thing you should know is that, according to our understanding today, fat and fasciae are poor electrical conductors, while the muscles are relatively good electrical conductors.[1, 2, 3] When these good and poor electrical materials are sandwiched together, they act like a battery. This is why, through up and down abdominal movements, the energy can be stored temporarily and generate warmth.

However, through nearly two thousand years of experience, Daoists have said that the front abdominal area is not the real *Dan Tian,* but is in fact a "False *Dan Tian*" (*Jia Dan Tian,* 假丹田). Their argument is that, although this Lower *Dan Tian* is able to generate *Qi* and build it up to a higher level, it does not store it for a long time. This is because the Lower *Dan Tian* is located on

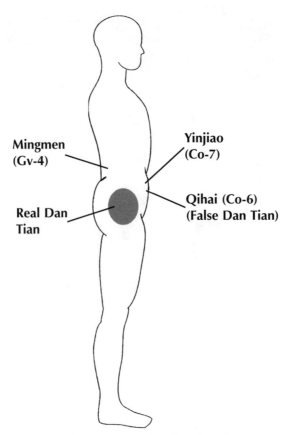

Figure 2–4. The Real Dan Tian and the False Dan Tian

the path of the Conception Vessel, so that whenever *Qi* is built up to a higher energy state, it will circulate in the Conception and Governing Vessels (please refer to Chapter 4 for a discussion of the eight vessels). This Lower *Dan Tian* therefore cannot be a battery as we understand the term. A real battery should be able to store the *Qi*. Where then, is the "Real *Dan Tian*" (*Zhen Dan Tian*, 眞丹田)?

Daoists teach that the Real *Dan Tian* is at the center of the abdominal area, at the physical center of the gravity located in the large and small intestines (Figure 2-4). Now, let us analyze this from two different points of view.

First, let us take a look of how a life is started. It begins with a sperm from the father entering an egg from the mother, thus forming the original human cell (Figure 2-5).[4] This cell next divides into two cells, then four cells, etc. When this group of cells adheres to the internal wall of the uterus, the umbilical cord starts to develop. Nutrition and energy for further cell multiplication is absorbed through the umbilical cord from the mother's body. The baby keeps growing until matured. During this nourishing and growing process, the baby's abdomen is moving up and down, acting like a pump drawing in nutrition and energy into his or her body. Later, immediately after the birth, air and nutrition are taken in from the nose and mouth through the mouth's sucking action and the lungs' breathing. As the child grows, it slowly forgets the natural movements of the abdomen. This is why the abdomen's up and down movement is called "back to the childhood breathing."

Think carefully: if your first human cell is still alive, where is this cell? Most likely, this cell has already died a long time ago. It is understood that approximately one trillion (10^{12}) cells die

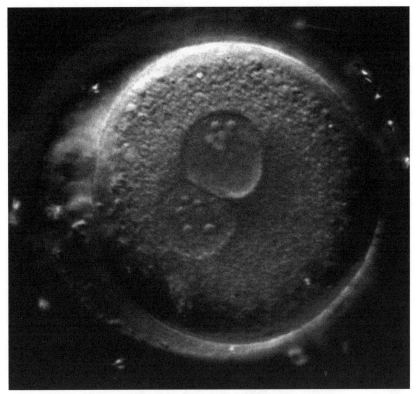

Figure 2–5. Original First Human Cell

in a human body each day.[5] However, if we assume that this first cell is still alive, then it should be located at our physical center, that is, our center of gravity. If we think carefully, we can see that it is from this center that the cells could multiply evenly outward until the body is completely constructed. In order to maintain this even multiplication physically, the energy or *Qi* must be centered at this point and radiate outward. When we are in an embryonic state, this is the gravity center and also the *Qi* center. As we grow after birth, this center remains.

The above argument adheres solely to the traditional point of view of the physical development of our body. Next, let us analyze this center from another point of view.

If we look at the physical center of gravity, we can see that the entire area is occupied by the Large and Small intestines (Figure 2-6). We know that there are three kinds of muscles existing in our body, and can examine them in ascending order of our ability to control them. The first kind is the heart muscle, in which the electrical conductivity among muscular groups is the highest. The heart beats all the time, regardless of our attention, and through practice and discipline, we are able only to regulate its beating, not start and stop it. If we supply electricity to even a small piece of this muscle, it will pump. The second category of muscles are those which contract automatically, but over which we can exert significant control if we make the effort. The diaphragm which controls breathing, our eyelids, and certain sexual responses are examples of this muscle type, and their electrical conductivity is lower than the first type. The third kind of muscles are those muscles which are directly controlled by our conscious mind. The electric conductivity of these muscles is the lowest of the three groups.

If you look at the structure of the Large and Small Intestines, the first thing you notice is that the total length of your Large and Small Intestines is approximately six times your body's height (Figure 2-7). With such long electrically conductive tissues sandwiched between all of the mesen-

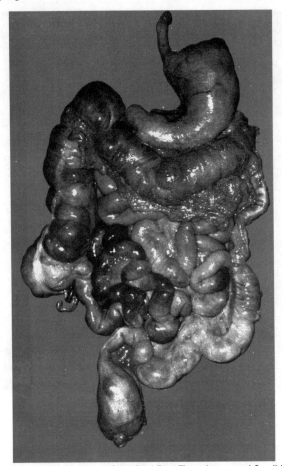

Figure 2–6. Anatomic Structure of the Real Dan Tian - Large and Small Intestines

tery, water, and outer casings (which it is reasonable to believe are poor electrical conductive tissues), it acts like a huge battery in our body (Figure 2-8).[6] From this, you can see that it makes sense both logically and scientifically that the center of gravity, rather than the false *Dan Tian,* is the real battery in our body.

Next, let us examine the structure of the Middle *Dan Tian* area. The Middle *Dan Tian* is located next to the diaphragm (Figure 2-9). We know that the diaphragm is a membranous muscular partition separating the abdominal and the thoracic cavities. It functions in respiration and is electrically conductive. On the top and the bottom of the diaphragm there is the fasciae, which isolates the internal organs from the diaphragm. We see now again a good electrical conductor isolated by a poor electrical conductor. That means that it is capable of storing electricity or *Qi.* Since this place is between the lungs and the stomach, and they absorb the Post-Birth essence (air and food) and convert it into energy, the *Qi* accumulated in the Middle *Dan Tian* is classified as Fire *Qi.* The reason for this name is that the *Qi* converted from the contaminated air and the food can affect *Qi* status and make it *Yang.* Naturally, this Fire *Qi* can also agitate your emotional mind.

Finally, let us analyze the brain, which is considered the Upper *Dan Tian.* We already know that the brain and the spinal cord are considered to be the central nervous system, in which the electrical conductivity is highest in our body. If we examine the brain's structure, we can see that it is segregated by the arachnoid mater (i.e., a delicate membrane of the spinal cord and brain, lying between the pia mater and dura mater) into separate portions (Figure 2-10). It is reasonable to assume that these materials are low electrically conductive tissues. Again, it is another giant

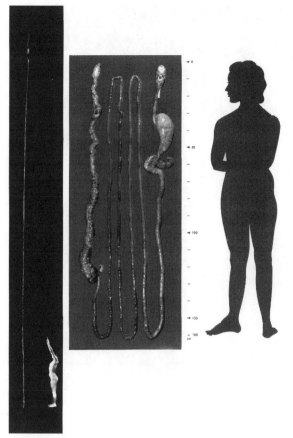

Figure 2–7. The Large and Small Intestines are About Six Times Your Height

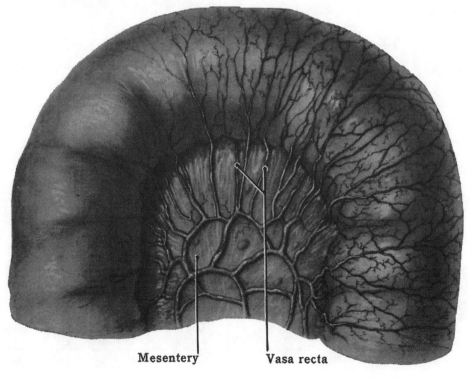

Mesentery   **Vasa recta**

Figure 2–8. Low Electrically Conductive Materials Such as Mesentery, Outer Casing,
and Water in and Around the Intestines Makes the Entire Area Act Like a Battery

(Used with permission: James E. Anderson, M.D., Grant's Atlas of Anatomy, 7th ed., ©Williams and Wilkins)

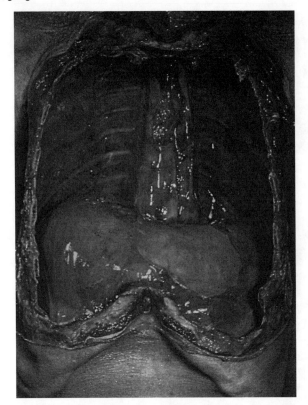

Figure 2–9. The Middle Dan Tian is Connected to the Diaphragm

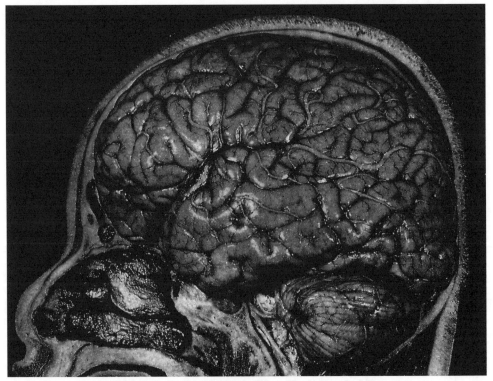

Figure 2–10. The Upper Dan Tian — The Human Brain

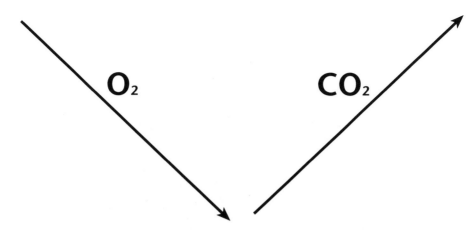

Figure 2–11. We Inhale to Absorb Oxygen and Exhale to Expel Carbon Dioxide

battery which consumes *Qi* in great amounts. However, since the brain does not produce *Qi* or bioelectricity, its function as a *Dan Tian* cannot be considered to be the same as the Lower *Dan Tian*.

From the above discussion, you may have gained a better idea of how we can link ancient experience together with modern scientific understanding. In order to make the scientific concept of *Qigong* even more clear, let us look at *Qigong* from another scientific point of view, this time chemical.

If we examine how we breath, we can see that we inhale to take in oxygen, and we exhale to expel carbon dioxide (Figure 2-11). From this, we can see that every minute we expel a great deal of carbon from our body through exhalation. Carbon is a material which can be seen. The question is, where is the carbon coming from in our body? Through breathing, how much carbon is actually processed out?

The first source of carbon is from the food (glucose) we eat. When this food is converted into energy through chemical reaction during our daily activities, carbon dioxide is produced.[7]

$$\text{glucose} + 6O_2 \longrightarrow 6\,CO_2 + 6H_2O$$
$$\Delta G^{\circ\prime} = -686 \text{ kcal}$$

The second source of this carbon is from the dead cells in our body. We already know that the majority of our body is constructed from the elements carbon (C), hydrogen (H_2), oxygen (O_2), and nitrogen (N_2), while other elements such as Calcium (Ca), Phosphorus (P), Chloride (Cl), Sulfur (S), Potassium (K), Sodium (Na), Magnesium (Mg), Iodine (I), and Iron (Fe) comprise much less of our body weight. This means that the cells in our body contain a great amount of carbon.

In addition, consider that every cell in our body has a life time. As many as a trillion (10^{12}) cells die in our body every 24 hours.[5] For example, we know that the life span of a skin cell is 28 days. Naturally, every living cell such as those of the bone, marrow, liver, etc. have their own individual lifetime. We rely on our respiration to bring the carbon (i.e., dead cells) out, and to supply living cells with new oxygen through inhalation, and new carbon sources, water, and other minerals from eating. All this aids in the formation of new cells and the continuation of life.

From the foregoing, we can conclude that the cell replacement process is ongoing at all times in our life. Health during our lifetime depends on how smoothly and how quickly this replacement process is carried out. If there are more new healthy cells to replace the old cells, you live and grow. If the cells replaced are as healthy as the original cells, you remain young. However, if there are fewer cells produced, or if the new cells are not as healthy as the original cells, then you age. Now, let us analyze *Qigong* from the point of view of cell replacement.

In order to produce a good, healthy cell, first you must consider the materials which are needed. From the structure of a cell, we know that we will need hydrogen, oxygen, carbon, and other minerals which we can absorb either from air or food. Therefore, air quality, water purity, and the choice of foods become critical factors for your health and longevity. Naturally, this has also been component of *Qigong* study.

However, we know that air and water quality today has been contaminated by pollution. This is especially bad in industrial areas. The quality of the food we have eaten depends on their source and processing methods. Naturally, it is not easy to find the same pristine environments as in ancient times. However, we must learn how to fit into our new environment and choose the way of our life wisely.

Since carbon comprises such a major part of our body, how to absorb good quality carbon is an important issue in modern health. You may obtain carbon from animal products or from plants. Generally speaking, the carbon taken from plants is more pure and clean than that taken from animals.

According to past experience and analysis, red meat is generally more contaminated than white meat, and is able to disturb and stimulate your emotional mind and confuse your thinking. Another source from which animal products can be obtained is fish. Again, some fish are good and others may be bad. For example, shrimp is high in cholesterol, which may increase the risk of high blood pressure.

Due to the impurities contained in most animal products, *Qigong* practitioners learned how to absorb protein from plants, especially from peas or beans. Soybean is one of the best of these sources; it is both inexpensive and easy to grow. However, if you are not a vegetarian originally, then it can be difficult for your body to produce the enzymes to digest an all-vegetable diet immediately. Humans evolved as omnivores, and the craving for meat can be strong. Even today, we all still have canine teeth, which were used to tear off raw meat in ancient times. Therefore, the natural enzymes existing in our body are more tailored to digesting meat. In an experiment, if we place a piece of meat and some corn in human digestive enzymes, we will see that the meat will be dissolved in a matter of minutes, while the corn will take many hours. This means it is generally easier for a human to absorb meat rather than plants as a protein source.

However, the above discussion does not mean we cannot absolutely absorb plant protein efficiently. The key is that if it is present to begin with, the **enzyme production can be increased within your body**, but it will take time. For example, if you cannot drink milk due to insufficient lactate in your stomach, you may start by drinking a little bit of milk every day, and slowly increase it as days pass by. You will realize that you are able to absorb milk six months later. This means that if you wish to become a vegetarian, you must reduce the intake of meat products slowly and allow your body to adjust to it; otherwise you may experience protein deficiency.

Other than a protein source, you must also consider minerals. Although they do not comprise a large proportion of our body, their importance in some ways is more significant than carbon. We know that calcium is an important element for bones, and iron is crucial for blood cells, etc. Therefore, when we eat we must consume a variety of foods instead of just a few. How to absorb nutrition from food has been an important part of Chinese *Qigong* study.

In order to produce healthy cells, other than the concerns of the material side, you must also consider energy. You should understand that when a person ages quickly, often it is not because he or she is malnourished, but instead is due to the weakening of their *Qi* storage and circulation. Without an abundant supply of *Qi* (bioelectricity), *Qi* circulation will not be regulated efficiently, and therefore your life force will weaken and the physical body will degenerate. In order to have abundant *Qi* storage, you must learn *Qigong* in order to build up the *Qi* in your eight vessels, and also to help you understand how to lead the *Qi* circulating in your body. This kind of *Qigong* training includes *Wai Dan* (external elixir) and *Nei Dan* (internal elixir) practice, which we will discuss in the next section.

Other than the concern for materials needed, and the *Qi* required for cell production and replacement, the next thing you should ask yourself is how this replacement process is carried out. Then, you will see that the entire replacement process depends on the blood cells. From western medicine, we know that a blood cell is the carrier of water, oxygen, and nutrients to everywhere in the body through the blood circulatory network. From arteries and capillaries, the components for new cells are brought to every tiny place in the body. The old cells then absorb everything required from the blood stream and divide to produce new cells. The dead cells are brought back through veins to the lungs. Through respiration, the dead cell materials are expelled as carbon dioxide.

However, there is one thing missing from the last process. This is the *Qi* or bioelectricity which is required for the biochemical process of cell division. It has been proven that every blood cell is actually like a dipole or a small battery, which is able to store bioelectricity and also to release it.[1] This means that each blood cell is actually a carrier of *Qi*. This is also understood in Chinese medicine. In Chinese medicine, the blood and the *Qi* are always together. Where there is blood, there is *Qi,* and where there is *Qi,* the blood will also be there. Therefore, the term *"Qi-Xue"* (i.e., *Qi*-blood)(氣血) is often used in Chinese medicine.

If you understand the above discussion, and if we take a look at our blood circulatory system, then we can see that the arteries are located deeply underneath the muscles, while the veins are situated near the skin's surface. The color of the blood is red in the arteries because of the presence of oxygen, and its color is blue in the veins both because of the absence of this oxygen and the presence of carbon. This implies that cell replacement actually happens from inside of the body, moving outward. This can also offer us a hint that, if we tense more, the blood circulation will be more stagnant, and cell replacement will be slower. We can also conclude that most cell replacement occurs in the night when we are at our most relaxed state during sleep. This can further lead one to conclude the importance of sleeping. We will discuss later how cell replacement is further related to our breathing.

If we already know that blood cells are the carriers of everything which is required for cell replacement, then we must also consider the healthy condition of our blood cells. If you have good health and a sufficient quantity of blood cells, then the nutrition and *Qi* can be carried to every part of the body efficiently. You will be healthy. However, if you do not have sufficient blood cells, or the quality of the cells is poor, then the entire cell replacement process will be stagnant. Naturally, you will degenerate swiftly.

According to modern medical science, blood cells also have a life span. When the old ones die, new ones must be produced from the bone marrow. Bone marrow is the major blood factory. From medical reports, we know that normally, after a person reaches thirty, the marrow near the end side of the bone cavity turns yellow. This indicates that fat has accumulated there. It also means that red blood cells are no longer being produced in the yellowed area (Figure 2-12).[8]

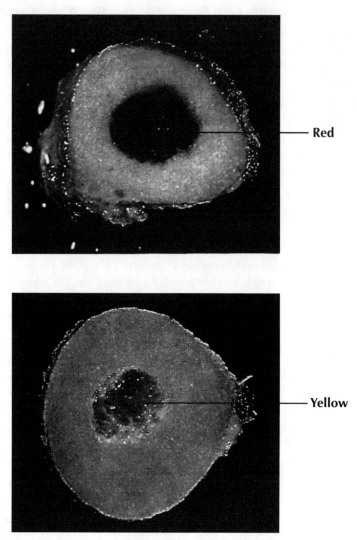

Figure 2-12. Structure of a Long Bone. Red Bone Marrow and Yellow Bone Marrow

Chinese *Qigong* practitioners believe that the degeneration of the bone marrow is due to insufficient *Qi* supply. Therefore, Bone Marrow Washing *Qigong* was developed. From experience, through marrow washing *Qigong* practice, health can be improved and life can be extended significantly. If you are interested in this subject, please read **Muscle/Tendon Changing and Marrow/Brain Washing Chi Kung**, by YMAA.

In addition to the above, the next thing which is highly important in human life is hormone production within your body. We already know from today's medical science that hormones act as a catalyst in the body. When the hormone levels are high, we are more energized and cell replacement can happen faster and more smoothly. When hormone production is slow and its level is low, then the cell replacement will be slow and we will age quickly. It was only in the last few years that scientists have discovered that by increasing the hormone levels in the body, we may be able to extend our life significantly.[9]

Maintenance of hormone production in a healthy manner has also been a major concern in Chinese *Qigong* practice. According to Chinese medicine, glands which produce hormones were recognized since ancient times. Hormones were not understood. However, throughout a thousand years of practice and experience, they understood that the essence of life is stored in the kidneys. Today, we know that this essence is actually the hormones produced from the adrenal glands on the top of the kidneys. The Chinese also believed that through stimulation of the testicles and ovaries, the life force could be increased. In addition, from still meditation practice, they learned how to lead the *Qi* to the brain and raise the "spirit of vitality." It has also been found that through practice, bioelectricity can be led to the pituitary gland to stimulate growth hormone production. All of these practices are believed to be effective paths to longevity.

From medical science, we know that our hormone levels are significantly reduced when the last pieces of our bones are completed, between ages 29 to 30. Theoretically, when our body has completed constructing itself, it somehow triggers the reduction of our hormone levels. From this, you can see that maintaining the hormone levels in our body may be a key to longevity.

Finally, in order to prevent ourselves from getting sick, we must also consider our immune system. According to Chinese medicine and *Qigong,* when *Qi* storage is abundant, you get sick less. If we take a careful look, we can realize that every white blood cell is just like a fighting soldier. If we do not have enough *Qi* to supply it, its fighting capability will be low. It is just like a soldier who needs food to maintain his strength. When the *Qi* is strong, the immune system is strong. Therefore, the skin breathing technique has been developed, which teaches a practitioner to lead the *Qi* to the surface of the skin to strengthen the "Guardian *Qi*" (*Wei Qi,* 衛氣) or an energetic component of the immune system near the skin surface.

From the foregoing, hopefully I have offered you a challenge for profound thought and understanding. Although most of these conclusions are drawn from my personal research, further study and verification is still needed. I deeply believe that if we can all open our minds and share our opinions together, we will be able to make our lives more healthy and meaningful.

2-3. Categories of Qigong

Often, people ask me the same question: Is jogging, weight lifting, or dancing a kind of Qigong practice? To answer this question, let us trace back *Qigong* history to before the Chinese Qin and Han dynastic periods (255 B.C.-223 A.D.). Then you can see that the origins of many *Qigong* practices were actually in dancing. Through dancing, the physical body was exercised and the healthy condition of the physical body was maintained. Also, through dancing and matching movements with music, the mind was regulated into a harmonious state. From this harmonious mind, the spirit could be raised to a more energized state, or could be calmed down to a peaceful level. This *Qigong* dancing later passed to Japan during the Chinese Han Dynasty, and became a very elegant, slow, and high style of dancing in the Japanese royal court. This *Taijiquan*-like dancing is still practiced in Japan today.

The ways of African or Native American dancing in which the body is bounced up and down is also known as a means of loosening up the joints and improving *Qi* circulation. Naturally, jogging, weight lifting, or even walking are a kind of *Qigong* practice. Therefore, we can say that **any activity which is able to regulate the *Qi* circulation** in the body is a *Qigong* practice.

Let us define it more clearly. In Figure 2-13, if the left vertical line represents the amount of usage of the physical body (*Yang*), and the right vertical line is the usage of the mind (*Yin*), then we can see that the more you practice toward the left, the more physical effort, and the less mind, is needed. This can be aerobic dancing, walking, or jogging in which the mind usage is relatively little compared to physical action. In this kind of *Qigong* practice, normally you do not need spe-

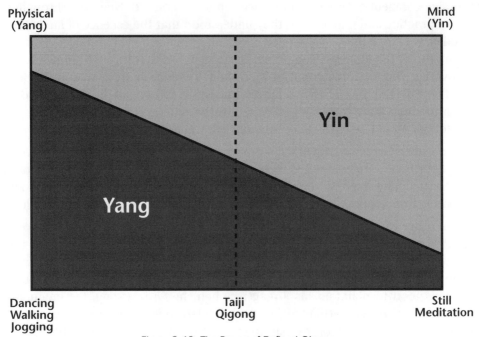

Figure 2–13. The Range of Defined Qigong

cial training, and it is classified as layman *Qigong*. In the middle point, the mind and the physical activity are almost equally important. This kind of *Qigong* will be the slow Moving *Qigong* commonly practiced, in which the mind is used to lead the *Qi* in coordination with the movements. For example, *Taiji Qigong,* The Eight Pieces of Brocade, The Five Animal Sports, and many others are very typical *Qigong* exercises, especially in Chinese medical and martial arts societies.

However, when you reach a profound level of *Qigong* practice, the mind becomes more important. When you reach this high level, you are dealing with your mind while you are sitting still. Most of this mental *Qigong* training was practiced by the scholars and religious *Qigong* practitioners. In this practice, you may have a little physical movement in the lower abdomen. However, the main focus of this *Qigong* practice is in the peaceful mind or spiritual enlightenment which originates from the cultivation of your mind. This kind of *Qigong* practice includes Sitting *Chan (Ren)* (坐禪，忍), Small Circulation Meditation (*Xiao Zhou Tian,* 小周天), Grand Circulation Meditation (*Da Zhou Tian,* 大周天), or Brain Washing Enlightenment Meditation (*Xi Sui Gong,* 洗髓功).

Theoretically speaking, in order to have good health, you will need to maintain your physical condition and also build up abundant *Qi* in your body. The best *Qigong* for health is actually located in the middle of our model, where you learn how to regulate your physical body and also your mind. From this *Yin* and *Yang* practice, your *Qi* can be circulated smoothly in the body.

Let us now review the traditional concepts of how *Qigong* was categorized. Generally speaking, all *Qigong* practices can be divided, according to their training theory and methods, into two general categories: *Wai Dan* (External Elixir, 外丹) and *Nei Dan* (Internal Elixir, 内丹. Understanding the differences between them will give you an overview of most Chinese *Qigong* practice.

External and Internal Elixirs

A. Wai Dan (External Elixir) 外丹

"Wai" means "external" or "outside," and *"Dan"* means "elixir." External here means the skin surface of the body or the limbs, as opposed to the torso or the center of the body, which includes all of the vital organs. Elixir is a hypothetical, life-prolonging substance for which Chinese Daoists have been searching for several millennia. They originally thought that the elixir was something physical which could be prepared from herbs or chemicals purified in a furnace. After thousands of years of study and experimentation, they found that the elixir is in the body. In other words, if you want to prolong your life, you must find the elixir in your body, and then learn to cultivate, protect, and nourish it. Actually, the elixir is what we have understood the inner energy or *Qi* circulating in the body to be.

There are many ways of producing elixir or *Qi* in the body. For example, in *Wai Dan Qigong* practice, you may exercise your limbs through dancing or even walking. As you exercise, the *Qi* builds up in your arms and legs. When the *Qi* potential in your limbs builds to a high enough level, the *Qi* will flow through the channels, clearing any obstructions and flowing into the center of the body to nourish the organs. This is the main reason that a person who works out, or has a physical job is, generally healthier than someone who sits around all day.

Naturally, you may simply massage your body to produce the *Qi*. Through massage, you may stimulate the cells of your body to a higher energized state and therefore the *Qi* concentration will be raised and the circulation enhanced. Then, after massage you relax, and the higher levels of *Qi* on the skin surface and muscles will flow into the center of the body and thereby improve the *Qi* circulatory conditions in your internal organs. This is the theoretical foundation of the *Tui Na Qigong* massage (pushing and grabbing massage, 推拿).

Through acupuncture, you may also bring the *Qi* level near the skin surface to a higher level and from this stimulation, the *Qi* condition of the internal organs can be regulated through *Qi* channels. Therefore, acupuncture can also be classified as *Wai Dan Qigong* practice. Naturally, the herbal treatments are a way of *Wai Dan* practice as well.

From this, we can briefly conclude that any possible stimulation or exercises which accumulate a high level of *Qi* on the surface of the body, and then flow inward toward the center of the body, can be classified as *Wai Dan* (external elixir) (Figure 2-14).

B. Nei Dan (Internal Elixir)

"Nei" means "internal" and *"Dan"* again means "elixir." Thus, *Nei Dan* means to build the elixir internally. Here, internally means in the body instead of in the limbs. Normally, the *Qi* is built on the *Qi* vessels instead of the primary *Qi* channels. Whereas in *Wai Dan* the *Qi* is built up in the limbs or skin surface and then moved into the body through primary *Qi* channels, **Nei Dan exercises build up *Qi* in the body and lead it out to the limbs** (Figure 2-15).

Generally, speaking, *Nei Dan* theory is deeper than *Wai Dan* theory, and it is more difficult to understand and practice. Traditionally, most of the *Nei Dan Qigong* practices have been passed down more secretly than those of the *Wai Dan*. This is especially true of the highest levels of *Nei Dan*, such as Marrow/Brain Washing, which were passed down to only a few trusted disciples.

Schools of Qigong Practice

We can also classify *Qigong* into four major categories according to the purpose or final goal of the training: A. maintaining health; B. curing sickness; C. martial arts; D. enlightenment or

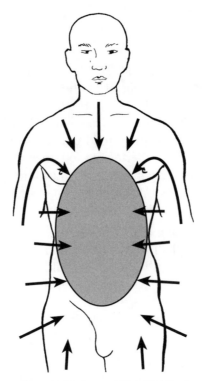

Figure 2–14. External Elixir (Wai Dan)

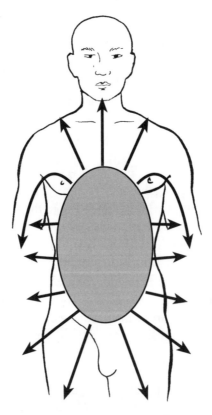

Figure 2–15 Internal Elixir (Nei Dan)

Buddhahood. This is only a rough breakdown, however, since almost every style of *Qigong* serves more than one of the above purposes. For example, although martial *Qigong* focuses on increasing fighting effectiveness, it can also improve your health. Daoist *Qigong* aims for longevity and enlightenment, but to reach this goal you need to be in good health and know how to cure sickness. Because of this multi-purpose aspect of the categories, it will be simpler to discuss their backgrounds rather than the goals of their training. Knowing the history and basic principles of each category will help you to understand their *Qigong* more clearly.

A. Scholar Qigong — for Maintaining Health

In China before the Han Dynasty, there were two major schools of scholarship. One of them was created by Confucius (551-479 B.C.)(孔子) during the Spring and Autumn period. Later, his philosophy was popularized and enlarged by Mencius (372-289 B.C.)(孟子) in the Warring States Period. The scholars who practice his philosophy are commonly called Confucians or Confucianists (*Ru Jia,* 儒家). The key words to their basic philosophy are **Loyalty** (*Zhong,* 忠), **Filial Piety** (*Xiao,* 孝), Humanity (*Ren,* 仁), **Kindness** (*Ai,* 愛), **Trust** (*Xin,* 信), **Justice** (*Yi,* 義), **Harmony** (*He,* 和), and **Peace** (*Ping,* 平). Humanity and human feelings are the main subjects of study. Ru Jia philosophy has become the center of much of Chinese culture.

The second major school of scholarship was called *Dao Jia* (Daoism)(道家) and was created by Lao Zi (老子) in the 6th century B.C. Lao Zi is considered to be the author of a book called the ***Dao De Jing*** (*Classic on the Virtue of the Dao*)(道德經) which describes human morality. Later, in the Warring States Period, his follower Zhuang Zhou (莊周) wrote a book called ***Zhuang Zi*** (莊子) which led to the forming of another strong branch of Daoism. Before the Han Dynasty, Daoism was considered a branch of scholarship. However, in the Han Dynasty, traditional Daoism was combined with the Buddhism imported from India by Zhang Dao-Ling (張道陵), and it began gradually to be treated as a religion. Therefore, the Daoism before the Han Dynasty should be considered scholarly Daoism rather than religious.

With regard to their contribution to *Qigong,* both schools emphasized maintaining health and preventing disease. They believed that many illnesses are caused by mental and emotional excesses. When a person's mind is not calm, balanced, and peaceful, the organs will not function normally. For example, depression can cause stomach ulcers and indigestion. Anger will cause the liver to malfunction. Sadness will cause stagnation and tightness in the lungs, and fear can disturb the normal functioning of the kidneys and bladder. They realized that if you want to avoid illness, you must learn to balance and relax your thoughts and emotions. This is called "regulating the mind" (*Tiao Xin,* 調心).

Therefore, the scholars emphasize gaining a peaceful mind through meditation. In their still meditation, the main part of the training is getting rid of thoughts so that the mind is clear and calm. When you become calm, the flow of thoughts and emotions slows down, and you feel mentally and emotionally neutral. This kind of meditation can be thought of as practicing emotional self-control. When you are in this **"no thought"** state, you become very relaxed, and can even relax deep down into your internal organs. When your body is this relaxed, your *Qi* will naturally flow smoothly and strongly. This kind of still meditation was very common in ancient Chinese scholar society.

In order to reach the goal of a calm and peaceful mind, their training focused on regulating the mind, body, and breath. They believed that as long as these three things were regulated, the *Qi* flow would be smooth and sickness would not occur. This is why the *Qi* training of the scholars is called *"Xiu Qi"* (修氣), which means "cultivating *Qi.*" *"Xiu"* in Chinese means to regulate, to cultivate, or to repair. It means to maintain in good condition. This is very different from the religious Daoist *Qi* training after the Han Dynasty which was called *"Lian Qi"* (練氣), which is translated "train *Qi*." *"Lian"* means to drill or to practice to make stronger.

Many of the *Qigong* documents written by the Confucians and Daoists were limited to the maintenance of health. The scholar's attitude in *Qigong* was to follow his natural destiny and maintain his health. This philosophy is quite different from that of the religious Daoist after the Han Dynasty, who believed that one's destiny could be changed. They believed that it is possible to train your *Qi* to make it stronger; and to extend your life. It is said in scholarly society: "in human life, seventy is rare."[10] You should understand that few of the common people in ancient times lived past seventy because of the lack of good food and modern medical technology. It is also said: "peace with Heaven and delight in your destiny" (安天樂命); and "cultivate the body and await destiny" (修身俟命). Compare this with the philosophy of the later Daoists, who said: "one hundred and twenty means dying young."[11] They believed and have proven that human life can be lengthened and destiny can be resisted and overcome.

Confucianism and Daoism were the two major scholarly schools in China, but there were many other schools which were also more or less involved in *Qigong* practices. We will not discuss them here because there is only a very limited number of *Qigong* documents from these schools.

B. Medical Qigong — for Healing

In ancient Chinese society, most emperors respected the scholars and were affected by their philosophy. Doctors were not regarded highly because they made their diagnosis by touching the patient's body, which was considered characteristic of the lower classes in society. Although the doctors developed a profound and successful medical science, they were commonly looked down on. However, they continued to work hard and study, and quietly passed down the results of their research to following generations.

Of all the groups studying *Qigong* in China, the doctors have been at it the longest. Since the discovery of *Qi* circulation in the human body about four thousand years ago, the Chinese doctors have devoted a major portion of their efforts to studying the behavior of *Qi*. Their efforts resulted in acupuncture, acupressure or Cavity Press massage, and herbal treatment.

In addition, many Chinese doctors used their medical knowledge to create different sets of *Qigong* exercises either for maintaining health or for curing specific illnesses. Chinese medical doctors believed that doing only sitting or still meditation to regulate the body, mind, and breathing as the scholars did was not enough to cure sickness. They believed that in order to increase the *Qi* circulation, you must move. Although a calm and peaceful mind was important for health, exercising the body was more important. They learned through their medical practice that people who exercised properly got sick less often, and their bodies degenerated less quickly than was the case with people who just sat around. They also realized that specific body movements could increase the *Qi* circulation in specific organs. They reasoned from this that these exercises could also be used to treat specific illnesses and to restore the normal functioning of these organs.

Some of these movements are similar to the way in which certain animals move. It is clear that in order for an animal to survive in the wild, it must have an instinct for how to protect its body. Part of this instinct is concerned with how to build up its *Qi*, and how to keep its *Qi* from being lost. We humans have lost many of these instincts over the years that we have been separating ourselves from nature.

Many doctors developed *Qigong* exercises which were modeled after animal movements to maintain health and cure sickness. A typical, well known set of such exercises is *"Wu Qin Shi"* (Five Animal Sports)(五禽戲) created by Dr. Jun Qing (君倩). Another famous set based on similar principles is called *"Ba Duan Jin"* (The Eight Pieces of Brocade)(八段錦). It was created by Marshal Yue Fei (岳飛) who, interestingly enough, was a soldier rather than a doctor.

In addition, using their medical knowledge of *Qi* circulation, Chinese doctors researched until they found which movements could help cure particular illnesses and health problems. Not surprisingly, many of these movements were not unlike the ones used to maintain health, since many illnesses are caused by unbalanced *Qi*. When an imbalance continues for a long period of time, the organs will be affected, and may be physically damaged. It is just like running a machine without supplying the proper electrical current — over time, the machine will be damaged. Chinese doctors believe that before physical damage to an organ shows up in a patient's body, there is first an abnormality in the *Qi* balance and circulation. **Abnormal *Qi* circulation is the very beginning of illness and organ damage**. When *Qi* is too positive (*Yang*) or too negative (*Yin*) in a specific organ's *Qi* channel, your physical organ is beginning to suffer damage. If you do not correct the *Qi* circulation, that organ will malfunction or degenerate. The best way to heal someone is to adjust and balance the *Qi* even before there is any physical problem. Therefore, correcting or increasing the normal *Qi* circulation is the major goal of acupuncture or acupressure treatments. Herbs and special diets are also considered important treatments in regulating the *Qi* in the body.

As long as the illness is limited to the level of *Qi* stagnation and there is no physical organ damage, the *Qigong* exercises used for maintaining health can be used to readjust the *Qi* circulation and treat the problem. However, if the sickness is already so serious that the physical organs have started to fail, then the situation has become critical and a specific treatment is necessary. The treatment can be acupuncture, herbs, or even an operation, as well as specific *Qigong* exercises designed to speed up the healing or even to cure the sickness. For example, ulcers and asthma can often be cured or helped by some simple exercises. Recently in both mainland China and Taiwan, certain *Qigong* exercises have been shown to be effective in treating certain kinds of cancer.

Over the thousands of years of observing nature and themselves, some *Qigong* practitioners went even deeper. They realized that the body's *Qi* circulation changes with the seasons, and that it is a good idea to help the body during these periodic adjustments. They noticed also that in each season different organs have characteristic problems. For example, in the beginning of Fall the lungs have to adapt to the colder air that you are breathing. While this adjustment is going on, the lungs are susceptible to disturbance, so your lungs may feel uncomfortable and you may catch colds easily. Your digestive system is also affected during seasonal changes. Your appetite may increase, or you may have diarrhea. When the temperature goes down, your kidneys and bladder will start to give you trouble. For example, because the kidneys are stressed, you may feel pain in the back. Focusing on these seasonal *Qi* disorders, the meditators created a set of movements which can be used to speed up the body's adjustment.

In addition to Marshal Yue Fei, many people who were not doctors also created sets of medical *Qigong*. These sets were probably originally created to maintain health, and later were also used for curing sickness.

C. Martial Qigong — for Fighting

Chinese martial *Qigong* was probably not developed until Da Mo wrote the ***Muscle/Tendon Changing Classic*** in the *Shaolin* Temple during the *Liang* Dynasty (502-557 A.D.). When *Shaolin* monks trained Da Mo's Muscle/Tendon Changing *Qigong*, they found that they could not only improve their health but also greatly increase the power of their martial techniques. Since then, many martial styles have developed *Qigong* sets to increase their effectiveness. In addition, many martial styles have been created based on *Qigong* theory. Martial artists have played a major role in Chinese *Qigong* society.

When *Qigong* theory was first applied to the martial arts, it was used to increase the power and efficiency of the muscles. The theory is very simple — **the mind (*Yi*) is used to lead *Qi* to the muscles to energize them so that they function more efficiently**. The average person generally uses his muscles at about 40% maximum efficiency. If one can train his concentration and use his strong *Yi* (the mind generated from clear thinking) to lead *Qi* to the muscles effectively, he will be able to energize the muscles to a higher level and, therefore, increase his fighting effectiveness.

As acupuncture theory became better understood, fighting techniques were able to reach even more advanced levels. Martial artists learned to attack specific areas, such as vital acupuncture cavities, to disturb the enemy's *Qi* flow and create imbalances which caused injury or even death. In order to do this, the practitioner must understand the route and timing of the *Qi* circulation in the human body. He also has to train so that he can strike the cavities accurately and to the correct depth. These cavity strike techniques are called *"Dian Xue"* (點穴)(Pointing Cavities) or *"Dian Mai"* (點脈)(Pointing Vessels).

Most of the martial *Qigong* practices help to improve the practitioner's health. However, there are other martial *Qigong* practices which, although they build up some special skill which is useful for fighting, also damage the practitioner's health. An example of this is Iron Sand Palm (*Tie Sha Zhang,* 鐵砂掌). Although this training can build up amazing destructive power, it can also harm your hands and affect the *Qi* circulation in the hands and internal organs.

As mentioned in Chapter 1, since the 6th century, many martial styles have been created which were based on *Qigong* theory. They can be roughly divided into external and internal styles.

The external styles emphasize building *Qi* in the limbs to coordinate with the physical martial techniques. They follow the theory of *Wai Dan* (External Elixir) *Qigong,* which usually generates *Qi* in the limbs through special exercises. The concentrated mind is used during the exercises to energize the *Qi.* This increases muscular strength significantly, and therefore increases the effectiveness of the martial techniques. *Qigong* can also be used to train the body to resist punches and kicks. In this training, *Qi* is led to energize the skin and the muscles, enabling them to resist a blow without injury. This training is commonly called "Iron Shirt" (*Tie Bu Shan,* 鐵布衫) or "Golden Bell Cover" (*Jin Zhong Zhao,* 金鐘罩). The martial styles which use *Wai Dan Qigong* training are normally called external styles (*Wai Jia,* 外家) or Hard *Qigong* training is called Hard Gong (*Ying Gong,* 硬功). *Shaolin Gongfu* is a typical example of a style which uses *Wai Dan* martial *Qigong.*

Although *Wai Dan Qigong* can help the martial artist increase his power, there is a disadvantage. Because *Wai Dan Qigong* emphasizes training the external muscles, it can cause over-development. This can cause a problem called "energy dispersion" (*San Gong,* 散功) when the practitioner gets older. In order to remedy this, when an external martial artist reaches a high level of external *Qigong* training he will start training internal *Qigong,* which specializes in curing the energy dispersion problem. That is why it is said: *"Shaolin Gongfu* from external to internal."

Internal Martial *Qigong* is based on the theory of *Nei Dan* (Internal Elixir). In this method, *Qi* is generated in the body instead of the limbs, and this *Qi* is then led to the limbs to increase power. In order to lead *Qi* to the limbs, the techniques must be soft and muscle usage must be kept to a minimum. The training and theory of *Nei Dan* martial *Qigong* is much more difficult than those of *Wai Dan* martial *Qigong*. Interested readers should refer to the author's book: ***Tai Chi Theory & Martial Power*** (Formerly *Advanced Yang Style Tai Chi Chuan, Vol. 1*).

Several internal martial styles were created in the *Wudang* (武當山) and *Emei* Mountains (峨嵋山). Popular styles are *Taijiquan, Baguazhang, Liu He Ba Fa,* and *Xingyiquan.* However, you should understand that even the internal martial styles, which are commonly called Soft Styles, must on some occasions use muscular strength while fighting. That means in order to have strong power in the fight, the *Qi* must be led to the muscular body and manifested externally. Therefore, once an internal martial artist has achieved a degree of competence in internal *Qigong*, he or she should also learn how to use harder, more external techniques. That is why it is said: "The internal styles are from soft to hard."

In the last fifty years, some of the *Taiji Qigong* or *Taijiquan* practitioners have developed training which is mainly for health, and is called *"Wuji Qigong"* (無極氣功) which means "no extremities *Qigong.*" *Wuji* is the state of neutrality which precedes Taiji, which is the state of complimentary opposites. When there are thoughts and feeling in your mind, there is *Yin* and *Yang,* but if you can still your mind you can return to the emptiness of *Wuji.* When you achieve this state your mind is centered and clear, your body relaxed, and your *Qi* is able to flow naturally and smoothly to reach the proper balance by itself. *Wuji Qigong* has become very popular in many parts of China, especially Shanghai and Canton.

You can see that, although *Qigong* is widely studied in Chinese martial society, the main focus of training was originally on increasing fighting ability rather than health. Good health was considered a by-product of training. It was not until this century that the health aspect of martial *Qigong* started receiving greater attention. This is especially true in the internal martial arts.

D. Religious Qigong — for Enlightenment or Buddhahood

Religious *Qigong,* though not as popular as other categories in China, is recognized as having achieved the highest accomplishments of all the *Qigong* categories. It used to be kept secret in the monastic society, and it is only in this century that it has been revealed to laymen.

In China, religious *Qigong* includes mainly Daoist and Buddhist *Qigong.* The main purpose of their training is striving for enlightenment, or what the Buddhists refer to as Buddhahood. They are looking for a way to lift themselves above normal human suffering, and to escape from the cycle of continual reincarnation. They believe that all human suffering is caused by the seven emotions and six desires (*Qi Qing Liu Yu,* 七情六慾). The seven emotions are **happiness** (*Xi,* 喜), **anger** (*Nu,* 怒), **sorrow** (*Ai,* 哀), **joy** (*Le,* 樂), **love** (*Ai,* 愛), **hate** (*Hen,* 恨), and **desire** (*Yu,* 慾). The six desires are the six sensory pleasures derived from the eyes, ears, nose, tongue, body, and mind. If you are still bound to these emotions and desires, you will reincarnate after your death. To avoid reincarnation, you must train your spirit to reach a very high stage where it is strong enough to be independent after your death. This spirit will enter the heavenly kingdom and gain eternal peace. This training is hard to do in the everyday world, so practitioners frequently flee society and move into the solitude of the mountains, where they can concentrate all of their energies on self-cultivation.

Religious *Qigong* practitioners train to strengthen their internal *Qi* to nourish their spirit (*Shen*) until the spirit is able to survive the death of the physical body. Marrow/Brain Washing *Qigong* training is necessary to reach this stage. It enables them to lead *Qi* to the forehead, where the spirit resides, and raise the brain to a higher energy state. This training used to be restricted to only a few priests who had reached an advanced level. Tibetan Buddhists were also involved heavily in this training. Over the last two thousand years the Tibetan Buddhists, the Chinese Buddhists, and the Daoists have followed the same principles to become the three major religious schools of *Qigong* training.

This religious striving toward enlightenment or Buddhahood is recognized as the highest and most difficult level of *Qigong*. Many *Qigong* practitioners reject the rigors of this religious striving, and practice Marrow/Brain Washing *Qigong* solely for the purpose of longevity. It was these people who eventually revealed the secrets of Marrow/Brain Washing to the outside world. If you are interested in knowing more about this training, you may refer to: "***Muscle/Tendon Changing and Marrow/Brain Washing Chi Kung***" by Dr. Yang.

From the above brief summary, you may obtain a general concept of how Chinese *Qigong* can be categorized. From the understanding of this general concept, you should not have further doubt about any *Qigong* you are training.

In the next section, we will discuss general *Qigong* training theory. This theoretical discussion of *Qigong* practice will offer you a foundation upon which to build your training. Without this scientific theoretical support, your mind will continue wondering and wandering. Understanding the theory is like learning how to read a map, which can direct you to the final goal of practice without confusion.

2-4. Qigong Training Theory

Many people think that *Qigong* is a difficult subject to comprehend. In some ways, this is true. However, you must understand one thing: regardless of how difficult the *Qigong* theory and practice of a particular style is, the basic theory and principles are very simple and remain the same for all *Qigong* styles. The basic theory and principles are the root of the entire *Qigong* practice. If you understand these roots, you will be able to grasp the key to the practice and grow. All of the *Qigong* styles originated from these roots, but each one has blossomed differently.

In this section we will discuss these basic *Qigong* training theories and principles. With this knowledge as foundation, you will be able to understand not only what you should be doing, but also why you are doing it. Naturally, it is impossible to discuss all of the basic *Qigong* ideas in such a short section. However, it will offer you the key to open the gate into the spacious, four thousand years old garden of Chinese *Qigong*. If you wish to know more about the theory of *Qigong,* please refer to ***The Root of Chinese Chi Kung,*** by Dr. Yang.

The Concept of Yin and Yang, Kan and Li

The concept of *Yin* (陰) and *Yang* (陽) is the foundation of Chinese philosophy. From this philosophy, Chinese culture was developed. Naturally, this includes Chinese medicine and *Qigong* practice. Therefore, in order to understand *Qigong,* first you should study the concept of Yin and *Yang*. In addition, you should also understand the concept of *Kan* (坎) and *Li* (離) which, unfortunately, has been confused with the concept of *Yin* and *Yang* even in China.

The Chinese have long believed that the universe is made up of two opposite forces — *Yin* and *Yang* — which must balance each other. When these two forces lose their balance, nature finds a way to re-balance them. If the imbalance is significant, disaster will occur. However, when these two forces interact with each other smoothly and harmoniously, they manifest power and generate the millions of living things.

As mentioned earlier, *Yin* and *Yang* theory is also applied to the three great natural powers: Heaven, Earth, and Man. For example, if the *Yin* and *Yang* forces of Heaven (i.e., energy which comes to us from the sky) are losing balance, there can be tornadoes, hurricanes, or other natural disasters. When the *Yin* and *Yang* forces lose their balance on earth, rivers can change their paths and earthquakes can occur. When the *Yin* and *Yang* forces in the human body lose their balance, sickness and even death can occur. Experience has shown that the *Yin* and *Yang* balance in Man is affected by the *Yin* and *Yang* balances of the Earth and Heaven. Similarly, the *Yin* and *Yang* balance of the Earth is influenced by the Heaven's *Yin* and *Yang*. Therefore, if you wish to have a healthy body and live a long life, you need to know how to adjust your body's *Yin* and *Yang*, and how to coordinate your *Qi* with the *Yin* and *Yang* energy of Heaven and Earth. The study of *Yin* and *Yang* in the human body is the root of Chinese medicine and *Qigong*.

Furthermore, the Chinese have also classified everything in the universe according to *Yin* and *Yang*. Even feelings, thoughts, strategy, and the spirit are covered. For example, female is *Yin* and male is *Yang*, night is *Yin* and day is *Yang*, weak is *Yin* and strong is *Yang*, backward is *Yin* and forward is *Yang*, sad is *Yin* and happy is *Yang*, defense is *Yin* and offense is *Yang*, and so on.

Practitioners of Chinese medicine and *Qigong* believe that they must seek to understand the *Yin* and *Yang* of nature and the human body before they can adjust and regulate the body's energy balance into a more harmonious state. Only then can health be maintained and the causes of sicknesses be corrected.

Another thing which you should understand is that the concept of *Yin* and *Yang* is relative instead of absolute. For example, the number seven is *Yang* compared with three. However, if seven is compared with ten, then it is *Yin*. That means in order to decide *Yin* or *Yang*, a reference point must first be chosen. Therefore, if five is the *Yin* and *Yang* balance number, then seven is *Yang* and three is *Yin*. If we choose zero as the *Yin* and *Yang* balance number, then any positive number is *Yang* and any negative number is *Yin*.

However, if what we are interested in is the most negative number, then we may choose the negative number as *Yang* and positive number as *Yin* with zero as the central number. For example, generally speaking in *Qigong*, techniques that can be seen physically and are the manifestation of *Qi* are considered *Yang*, and the techniques that cannot be seen but can be felt are treated as *Yin*. When the *Yin* and *Yang* concept is applied in Chinese medicine, since the *Qi* is the major concern and plays the main role in medicine, it is considered *Yang*, while the blood (physical) is considered *Yin*.

Now let us discuss how the concept of *Yin* and *Yang* is applied to the *Qi* circulating in the human body. Many people, even some *Qigong* practitioners, are still confused by this. When it is said that *Qi* can be either *Yin* or *Yang*, it does not mean that there are two different kinds of *Qi* like male and female, fire and water, or positive and negative charges. *Qi* is energy, and energy itself does not have *Yin* and *Yang*. It is like the energy which is generated from the sparking of negative and positive charges. Charges have the potential for generating energy, but are not the energy itself.

When it is said that *Qi* is *Yin* or *Yang*, it means that the *Qi* is too strong or too weak for a particular circumstance. Again, it is relative and not absolute. Naturally, this implies that the potential which generates the *Qi* is strong or weak. For example, the *Qi* from the sun is *Yang Qi*, and *Qi* from the moon is *Yin Qi*. This is because the sun's energy is Yang in comparison to Human *Qi*, while the moon's is *Yin*. In any discussion of energy where people are involved, Human *Qi* is used as the standard. People are always especially interested in what concerns them directly, so it is natural that we are interested primarily in Human *Qi* and tend to view all *Qi* from the perspective of Human *Qi*. This is not unlike looking at the universe from the physical perspective of the Earth.

When we look at the *Yin* and *Yang* of *Qi* within the human body, however, we must redefine our point of reference. For example, when a person is dead, his residual Human *Qi* (*Gui Qi* or ghost *Qi*, 鬼氣) is weak compared to a living person's. Therefore, the ghost *Qi* is *Yin* as it dissipates, while the living person's *Qi* is *Yang*. When discussing *Qi* within the body, in the Lung Channel for example, the reference point is the normal, healthy status of the *Qi* there. If the *Qi* is stronger than it is in the normal state, it is *Yang*, and, naturally, if it is weaker than this, it is *Yin*. There are twelve parts of the human body that are considered organs in Chinese medicine, six of them are *Yin* and six are *Yang*. The *Yin* organs are the **Heart**, **Lungs**, **Kidneys**, **Liver**, **Spleen**, and **Pericardium**, and the Yang organs are **Large Intestine**, **Small Intestine**, **Stomach**, **Gall Bladder**, **Urinary Bladder**, and **Triple Burner**. General speaking, the *Qi* level of the *Yin* organs is lower than that of the *Yang* organs. The *Yin* organs store Original Essence and process the Essence obtained from food and air, while the *Yang* organs handle digestion and excretion.

When the *Qi* in any of your organs is not in its normal state, you feel uncomfortable. If it is very much off from the normal state, the organ will start to malfunction and you may become sick. When this happens, the *Qi* in your entire body will also be affected and you will feel too *Yang*, perhaps feverish, or too *Yin*, such as the weakness after diarrhea.

Your body's *Qi* level is also affected by your natural environment, such as the weather, climate, and seasonal changes. Therefore, when the body's *Qi* level is classified, the reference point is the level which feels most comfortable for those particular circumstances. Naturally, each of us is a little bit different, and what feels best and most natural for one person may be a bit different from what is right for another person. That is why the doctor will usually ask "how do you feel?" It is according to your own standard that you are judged.

Breathing is closely related to the state of your *Qi*, and is therefore also considered *Yin* or *Yang*. When you exhale you expel air from your lungs, your mind moves outward, and the *Qi* around the body expands. In the Chinese martial arts, the exhale is generally used to expand the *Qi* to energize the muscles during an attack. Therefore, you can see that the exhale is *Yang* - it is expanding, offensive, and strong. Naturally, based on the same theory, the inhale is considered *Yin*.

Your breathing is closely related to your emotions. When you lose your temper, your breathing is short and fast, i.e., *Yang*. When you are sad, your body is more *Yin*, and you inhale more than you exhale in order to absorb *Qi* from the air to balance the body's *Yin* and bring the body back into balance. When you are excited and happy your body is *Yang*, and your exhale is longer than your inhale to get rid of the excess *Yang* which is caused by the excitement.

As mentioned before, your mind is also closely related to your *Qi*. Therefore, when your *Qi* is *Yang*, your mind is usually also *Yang* (excited) and vice versa. The mind can also be classified according to the *Qi* which generated it. The mind (*Yi*) which is generated from the calm and peaceful *Qi* obtained from the Original Essence is considered *Yin*. The mind (*Xin*) which originates with the food and air Essence is emotional, scattered, and excited, and it is considered *Yang*. The spirit, which is related to the *Qi*, can also be classified as *Yang* or *Yin* based on its origin.

Do not confuse *Yin Qi* and *Yang Qi* with Fire *Qi* and Water *Qi*. When the *Yin* and *Yang* of *Qi* are mentioned, it refers to the level of *Qi* according to some reference point. However, when Water and Fire *Qi* are mentioned, it refers to the quality of the *Qi*. If you are interested in reading more about the *Yin* and *Yang* of *Qi*, please refer to the Book: ***The Root of Chinese Chi Kung and Muscle/Tendon Changing and Marrow/Brain Washing Chi Kung***, by YMAA.

The terms *Kan* and *Li* occur frequently in *Qigong* documents. In the Eight Trigrams *Kan* represents "Water" while *Li* represents "Fire." However, the everyday terms for water and fire are also often used. *Kan* and *Li* training has long been of major importance to *Qigong* practitioners. In order to understand why, you must understand these two words, and the theory behind them.

First you should understand that though *Kan-Li* and *Yin-Yang* are related, *Kan* and *Li* are not *Yin* and *Yang*. **Kan is Water, which is able to cool your body down and make it more Yin, while Li is Fire, which warms your body and makes it more *Yang*. Kan and *Li* are the methods or causes, while *Yin* and *Yang* are the results**. When *Kan* and *Li* are adjusted and regulated correctly, *Yin* and *Yang* will be balanced and interact harmoniously.

Qigong practitioners believe that your body is always too *Yang,* unless you are sick or have not eaten for a long time, in which case your body may be more *Yin.* Since your body is always *Yang,* it is degenerating and burning out. It is believed that this is the cause of aging. If you are able to use Water to cool down your body, you will be able to slow down the degeneration process and thereby lengthen your life. This is the main reason why **Chinese *Qigong* practitioners have been studying ways of improving the quality of the Water in their bodies, and of reducing the quantity of the Fire**. I believe that as a *Qigong* practitioner you should always keep this subject at the top of your list for study and research. If you earnestly ponder and experiment, you will be able to grasp the trick of adjusting them.

If you want to learn how to adjust them, you must understand that Water and Fire mean many things in your body. The first concerns your *Qi.* As mentioned earlier, *Qi* is classified as Fire and Water. When your *Qi* is not pure and causes your physical body to heat up and your mental/spiritual body to become unstable (*Yang*), it is classified as Fire *Qi.* The *Qi* which is pure and is able to cool both your physical and spiritual bodies (make them more Yin) is considered Water *Qi.* However, you body can never be purely Water. Water can cool down the Fire, but it must never totally quench it, because then you would be dead. It is also said that Fire *Qi* is able to agitate and stimulate the emotions, and from these emotions generate a "mind." This mind is called *Xin* (心), and is considered the Fire mind, *Yang* mind, or emotional mind. On the other hand, the mind that Water *Qi* generates is calm, steady, and wise. This mind is called *Yi* (意), and is considered to be the Water mind or wisdom mind. If your spirit is nourished by the Fire *Qi,* although your spirit may be high, it will be scattered and confused (a *Yang* spirit). Naturally, if the spirit is nourished and raised by Water *Qi,* it will be firm and steady (a *Yin* mind). When your *Yi* is able to govern your emotional *Xin* effectively, your will (strong emotional intention) can be firm.

You can see from this discussion that your *Qi* is the main cause of the *Yin* and *Yang* of your physical body, your mind, and your spirit. To regulate your body's *Yin* and *Yang,* you must learn how to regulate your body's Water and Fire *Qi,* but in order to do this efficiently you must know their sources.

Once you have grasped the concepts of *Yin-Yang* and *Kan-Li,* then you have to think about how to adjust *Kan* and *Li* so that you can balance the *Yin* and *Yang* in your body.

Theoretically, a *Qigong* practitioner would like to keep his body in a state of *Yin-Yang* balance, which means the "center" point of the *Yin* and *Yang* forces. This center point is commonly called "*Wuji*" (無極)(no extremities). It is believed that Wuji is the original, natural state where *Yin* and *Yang* are not distinguished. In the *Wuji* state, nature is peaceful and calm. In the *Wuji* state, all of the *Yin* and *Yang* forces have gradually combined harmoniously and disappeared. When this *Wuji* theory is applied to human beings, it is the final goal of *Qigong* practice where your mind is neutral and absolutely calm. The *Wuji* state makes it possible for you to find the origin of your life, and to combine your *Qi* with the *Qi* of nature.

The ultimate goal and purpose of *Qigong* practice is to find this peaceful and natural state. In order to reach this goal, you must first understand your body's *Yin* and *Yang* so that you can balance them by adjusting your *Kan* and *Li.* Only when your *Yin* and *Yang* are balanced will you be able to find the center balance point, the *Wuji* state.

Theoretically, between the two extremes of *Yin* and *Yang* are millions of paths (i.e., different *Kan* and *Li* methods) which can lead you to the neutral center. This accounts for the hundreds of different styles of *Qigong* which have been created over the years. You can see that the theory of *Yin* and *Yang* and the methods of *Kan* and *Li* are the root of training all Chinese *Qigong* styles. Without this root, the essence of *Qigong* practice would be lost.

Three Treasures — Jing, Qi, and Shen (三寶 - 精、氣、神)

Before you start any *Qigong* training you must also understand the three treasures of your body (*San Bao,* 三寶): **Jing** (Essence, 精), **Qi** (Internal Energy, 氣), and **Shen** (Spirit, 神). They are also called the three origins or the three roots (*San Yuan,* 三元), because they are considered the origins and roots of your life. *Jing* means Essence, the most original and refined part. *Jing* is the original source and most basic part of every living thing, and determines its nature and characteristics. It is the root of life. Sperm is called *Jing Zi* (精子), which means "Essence of the Son," because it contains the *Jing* of the father which is passed on to his son (or daughter) and becomes the son's *Jing.*

Qi, known as bioelectricity today, is the internal energy of your body. It is like the electricity which passes through a machine to keep it running. *Qi* comes either from the conversion of the *Jing* which you have received from your parents, or from the food you eat and the air you breathe.

Shen is the center of your mind and being. It is what makes you human, because animals do not have a *Shen.* The *Shen* in your body must be nourished by your *Qi* or energy. When your *Qi* is full, your *Shen* will be enlivened.

Chinese meditators and *Qigong* practitioners believe that the body contains two general types of *Qi*. The first type is called **Pre-Birth Qi** or **Pre-Heaven Qi** (*Xian Tian Qi,* 先天氣), and it comes from converted Original *Jing* (*Yuan Jing,* 元精), which you get from your parents at conception. The second type, which is called **Post-Birth Qi** or **Post Heaven Qi** (*Hou Tian Qi,* 後天氣), is drawn from the *Jing* of the food and air we take in. When this *Qi* flows or is led to the brain, it can energize the *Shen* and soul. This energized and raised *Shen* is able to govern and lead the *Qi* to the entire body.

Each one of these three elements or treasures has its own root. You must know the roots so that you can strengthen and protect your three treasures.

1. Your body requires many kinds of *Jing.* Except for the *Jing* which you inherit from your parents, which is called Original *Jing* (*Yuan Jing,* 元精), all other Jings must be obtained from food and air. Among all of these *Jings,* Original *Jing* is the most important one. It is the root and the seed of your life, and your basic strength. If your parents were strong and healthy, your Original *Jing* will be strong and healthy, and you will have a strong foundation on which to grow. The Chinese people believe that in order to stay healthy and live a long life, you must protect and maintain this *Jing.*

According to Chinese medicine, the root of Original *Jing* before your birth was in your parents. After birth this Original *Jing* stays in its residence — the kidneys, which are considered the root of your *Jing.* When you keep this root strong, you will have sufficient Original *Jing* to supply to your body. Although you cannot increase the amount of Original *Jing* you have, *Qigong* training can improve the quality of your *Jing. Qigong* can also teach you how to convert your *Jing* into Original *Qi* more efficiently, and how to use this *Qi* effectively.

If we analyze the concept of *Jing* from a modern physical scientific point of view, we might postulate that *Jing* is in the genetic material which we inherited from our parents. From this material, the structure and healthy condition of one person is different from all others. From different genes, the different levels of hormones in different people are controlled. When Chinese medicine says that the Original *Jing* is stored in the kidneys, it implies the hormones which are produced in the adrenal glands. According to Chinese medicine, there is no record of the endocrine glands. This implies that Chinese medicine has never understood the function of the endocrine. In my opinion, the *Jing* (essence) is stored in all of the endocrine glands. I believe that the most significant gland which stores the essence and affects the level of the entire body's *Jing* (hormone production) is the pituitary gland (corresponding to the Upper *Dan Tian*).

2. According to Chinese medicine and *Qigong*, *Qi* is converted both from the *Jing* which you have inherited from your parents and from the *Jing* which you draw from the food and air you take in. *Qi* that is converted from the Original *Jing* which you inherited is called Original *Qi* (*Yuan Qi*, 元氣).[12] Just as Original *Jing* is the most important type of *Jing*, Original *Qi* is the most important type of *Qi*. It is pure and of high quality, while the *Qi* from food and air may make your body too positive or too negative, depending on how and where you absorb it. When you retain and protect your Original *Jing*, you will be able to generate Original *Qi* in a pure, continuous stream. As a *Qigong* practitioner, you must know how to convert your Original *Jing* into Original *Qi* in a smooth, steady stream.

Since your Original *Qi* comes from your Original *Jing*, they both have the kidneys for their root. When your kidneys are strong, the Original *Jing* is strong, and the Original *Qi* converted from this Original *Jing* will also be full and strong. This *Qi* resides in the Lower *Dan Tian* in your abdomen. Once you learn how to convert your Original Jing, you will be able to supply your body with all the *Qi* it needs.

Again, if we analyze the above concepts, we can see that the essence here means the hormone level which is produced from the adrenal glands on the top of your kidneys. In fact, we have already seen that the pituitary gland is considered the master of the glands, and when the hormone production in this gland is high, the hormone production of all other Endocrine Glands will also be high. When the hormone level of the body is high, the *Qi* is abundant and the circulation is smooth. When the hormone production level is high in the pituitary gland, the spirit (*Shen*, 神) residing in the center of your brain will be high. When the spirit is high, it is able to strongly and smoothly direct the *Qi* circulating in the body for function, repair and healing. This results in the development of spiritual healing science.

3. *Shen* (i.e., spirit, 神) is the force which keeps you alive. It has no substance, but it gives expression and appearance to your *Jing*. *Shen* is also the control tower for the *Qi*. When your *Shen* is strong, your *Qi* is strong and you can lead it efficiently. The root of *Shen* (Spirit) is your mind (*Yi*, or intention). When your brain is energized and stimulated, your mind will be more aware and you will be able to concentrate more intensely. Also, your *Shen* will be raised. Advanced *Qigong* practitioners believe that your brain must always be sufficiently nourished by your *Qi*. It is the *Qi* which keeps your mind clear and concentrated. With an abundant *Qi* supply, the mind can be energized, and can raise the *Shen* and enhance your vitality.

The deeper levels of *Qigong* training include the conversion of *Jing* into *Qi* (*Lian Jing Hua Qi*, 練精化氣), which is then led to the brain to raise the *Shen* (*Lian Qi Hua Shen*, 練氣化神). This process is called *"Huan Jing Bu Nao"* (還精補腦) and means "return the *Jing* to nourish the brain." When *Qi* is led to the head, it stays at the Upper *Dan Tian* (at the center of the forehead), which is the residence of your *Shen*. *Qi* and *Shen* are mutually related. When your *Shen* is weak, your *Qi* is weak, and your body will degenerate rapidly. *Shen* is the headquarters of *Qi*. Likewise, *Qi* supports the *Shen,* energizing it and keeping it sharp, clear, and strong. If the *Qi* in your body is weak, your *Shen* will also be weak.

Scientifically, in order to maintain a high hormone production level, you must continue to supply bioelectricity to the pituitary gland. Without this basic energy, the gland will function inadequately. Therefore, one of the main *Qigong* practices is learning, through meditation, how to lead the *Qi* to the brain and nourish the pituitary gland.

From the above discussion, you can see that in order to have a healthy and strong body, you must first learn how to keep the *Yin* and *Yang* balance in your body. In addition, you should also learn how to adjust or regulate your body, allowing you to fit in the natural environment more harmoniously. Furthermore, you should learn how to **retain and generate your *Jing*, strengthen and smooth your *Qi* flow**, and **enlighten your *Shen*.** That means you should learn how to maintain the hormone production of your body, how to store the *Qi* in your Lower *Dan Tian* (battery) and smoothly circulate it in your body, and how to lead the *Qi* to the brain to nourish your Spirit. If you are interested in the further pursuit of enlightenment, then you must learn how to regulate your mind to a neutral state and build up a Spiritual Embryo (*Sheng Tai,* 聖胎). From the cultivation of this spiritual embryo, you will be able to separate your spiritual body and your physical body. If you are interested in this subject, please refer to ***Muscle/Tendon Changing and Marrow/Brain Washing Chi Kung***, by YMAA.

Qigong Training Theory

Every *Qigong* form or practice has its special training purpose and theory. If you do not know the purpose and theory, you have lost the root (meaning) of the practice. Therefore, as a *Qigong* practitioner, you must continue to ponder and practice until you understand the root of every set or form.

Remember that getting the gold is not enough. Like the boy in the old Chinese story, you should concern yourself with learning the trick of turning the rock into gold. You can see that getting the gold is simply gaining the flowers and branches, and there can be no growth. However, if you have the trick which is the theory, then you will have the root, and you may continue to grow by yourself.

Now that you have learned the basic theory of the *Qigong* practice, let us discuss the general training principles. In Chinese *Qigong* society, it is commonly known that in order to reach the goal of *Qigong* practice, you must learn how to **regulate the body** (*Tiao Shen,* 調身), **regulate the breathing** (*Tiao Xi,* 調息), **regulate the emotional mind** (*Tiao Xin,* 調心), **regulate the Qi** (*Tiao Qi,* 調氣), and **regulate the spirit** (*Tiao Shen,* 調神). *Tiao* in Chinese is constructed from two words, "言" (*Yan,* means speaking or talking) and "周" (*Zhou,* means round or complete). That means the roundness (i.e., harmony) or the completeness is accomplished by negotiation. Like an out of tune piano, you must adjust it and make it harmonize with others. This implies that, when you are regulating one of the above five processes, you must also coordinate and harmonize the other four regulating elements.

Regulating the body includes understanding how to find and build the root of the body, as well as the root of the individual forms you are practicing. To build a firm root, you must know how to keep your center, how to balance your body, and most important of all, how to relax so that the *Qi* can flow.

To regulate your breathing, you must learn how to breathe so that your respiration and your mind mutually correspond and cooperate. When you breathe this way, your mind will be able to attain peace more quickly, and therefore concentrate more easily on leading the *Qi*.

Regulating the mind involves learning how to keep your mind calm, peaceful, and centered, so that you can judge situations objectively and lead *Qi* to the desired places. The mind is the main key to success in *Qigong* practice.

Regulating the *Qi* is one of the ultimate goals of *Qigong* practice. In order to regulate your *Qi* effectively you must first have regulated your body, breathing, and mind. Only then will your mind be clear enough to sense how the *Qi* is distributed in your body, and understand how to adjust it.

For Buddhist and Daoist priests, who seek enlightenment or Buddhahood, regulating the spirit (*Shen*) is the final goal of *Qigong*. This enables them to maintain a neutral, objective perspective of life, and this perspective is the eternal life of the Buddha. The average *Qigong* practitioner has lower goals. He raises his spirit in order to increase his concentration and enhance his vitality. This makes it possible for him to lead *Qi* effectively throughout his entire body so that it carries out the managing and guarding duties. This maintains health and slows the aging process.

If you understand these few things you will be able to quickly enter into the field of *Qigong*. Without all of these important elements, your training will be ineffective and your time will be wasted.

Before you start training, you must first understand that all of the training originates in your mind. You must have a clear idea of what you are doing, and your mind must be calm, centered, and balanced. This also implies that your feeling, sensing, and judgment must be objective and accurate. This requires emotional balance and a clear mind. This takes a lot of hard work, but once you have reached this level you will have built the root of your physical training, and your *Yi* (mind) will be able to lead your *Qi* throughout your physical body.

1. Regulating the Body (*Tiao Shen*, 調身)

When you learn any Qigong, either moving or still, the first step is to learn the correct postures or movements. After you have learned the postures and movements, learn how to improve them until you are able to perform them accurately. Then, you start to regulate your body until it has reached the stage which could provide the best condition for the *Qi* to build up or to circulate.

In Still *Qigong* practice or Soft *Qigong* movement, this means to adjust your body until it is in the most **comfortable** and **relaxed** state. This implies that your body must be **centered** and **balanced.** If it is not, you will be tense and uneasy, and this will affect the judgment of your *Yi* and the circulation of your *Qi*. In Chinese medical society it is said: "(When) shape (body's posture) is not correct, then the *Qi* will not be smooth. (When) the *Qi* is not smooth, the *Yi* (wisdom mind) will not be peaceful. (When) the *Yi* is not peaceful, then the *Qi* is disordered."[13] You should understand that the relaxation of your body originates with your *Yi*. Therefore, before you can relax your body, you must first relax or regulate your mind (*Yi*). This is called *"Shen Xin Ping Heng,"* (身心平衡) which means "Body and heart (i.e., mind) balanced." The body and the mind are mutually related. A relaxed and balanced body helps your *Yi* to relax and concentrate. When your *Yi* is at peace and can judge things accurately, your body will be relaxed, balanced, centered, and rooted. Only when you are rooted, then you will be able to raise up your spirit of vitality.

Relaxation

Relaxation is one of the major keys to success in *Qigong*. You should remember that **only when you are relaxed will all your *Qi* channels be open**. In order to be relaxed, your *Yi* must first be relaxed and calm. When the *Yi* coordinates with your breathing, your body will be able to relax.

In *Qigong* practice there are three levels of relaxation. The first level is the external physical relaxation, or postural relaxation. This is a very superficial level, and almost anyone can reach it. It consists of adopting a comfortable stance and avoiding unnecessary strain in how you stand and move. The second level is the relaxation of the muscles and tendons. To do this your *Yi* must be directed deep into the muscles and tendons. This relaxation will help open your *Qi* channels, and will allow the *Qi* to sink and accumulate in the *Dan Tian.*

The final stage is the relaxation which reaches the internal organs and the bone marrow. Remember, **only if you can relax deep into your body will your mind be able to lead the *Qi* there**. Only at this stage will the *Qi* be able to reach everywhere. Then you will feel transparent - as if your whole body had disappeared. If you can reach this level of relaxation, you will be able to communicate with your organs and use *Qigong* to adjust or regulate the *Qi* disorders which are giving you problems. You will also be able to protect your organs more effectively, and therefore slow down their degeneration.

Rooting

In all *Qigong* practice it is very important to be rooted. Being rooted means to be stable and in firm contact with the ground. If you want to push a car, you have to be rooted so the force you exert into the car will be balanced by a force into the ground. If you are not rooted, when you push the car you will only push yourself away, and not move the car. Your root is made up of your body's root, center, and balance.

Before you can develop your root, you must first relax and let your body "settle." As you relax, the tension in the various parts of your body will dissolve, and you will find a comfortable way to stand. You will stop fighting the ground to keep your body up, and will learn to rely on your body's structure to support itself. This lets the muscles relax even more. Since your body isn't struggling to stand up, your *Yi* won't be pushing upward, and your body, mind, and *Qi* will all be able to sink. If you let dirty water sit quietly, the impurities will gradually settle down to the bottom, leaving the water above it clear. In the same way, if you relax your body enough to let it settle, your *Qi* will sink to your *Dan Tian* and the Bubbling Wells (*Yongquan,* K-1, 湧泉) in your feet, and your mind will become clear. Then you can begin to develop your root.

To root your body you must imitate a tree and grow an invisible root under your feet. This will give you a firm root to keep you stable in your training. **Your root must be wide as well as deep**. Naturally, your *Yi* must grow first, because it is the *Yi* which leads the *Qi*. Your *Yi* must be able to lead the *Qi* to your feet, and be able to communicate with the ground. Only when your *Yi* can communicate with the ground will your *Qi* be able to grow beyond your feet and enter the ground to build the root. The Bubbling Well cavity is the gate which enables your *Qi* to communicate with the ground.

After you have gained your root, you must learn how to keep your center. A stable center will make your *Qi* develop evenly and uniformly. If you lost this center, your *Qi* will not be led evenly. In order to keep your body centered, you must first center your *Yi,* and then match your body to it. Only under these conditions will the *Qigong* forms you practice have their root. Your mental and physical centers are the keys which enable you to lead your *Qi* beyond your body.

Balance is the product of rooting and centering. Balance includes balancing the *Qi* and the physical body. It does not matter which aspect of balance you are dealing with, first you must balance your *Yi,* and only then can you balance your *Qi* and your physical body. If your *Yi* is balanced, it can help you to make accurate judgments, and therefore to correct the path of the *Qi* flow.

Rooting includes not just rooting the body, but also the form or movement. The root of any form or movement is found in its purpose or principle. For example, in certain *Qigong* exercises you want to lead the *Qi* to your palms. In order to do this you may imagine that you are pushing an object forward while keeping your muscles relaxed. In this exercise, your elbows must be down to build the sense of root for the push. If you raise the elbows, you lose the sense of "intention" of the movement, because the push would be ineffective if you were pushing something for real. Since the intention or purpose of the movement is its reason for being, you now have a purposeless movement, and you have no reason to lead *Qi* in any particular way. Therefore, in this case, the elbow is the root of the movement.

2. Regulating the Breath (*Tiao Xi*, 調息)

Regulating the breath means to regulate your breathing until it is calm, smooth, and peaceful. Only when you have reached this point will you be able to make the breathing **deep**, **slender**, **long**, and **soft**, which is required for successful *Qigong* practice.

Breathing is affected by your emotions. For example, when you are angry or excited you exhale more strongly than you inhale. When you are sad, you inhale more strongly than you exhale. When your mind is peaceful and calm, your inhalation and exhalation are relatively equal. In order to keep your breathing calm, peaceful, and steady, your mind and emotions must first be calm and neutral. Therefore, in order to regulate your breathing, you must first regulate your mind.

The other side of the coin is that you can use your breathing to control your *Yi*. When your breathing is uniform, it is as if you were hypnotizing your *Yi*, which helps to calm it. You can see that *Yi* and breathing are interdependent, and that they cooperate with each other. Deep and calm breathing relaxes you and keeps your mind clear. It fills your lungs with plenty of air, so that your brain and entire body have an adequate supply of oxygen. In addition, deep and complete breathing enable the diaphragm to move up and down, which massages and stimulates the internal organs. For this reason, deep breathing exercises are also called "internal organ exercises."

Deep and complete breathing does not mean that you inhale and exhale to the maximum. This would cause the lungs and the surrounding muscles to tense up, which in turn would keep the air from circulating freely, and hinder the absorption of oxygen. Without enough oxygen, your mind becomes scattered, and the rest of your body tenses up. In correct breathing, you inhale and exhale to about 70% or 80% of capacity, so that your lungs stay relaxed.

You can conduct an easy experiment. Inhale deeply so that your lungs are completely full, and time how long you can hold your breath. Then try inhaling to only about 70% of your capacity, and see how long you can hold your breath. You will find that with the latter method you can last much longer than the first one. This is simply because the lungs and the surrounding muscles are relaxed. When they are relaxed, the rest of your body and your mind can also relax, which significantly decreases your need for oxygen. Therefore, when you regulate your breathing, the first priority is to keep your lungs relaxed and calm.

When training, your mind must first be calm so that your breathing can be regulated. When the breathing is regulated, your mind is able to reach a higher level of calmness. This calmness can again help you to regulate the breathing, until your mind is deep. After you have trained for a long time, your breathing will be full and slender, and your mind will be very clear. It is said: "*Xin Xi Xiang Yi,*" (心息相依) which means "Heart (Mind) and breathing (are) mutually dependent." When you reach this meditative state, your heartbeat slows down, and your mind is very clear: you have entered the sphere of real meditation.

An Ancient Daoist named Li Ching-Yen said: "Regulating breathing means to regulate the real breathing until (you) stop."[14] This means that **correct regulating means regulating is no longer necessary. Real regulating is no longer a conscious process, but has become so natural that it can be accomplished without conscious effort**. In other words, although you start by consciously regulating your breath, you must get to the point where the regulating happens naturally, and you no longer have to think about it. When you breathe, if you concentrate your mind on your breathing, then it is not true regulating, because the *Qi* in your lungs will become stagnant. When you reach the level of true regulating, you don't have to pay attention to it, and you can use your mind efficiently to lead the *Qi*. Remember, **wherever the *Yi* is, there is the *Qi*. If the *Yi* stops in one spot, the *Qi* will be stagnant. It is the *Yi* which leads the *Qi* and makes it move**. Therefore, when you are in a state of correct breath regulation, your mind is free. There is no sound stagnation, urgency, or hesitation, and you can finally be calm and peaceful.

You can see that when the breath is regulated correctly, the *Qi* will also be regulated. They are mutually related and cannot be separated. This idea is explained frequently in the Daoist literature. The Daoist Goang Cheng Zi said: "One exhale, the Earth *Qi* rises; one inhale, the Heaven *Qi* descends; real man's (meaning one who has attained the real *Dao*) repeated breathing at the navel, then my real *Qi* is naturally connected."[15] This says that when you breathe you should move your abdomen, as if you were breathing from your navel. The earth *Qi* is the negative (*Yin*) energy from your kidneys, and the sky *Qi* is the positive (*Yang*) energy which comes from the food you eat and the air you breathe. When you breathe from the navel, these two *Qis* will connect and combine. Some people think that they know what *Qi* is, but they really don't. Once you connect the two *Qis*, you will know what the "real" *Qi* is, and you may become a "real" man, which means to attain the *Dao*.

The Daoist book ***Chain Dao Zhen Yen (Sing (of the) Dao (with) Real Words)*** says: "One exhale one inhale to communicate *Qi*'s function, one movement one calmness is the same as (i.e., is the source of) creation and variation."[16] The first part of this statement again implies that the functioning of *Qi* is connected with the breathing. The second part of this sentence means that all creation and variation come from the interaction of movement (*Yang*) and calmness (*Yin*). *Huang Ting Ching* (*Yellow Yard Classic*) says: "Breathe Original *Qi* to seek immortality."[17] In China, the traditional Daoists wore yellow robes, and they meditated in a "yard" or hall. This sentence means that in order to reach the goal of immortality, you must seek to find and understand the Original *Qi* which comes from the *Dan Tian* through correct breathing.

Moreover, the Daoist Wu Zhen Ren said: "Use the Post-Birth breathing to look for the real person's (i.e. the immortal's) breathing place."[18] In this sentence it is clear that in order to locate the immortal breathing place (the *Dan Tian*), you must rely on and know how to regulate your Post-Birth, or natural, breathing. Through regulating your Post-Birth breathing you will gradually be able to locate the residence of the *Qi* (the *Dan Tian*), and eventually you will be able to use your *Dan Tian* to breath like the immortal Daoists. Finally, in the Daoist song *Ling Yuan Da Dao Ge* (*The Great Daoist Song of the Spirit's Origin*) it is said: "The Originals (Original *Jing, Qi,* and *Shen*) are internally transported peacefully, so that you can become real (immortal); (if you) depend (only) on external breathing (you) will not reach the end (goal)."[19] From this song, you can see the internal breathing (breathing at the *Dan Tian*) is the key to training your three treasures and finally reaching immortality. However, you must first know how to regulate your external breathing correctly.

All of these emphasize the importance of breathing. There are eight key words for breathing which a *Qigong* practitioner should follow during his practice. Once you understand them you will be able to substantially shorten the time needed to reach your *Qigong* goals. These eight key words are: 1. Calm (*Jing,* 靜); 2. Slender (*Xi,* 細); 3. Deep (*Shen,* 深); 4. Long (*Chang,* 長); 5. Continuous (*You,* 悠); 6. Uniform (*Yun,* 勻); 7. Slow (*Huan,* 緩), and 8. Soft (*Mian,* 綿). These key words are self-explanatory, and with a little thought you should be able to understand them.

3. Regulating the Mind (*Tiao Xin,* 調心)

It is said in Daoist society that: "(When) large *Dao* is taught, first stop thought; when thought is not stopped, (the lessons are) in vain."[20] This means that when you first practice *Qigong,* the most difficult training is to stop your thinking. The final goal for your mind is "the thought of no thought" (無念之念). Your mind does not think of the past, the present, or the future. Your mind is completely separated from influences of the present such as worry, happiness, and sadness. Then your mind can be calm and steady, and can finally gain peace. Only when you are in the state of "the thought of no thought" will you be relaxed and able to sense calmly and accurately.

Regulating your mind means using your consciousness to stop the activity in your mind in order to set it free from the bondage of ideas, emotion, and conscious thought. When you reach this level your mind will be calm, peaceful, empty, and light. Then your mind has really reached the goal of relaxation. Only when you reach this stage will you be able to relax deep into your marrow and internal organs. Only then will your mind be clear enough to see (feel) the internal *Qi* circulation and to communicate with your *Qi* and organs. In Daoist society it is called, *"Nei Shi Gongfu"* (內視功夫) which means the *Gongfu* of internal vision.

When you reach this real relaxation you may be able to sense the different elements which make up your body: solid matter, liquids, gases, energy, and spirit. You may even be able to see or feel the different colors that are associated with your five organs — green (liver), white (lungs), black (kidneys), yellow (spleen), and red (heart).

Once your mind is relaxed and regulated and you can sense your internal organs, you may decide to study the five element theory. This is a very profound subject, and it is sometimes interpreted differently by Oriental physicians and *Qigong* practitioners. When understood properly, it can give you a method of analyzing the interrelationships between your organs and help you devise ways to correct imbalances.

For example, the lungs correspond to the element Metal, and the heart to the element Fire. Metal (the lungs) can be used to adjust the heat of the Fire (the heart), because metal can take a large quantity of heat away from fire, (and thus cool down the heart). When you feel uneasy or have heartburn (excess fire in the heart), you may use deep breathing to calm down the uneasy emotions or cool off the heartburn.

Naturally, it will take a lot of practice to reach this level. In the beginning, you should not have any ideas or intentions, because they will make it harder for your mind to relax and empty itself of thoughts. Once you are in a state of "no thought," place your attention on your *Dan Tian.* It is said *"Yi Shou Dan Tian"* (意守丹田) which means "The Mind is kept on the *Dan Tian."* The *Dan Tian* is the origin and residence of your *Qi.* Your mind can build up the *Qi* here (start the fire, *Qi Huo,* 起火), then lead the *Qi* anywhere you wish, and finally lead the *Qi* back to its residence. When your mind is on the *Dan Tian,* your *Qi* will always have a root. When you keep this root, your *Qi* will be strong and full, and it will go where you want it to. You can see that when you practice *Qigong,* your mind cannot be completely empty and relaxed. You must find the firmness within the relaxation, then you can reach your goal.

In *Qigong* training, it is said: "Use your *Yi* (Mind) to **lead** your *Qi*" (*Yi Yi Yin Qi,* 以意引氣). Notice the word **lead**. *Qi* behaves like water — it cannot be pushed, but it can be led. When *Qi* is led, it will flow smoothly and without stagnation. When it is pushed, it will flood and enter the wrong paths. Remember wherever your *Yi* goes first, the *Qi* will naturally follow. For example, if you intend to lift an object, this intention is your *Yi*. This *Yi* will lead the *Qi* to the arms to energize the physical muscles, and then the object can be lifted.

It is said: "Your *Yi* cannot be on your *Qi*. Once your *Yi* is on your *Qi*, the *Qi* is stagnant."[21] When you want to walk from one spot to another, you must first mobilize your intention and direct it to the goal, then your body will follow. The mind must always be ahead of the body. If your mind stays on your body, you will not be able to move.

In *Qigong* training, the first thing is to know what *Qi* is. If you do not know what *Qi* is, how will you be able to lead it? Once you know what *Qi* is and experience it, then your *Yi* will have something to lead. The next thing in *Qigong* training is knowing how your *Yi* communicates with your *Qi*. That means that your *Yi* should be able to sense and feel the *Qi* flow and understand how strong and smooth it is. In *Taiji Qigong* society, it is commonly said that your *Yi* must "listen" to your *Qi* and "understand" it. Listen means to pay careful attention to what you sense and feel. The more you pay attention, the better you will be able to understand. Only after you understand the *Qi* situation will your *Yi* be able to set up the strategy. In *Qigong* your mind or *Yi* must generate the idea (visualize your intention), which is like an order to your *Qi* to complete a certain mission.

The more your *Yi* communicates with your *Qi*, the more efficiently the *Qi* can be led. For this reason, as a *Qigong* beginner you must first learn about *Yi* and *Qi*, and also learn how to help them communicate efficiently. *Yi* is the key in *Qigong* practice. Without this *Yi* you would not be able to lead your *Qi*, let alone build up the strength of the *Qi* or circulate it throughout your entire body.

Remember **when the *Yi* is strong, the *Qi* is strong, and when the *Yi* is weak, the *Qi* is weak**. Therefore, the first step of *Qigong* training is to develop your *Yi*. The first secret of a strong *Yi* is **calmness**. When you are calm, you can see things clearly and not be disturbed by surrounding distractions. With your mind calm, you will be able to concentrate.

Confucius said: "First you must be calm, then your mind can be steady. Once your mind is steady, then you are at peace. Only when you are at peace are you able to think and finally gain."[22] This procedure is also applied in meditation or *Qigong* exercise: First Calm, then Steady, Peace, Think, and finally Gain. When you practice *Qigong,* first you must learn to be emotionally calm. Once calm, you will be able to see what you want and firm your mind (steady). This firm and steady mind is your intention or *Yi* (it is how your *Yi* is generated). Only after you know what you really want will your mind gain peace and be able to relax emotionally and physically. Once you have reached this step, you must then concentrate or think in order to execute your intention. Under this thoughtful and concentrated mind, your *Qi* will follow and you will be able to gain what you wish.

However, the most difficult part of regulating the mind is learning how to neutralize the thoughts which keep coming back to bother you. This is especially true in still meditation practice. In still meditation, once you have entered a deep, profound meditative state, new thoughts, fantasies, your imagination, or any guilt from what you have done in the past that is hidden behind your mask will emerge and bother you. Normally, the first step of the regulating process is to stop new fantasies and images. Then, you must deal with your conscious mind. That means you must learn how to remove the mask from your face. Only then will you see yourself clearly. Therefore, the first step is to know yourself. Next, you must learn how to handle the problem instead of continuing to avoid it.

There are many ways of regulating your mind. However, the most important key to success is to use your wisdom mind to analyze the situation and find the solution. Do not let your emotional mind govern your thinking. Here, I would like to share with you a few stories about regulating the mind. Hopefully these stories can provide you with a guideline for your own regulation.

In China many centuries ago, two monks were walking side by side down a muddy road when they came upon a large puddle which completely blocked the road. A very beautiful lady in a lovely gown stood at the edge of the puddle, unable to go further without spoiling her clothes.

Without hesitation, one of the monks picked her up and carried her across the puddle, set her down on the other side, and continued on his way. Many hours later when the two monks were preparing to camp for the night, the second monk turned to the first and said, "I can no longer hold this back, I'm quite angry at you! We are not supposed to look at women, particularly pretty ones, never mind touch them. Why did you do that?" The first monk replied, "Brother, I left the woman at the mud puddle; why are you still carrying her?"

From this story, you can see that often, the thought which bothers you is created by nobody but yourself. If you are able to use your wisdom mind to govern yourself, many times you can set your mind free from emotional bondage regardless of the situation.

It is true that frequently the mind bothers or enslaves you to the desire for material enjoyment or money. From this desire, you misunderstand the meaning of life. **A really happy life comes from satisfaction of both material and spiritual needs.**

Have you ever thought about what the real meaning of your life is? What is the real goal for your life? Are you enslaved by money, power or love? What will make you truly happy?

I remember a story one of my professors at Taiwan University told me: "There was a jail with a prisoner in it," he said, "who was surrounded by mountains of money. He kept counting the money and feeling so happy about his life, thinking that he was the richest man in the whole world. A man passing by saw him and said through the tiny window: 'Why are you so happy, you are in prison?' Do you know that? The prisoner laughed: "No! No! It is not that I am inside the jail, it is that you are outside of the jail!"

How do you feel about this story? Do you want to be a prisoner and a slave to money, or do you want to be the real you and feel free internally? Think and be happy.

There is another story which was told to me by one of my students. Since I heard this story, it has always offered me a new guideline for my life. This new guideline is to appreciate what you have; only then will you have a peaceful mind. This does not mean you should not be aggressive in pursuing a better life. Keep pursuing by creating a new target and a new path for your life. It is *Yang*. However, often you will be depressed and discouraged from obstacles on this path. Therefore, you must also learn how to comfort yourself and appreciate what you already have. This is *Yin*. Only if you have both *Yin* and *Yang* can your life be happy and meaningful.

Long ago, there was a servant who served a bad tempered and impatient master. It did not matter how he tried, he was always blamed and beaten by this master. However, it was the strange truth that the servant was always happy, and his master was always sad and depressed.

One day, there was a kind man who could not understand this phenomena, and finally decided to ask this servant why he was always happy even though he was treated so badly. The servant replied: "Everyone has one day of life each day; half of the day is spent awake and the other half is spent sleeping. Although in the daytime, I am a servant and my master treats me badly, in the nighttime, I always dream that I am a king and there are thousands of servants serving me luxuriously. Look at my master: In the daytime, he is mad, depressed, greedy, and unhappy. In the nighttime, he has nightmares and cannot even have one night of nice rest. I really feel sorry for my master. Comparing me to him, I am surely happier than he is."

Friends, what do you think about this story? You are the only one responsible for your happiness. If you are not satisfied, and always complain about what you have obtained, you will be on the course of forever-unhappiness. It is said in the western society: "If you smile, the whole world smiles with you, but if you cry, you cry alone." What an accurate saying!

4. Regulating the Qi (*Tiao Qi,* 調氣)

Before you can regulate your *Qi* you must first regulate your body, breath, and mind. If you compare your body to a battlefield, then your mind is like the general who generates ideas and controls the situation, and your breathing is the strategy. Your *Qi* is like the soldiers who are led to the most advantageous places on the battlefield. All four elements are necessary and all four must be coordinated with each other if you are to win the war against sickness and aging.

If you want to arrange your soldiers most effectively for battle, you must know which area of the battlefield is most important, and where you are weakest (where your *Qi* is deficient) and need to send reinforcements. If you have more soldiers than you need in one area (excessive *Qi*), then you can send them somewhere else where the ranks are thin. As a general, you must also know how many soldiers are available for the battle, and how many you will need for protecting yourself and your headquarters. To be successful, not only do you need good strategy (breathing), but you also need to communicate and understand the situation effectively with your troops, or all of your strategy will be in vain. When your *Yi* (the general) knows how to regulate the body (knows the battlefield), how to regulate breathing (set up the strategy), and how to effectively regulate *Qi* (direct your soldiers), you will be able to reach the final goal of *Qigong* training.

In order to regulate your *Qi* so that it moves smoothly in the correct paths, you need more than just efficient *Yi-Qi* communication. You also need to know how to generate *Qi*. If you do not have enough *Qi* in your body, how can you regulate it? In a battle, if you do not have enough soldiers to set up your strategy, you have already lost.

When you practice *Qigong,* you must first train to make you *Qi* flow naturally and smoothly. There are some *Qigong* exercises in which you intentionally hold your *Yi,* and thus hold your *Qi,* in a specific area. As a beginner, however, you should first learn how to make the *Qi* flow smoothly instead of building a *Qi* dam, which is commonly done in external martial *Qigong* training.

In order to make *Qi* flow naturally and smoothly, your *Yi* must first be relaxed. Only when your *Yi* is relaxed will your body be relaxed and the *Qi* channels open for the *Qi* to circulate. Then you must coordinate your *Qi* flow with your breathing. Breathing regularly and calmly will make your *Yi* calm, and allow your body to relax even more.

5. Regulating the Spirit (*Tiao Shen,* 調神)

There is one thing that is more important than anything else in a battle, and that is fighting spirit. You may have the best general, who knows the battlefield well and is also an expert strategist, but if his soldiers do not have a high fighting spirit (morale), he might still lose. Remember, **spirit is the center and root of a fight**. When you keep this center, one soldier can be equal to ten soldiers. When his spirit is high, a soldier will obey his orders accurately and willingly, and his general will be able to control the situation efficiently. In a battle, in order for a soldier to have this kind of morale, he must know why he is fighting, how to fight, and what he can expect after the fight. Under these conditions, he will know what he is doing and why, and this understanding will raise his spirit, strengthen his will, and increase his patience and endurance.

Shen, which is the Chinese term for spirit, originates from the *Yi* (the general). When the *Shen* is strong, the *Yi* is firm. When the *Yi* is firm, the *Shen* will be steady and calm. **The *Shen* is the mental part of a soldier. When the *Shen* is high, the *Qi* is strong and easily directed. When the *Qi* is strong, the *Shen* is also strong.**

To the religious *Qigong* practitioners, the goal of regulating the spirit is to set the spirit free from the bondage of the physical body, and thus reach the stage of Buddhahood or enlightenment. To the layman practitioners, the goal of regulating the spirit is to keep the spirit of living high to prevent the body from getting sick and degenerating. It is often seen that, before a person retires, he has good health. However, once retired, he will get sick easily and his physical condition will deteriorate quickly. When you are working, your spirit remains high and alert. This keeps the *Qi* circulating smoothly in the body.

All of these training concepts and procedures are common to Chinese *Qigong*. To reach a deep level of understanding and penetrate to the essence of any *Qigong* practice, you should always keep these five training criteria in mind and examine them for deeper levels of meaning. This is the only way to gain the real mental and physical health benefits from your training. Always remember that *Qigong* training is not just the forms. Your feelings and comprehension are the essential roots of the entire training. This *Yin* side of the training has no limit, and the deeper you understand, the better you will see how much more there is to know. We will discuss how these five regulating criteria fit into martial *Qigong* practice in Chapter 4.

References

1. **"Life's Invisible Current"** by Albert L. Huebner, *East West Journal,* June 1986.

2. **The Body Electric**, by Robert O. Becker, M.D. and Gary Selden, Quill, William Morrow, New York, 1985.

3. **"Healing with Nature's Energy"** by Richard Leviton, *East West Journal,* June 1986.

4. **A Child is Born,** by Lennart Nilsson, A DTP/Seymour Lawrence Book, 1990.

5. 解剖生理學 (**A Study of Anatomic Physiology**) 李文森編著。華杏出版股份有限公司。Taipei, 1986.

6. **Grant's Atlas of Anatomy**, James E. Anderson, 7th Edition, Williams & Wilkins Co., 9-92, 1978.

7. **Bioenergetics**, by Albert L. Lehninger, pp. 5-6, W. A, Benjamin, Inc. Menlo Park, California, 1971.

8. **Photographic Anatomy of the Human Body**, by J. W. Rohen, 邯鄲出版社 Taipei, Taiwan, 1984.

9. **"Restoring Ebbing Hormones May Slow Aging,"** by Jane E. Brody, *The New York Times,* July 18, 1995.

10. 人生七十古來稀。

11. 一百二十謂之天。

12. Before birth, you have no *Qi* of your own, but rather you use your mother's *Qi*. When you are born, you start creating *Qi* from the Original Essence (*Yuan Jing*) which you received from your parents. This *Qi* is called Pre-Birth *Qi*, as well as Original *Qi*. It is also called Pre-Heaven *Qi* (*Xian Tian Qi*) because it comes from the Original *Jing* which you received before you saw the heavens (which here means the sky), i.e., before your birth.

13. 形不正，則氣不順。氣不順，則意不寧。意不寧，則氣散亂。

14. 調息要調無息息。

15. 廣成子曰：一呼則地氣上升，一吸則天氣下降，人之反覆呼吸於蒂， 則我之真氣自然相接。

16. 唱道真言曰：一呼一吸通乎氣機，一動一靜同乎造化。

17. 黃庭經曰：呼吸元氣以求仙。

18. 伍真人曰：用後天之呼吸，尋真人呼吸處。

19. 靈源大道歌曰：元和內運即成真，呼吸外求終未了。

20. 大道教人先止念，念頭不住亦徒然。

21. 意不在氣，在氣則滯。

22. 孔子曰：先靜爾后有定，定爾后能安，安爾后能慮，慮爾后能得。

Chapter 3

About White Crane Martial Arts

白鶴拳介紹

3-1. Introduction

From the last two chapters, you have seen that White Crane is only one of hundreds of Chinese martial styles. Even within the White Crane style itself, divisions can be made into many different schools, with each school having its own characteristics and special emphasis in training. Because of this and my personally limited knowledge, it is nearly impossible to cover all White Crane styles in one book. However, you should know that the root of all White Crane styles remains the same. Therefore, if you are able to ponder and study hard from this book, you will be able to grasp the essence of most White Crane styles.

In this chapter, I would first like to summarize all of the Chinese martial styles which are related to White Crane fighting techniques. From this brief historical survey, you will be able to trace back the origin of a style. Next, in section 3-3, the theoretical root and training principles of Southern White Crane will be discussed. From this section, you will be able to understand the root of White Crane practice. Then, I will list the training contents of Southern White Crane style in section 3-4. In fact, due to such a wide and long history of development during the last nine hundred years of the White Crane style, it is impossible to list all the possible contents or sequences which have been created. What I have listed in this section is only from the *Zong He* Crane style that I have learned. Finally, in the last section, I would like to discuss how to read and use this book.

3-2. Chinese Martial Arts Related to White Crane Styles

In this section, I would like to summarize the historical information which I could find related to White Crane Styles. In addition, in order to have an accurate sense and concept of the different styles, the special training theory and contents of each related style will be discussed.

In China, most martial arts styles seldom kept formal, official records. Instead, the history of each style was passed down orally from generation to generation. After being passed down for many years, with new stories being added occasionally, the history eventually turned into a story. In many instances, a more accurate record can actually be obtained from martial novels written at that time, since they were based on the customs and actual events of the time. For example, the novels ***Historical Drama of Shaolin*** (*Shaolin Yan Yi, 少林演義*) by Shao, Yu-Sheng (*少餘生*), and ***Qian Long Visits South of the River*** (*Qian Long Xia Jiang Nan, 乾隆下江南*) by an unknown author, were written during the Qing Dynasty, about two hundred years ago. In these novels, the characters and background are all based on real people and events of the time. Of course, some liberties were taken with the truth, but since the novels were meant to be read by the public at that time, they have to be based very strongly on fact. Because of these and other similar novels, most martial arts styles are able to trace back their histories with some degree of accuracy.

This is the case with the history of the White Crane style. Except for some valuable information which can be obtained from the book ***Historical Record of Shaolin Temple*** (*Shaolin Si Zhi, 少林寺志*), most other information is vague. You may therefore treat the following historical survey as a story, or as an informal history. Actually, no one can be sure how accurate it is. The history described here is based on the book ***Historical Record of Shaolin Temple*** (*Shaolin Si Zhi, 少林寺志*), the ancient novels (mainly from ***Historical Drama of Shaolin***, *Shaolin Yan Yi, 少林演義*), ***Chinese Wushu Great Dictionary*** (*Zhong Guo Wushu Da Ci Dian, 中國武術大辭典*), ***Zhongguo Wushu*** (*Zhong Guo Wushu Shi Yong Da Quan, 中國武術實用大全*), a few other random sources, and the oral traditions of my White Crane Master.

Histories Related to White Crane Styles

1. Five Shape Fists (or Five Animal Patterns) *(Wuxing Quan, 五形拳)*

The exact date when White Crane style was created is not clear. One legend is that there were Five Shape Fists (*Wuxing Quan, 五形拳*) already practiced when Da Mo retired to the *Shaolin* Temple (527-536 A.D.). The five shapes include the shapes of the Dragon (*Long, 龍*), Tiger (*Hu, 虎*). Panther (*Bao, 豹*), Snake (*She, 蛇*), and Crane (*He, 鶴*). If this legend is accurate, then the earliest history of White Crane style should begin during this period.

However, in the book ***Historical Record of Shaolin Temple*** (*Shaolin Si Zhi, 少林寺志*), it is mentioned that during the Song Dynasty (960-1278 A.D.) a *Shaolin* monk named Qiu Yue Chan Shi (*秋月禪師*) compiled the techniques of the Five Shape Fists and wrote a book, ***The Essence of the Five Shape Fists*** (*五拳精要*).[1] Qiu Yue Chan Shi's name is Bai Yu-Feng (*白玉峰*) and he came from Taiyuan county, Shanxi Province (*山西太原*). Later, he joined the *Shaolin* Temple and became a monk. From these records, we can see that the Five Shape Fists already existed and were being practiced in the *Shaolin* Temple for quite some time.

The differences among the Fist Shapes were recorded in the book ***Shaolin Ancestral Techniques*** (*Shaolin Zong Fa, 少林宗法*). It said:[2]

龍拳練神，虎拳練骨，豹拳練力，蛇拳練氣，鶴拳練精。五拳學之能
精，則身堅氣壯，手靈足穩，眼銳膽壯。

Dragon Fist trains spirit, Tiger Fist trains bones, Panther Fist trains power, Snake Fist trains *Qi*, and the Crane Fist trains essence. If the practice of the Fists can be refined, then the body is strong and the Qi is abundant. The hands are agile and feet are firmed. Eyes are sharp and the Gall Bladder is strong (i.e., can be brave).

The Five Shape Fists training adopts the spirit of the dragon. It is believed that the dragon's spirit is the highest among the animals. Therefore, it can move nimbly and swiftly in the water and in the sky. The Tiger is known as a strong animal. Chinese believe that this is because the bones of the tiger are strong. Only when the bones are strong can the physical body have a firm support. The firm structure of the physical body is the most basic requirement of a strong body. The Fists also adopt the strength of the panther, which has strong muscular power. Other than these three important factors which are required to be a strong, highly spiritual martial artist, in order to make the physical body manifest to its maximal capability, you must also learn how to conserve and build up the *Qi*. Therefore, the Five Shape Fists adopts the way of a snake preserving its *Qi*. Finally, you must know how to conserve your essence. If you have abused the use of your essence, you will not live long. It is believed that White Cranes can live for a long time because they know how to protect and conserve the essence of the body.

To help you understand the essence of the Five Shape Fists more clearly, I will here list their key training points:

Dragon:

兩肩沈靜，五心相印，氣注丹田，用意不用力。

Two shoulders are sunk and firmed, five centers are corresponding with each other, Qi is sunk to the Lower *Dan Tian*, using *Yi* and not using *Li*.

Dragon Fist is considered a Soft-Hard Style. When it is necessary to be soft, it is soft, and when it is necessary to be hard, it is hard. The key to reaching this goal is that the two shoulders are sunk, relaxed, and calm. In this case, shoulder power is rooted. The five centers are the centers of the two hands, two soles of the feet, and the head. In order to make the mind control the limbs efficiently, these five centers must act as one and correspond with each other skillfully. In order to have a high spirit, you must first have an abundant store of *Qi* in the Lower *Dan Tian*. When the *Qi* in the Lower *Dan Tian* is full, then you will be able to lead it to the brain to energize the spirit. The trick to manifesting the power is to use the *Yi* (i.e., wisdom mind) instead of dull muscular power.

Tiger:

鼓全身之氣，臂堅腰實，腋力充沛，努目強項，一氣相貫。

Expanding the entire body's *Qi*, the arms are strong and the waist is firm. The *Li* (i.e., muscular power) from the armpit area is full and abundant. Open the eyes with effort and strengthen the neck strongly, a single *Qi* is threaded (through the entire body).

The tiger is a muscular, strong animal and therefore, it will take advantage of its muscular strength. In order to energize the entire physical body to its maximum strength, you must first lead the *Qi* throughout the entire body. This enables the arms to be strong and the waist firm. In addition, in order to make the arms' power strong, the muscles in the armpit area must also be strong. You should open your eyes widely to show the fiery spirit. The head is upright and firm. All of these things should be done with the sole *Qi* in the body.

Panther:

全身鼓力，兩拳緊握，五指如鉤銅曲鐵。

The entire body is filled with *Li* (i.e., muscular power). Two fists are holding tightly. Five fingers are as (strong as) hooked copper and bent iron.

The panther is also a strong animal, and therefore it also takes advantage of using its entire body's muscular strength. However, the difference between panther and the tiger is that the panther has strong claws (panthers can climb trees). Therefore, when the fingers are holding tight the fists are strong, and when they are opened they are as powerful as metal hooks.

Snake:

注意氣之吞吐仰揚，以沈靜柔實爲主。

Pay attention to the breathing's in and out and (the head's) raising. Use sinking, calmness, softness, and solid (i.e., firm) as the major (training concerns).

When a snake martial artist is fighting, his or her postures are low. You must be able to breath softly and smoothly while your head is facing slightly upward to watch your opponent. In addition, because the snake is a weak animal, you must use defense as an offense. Therefore, you must be calm and the postures must be sunk. Not only that, the movements must be soft yet firm.

Crane:

凝精鑄神，舒臂運氣，以緩急適中爲得宜。

Condense the essence (*Jing*) and concentrate the spirit. Soothe the arms and transport the *Qi*. (The actions) should be neither too slow nor too urgent; it is appropriate to choose the proper (speed).

Jing is the essence of our body and is the most essential and refined part of our life. It is believed that the White Crane has longevity because it knows how to conserve and protect its essence. When this essence is conserved, the spirit of vitality can then be raised. When you move, the arms should be comfortable and opened, which allows the *Qi* to circulate smoothly. All the actions in the movements should coordinate with the timing and strategies. When it is necessary to be slow, then be slow, and when it is necessary to be fast, act fast.

The above descriptions of each style can provide you with a better idea of one of the most comprehensive foundations of *Shaolin* martial arts as they developed during this time. It is said that later, in the beginning of the Qing Dynasty (清朝, 1644 A.D.), a monk named "Xinglong" (星龍) who specialized in the Crane style was sent by the *Shaolin* Temple to Tibet to study Tibetan Buddhism. Before he died there, he passed down Crane style, which became known as *"La Ma,"* (喇嘛) or the "Northern White Crane" system. After a few hundred years of separate development in the Tibetan region, Northern White Crane has evolved its own characteristics and expertise, which are somewhat different from those of the Southern White Crane styles. Unfortunately, I am currently unable to find more information on either the history or training of the Northern White Crane style in Tibet.

Later, a martial artist during the Qing Dynasty (1644-1911 A.D.), Tang, Hao (唐豪), believed that *Hong Quan* (*Hong* Fist, 洪拳) was created based on the five animal patterns. This was corroborated by Chen, Tie-Sheng (陳鐵生) in his article, ***Martial Treasury*** (*Wuku,* 武庫), which said: "After viewing the illustrations and hand techniques of this book (i.e., ***Shaolin Zong Fa***), it is purely the *Hong* Fist from Canton."[2] From this, we can see that the well-known *Hong Jia* Tiger Claw martial arts may be rooted in the Five Shape Fists.

The Five Shape Fists were later mixed with the following five palms techniques: raising (托), pushing (推), horizontal circle (雲), expelling (撞), and rubbing (摩); together with five *Gongs* (i.e., *Qigong* training): lying cow *Gong* (臥牛功), hemp pigtail *Gong* (麻辮功), wood ball *Gong* (木球功), wood board *Gong* (木板功), hanging bag *Gong* (吊袋功). Together, these techniques and *Gongs* became a new style called **Shaolin Five Phases Soft Techniques** (少林五行柔術).[3] Its theory is very similar to that of *Xingyiquan* (形意拳). This new style was introduced to the general public by Li Zhi-Ying (李志英) in his book: ***Shaolin Five Phases Soft Techniques Illustrations*** (少林五行柔術譜) in 1925. According to this book, Li Zhi-Ying's grandfather learned this fist technique from a *Shaolin* monk, Miao Dan (妙丹禪師), during the Qing Qian Long period (清乾隆, 1736-1796 A.D.). This means this new style was developed before 1796 A.D. in the *Shaolin* Temple.

In addition, *Shaolin* Five Shape Fists were also mixed with eight training techniques and became a new *Shaolin* martial style called **Shaolin Five Phases Eight Technique Fist** (少林五形八法拳). The eight techniques are: Internal *Gong* Technique (內功法), External *Gong* Technique (外功法), Concentrating Technique (*Yi* and *Nian* Technique, 意念法), Fist Technique (拳法), Leg Technique (腿法), Seizing and Wrestling Technique (擒摔法), Body-Stepping Technique (身步法), and Emitting Sound Utilizing *Qi* Technique (發聲用氣法). This style is still practiced today.

2. Southern White Crane Style *(Nan Bai He Quan, 南白鶴拳)*[2 & 4]

It is said that this style was created by a lady named Fang, *Qi*-Niang (方七娘) during the early Qing Kangxi period (清康熙, 1662-1723 A.D.). According to the book, ***Thesis of White Crane Fist*** *(Bai He Quan Lun, 白鶴拳論)*, during the Qing Kangxi period, there was an old martial arts master named Fang, Zhen-Dong (方振東) (also called Fang, Zhang-Guang, 方掌光) in Lishui of Zhejiang Province (浙江，麗水) who taught his daughter, Fang, Qi-Niang, martial arts. Fang, Qi-Niang always went to the river near her house to watch the Cranes hunt for food, play in the water, jump, shake, shout, stand, sleep, etc. From these observations, she combined what she had learned from the Cranes' movements into her father's style, and so invented the Southern White Crane style. According to the book, ***Yongchun County Recording: Number 24, the Local Skills*** *(Yongchun Xian Zhi, 24 Juan, Fang Ji Zhuan, 永春縣志，二十四卷方技傳)*, Crane style was passed down to Zheng, Li (鄭里) in Yongchun county by Fang Qi-Niang, and since then continued to spread out and be popularly practiced in Southeast China, especially in Fuzhou (福州), Yongchun (永春), Fuqing (福清), Changle (長樂), and Putian (浦田) of Fujian Province (福建). It has also spread to Taiwan Province (台灣), and to Southeast Asia.

I personally believe that Fang Qi-Niang used her heritage as a foundation, which most likely included some Crane foundation, and combined it with the Crane movements she had comprehended to form a new style. The reason for this is that the *Shaolin* Five Shape Fists were popularly spread and practiced in her area at that time, and Crane was one of them.

After so many years of spreading and development, today there are four common White Crane Styles. These four styles are: ***Zong He Quan*** (Ancestral Crane Fist, 宗鶴拳), ***Shi He Quan*** (Eating Crane Fist, 食鶴拳), ***Fei He Quan*** (Flying Crane Fist, 飛鶴拳), and ***Ming He Quan*** (Shouting Crane Fist, 鳴鶴拳). It is said about these four styles:

飛如大鵬展翅之壯，鳴如伸頸歌聲之意，宿如大熊初醒之態，食如白
鶴啄物之形。

Flying as splendidly as a great roc extending its wings, Shouting as meaningful as extending the neck to sing, Sleeping in the manner of a great bear just waking up,

and Eating like the shape of a Crane's pecking.

The roc is a legendary great bird from Chinese ancient times. When performing the Flying Crane style, your arms' actions are as splendid as a great bird's flapping: strong and powerful. When you perform the Shouting Crane and use the shouting in actions, it has a deep meaning. Shouting is not only used to lead the *Qi* outward, but also to soothe breathing. When you are performing the Sleeping Crane (i.e., Ancestral Crane Fist), it is like a large bear just waking up, slow but powerful. When practicing the Eating Crane, you use the beak to peck and attack the opponent.

Next, I would like to summarize the background of these four styles. Before we discuss them, you should understand one fact. Most Chinese people in ancient times were illiterate. Often, only the sounds and the meanings were passed down from generation to generation. Later when these sounds and meanings were translated into the Mandarin language from Fujian dialect, many possible options for translation could be found. Consequently, there are several possible translations within the style. I have been able to figure out the meaning of some of the names. However, I still have difficulty in connecting the name and the styles for some other translations.

A. Zong He Quan (宗鶴拳) (or Zhan He Quan, 顫鶴拳) (or Z'ong He Quan, 縱鶴拳) (or Su He Quan, 宿鶴拳)[2 & 4]

Zong He Quan means "Ancestral Crane Fist." From this, you can see that this style can be considered the most original style of Southern White Crane. It is also called *Zhan He Quan*, which can be translated as "Shaking or Trembling Crane Fist." The *Jin* generated in this White Crane style imitates the shaking or trembling power of Crane shaking water from its body after a rain or hunting in the water. This kind of shaking power can commonly be seen in other animals as well. *Z'ong He Quan* means "Jumping Crane." The reason for this name is that when a White Crane fights, it often jumps around. Finally, *Su He Quan* means "Sleeping Crane." I don't know exactly why, but this style is also called "Sleeping Crane." The only explanation I have is that the White Crane uses defense as offense. This means that if the opponent does not move, the defender also will not move. However, if the opponent moves slightly, then the defender moves first. This implies the calmness of the Crane as it sleeps. In Taiwan, this style has been practiced in the Xinzhu (新竹), Zhunan (竹南), Xiangshan (香山), and Zhudong areas (竹東). This branch of Zong He Quan was passed down by Jin, Shao-Feng (金紹峰) in the 1930's. Master Jin was originally from Fujian Province, China.

Since this style is so ancestral and original, it embodies almost all of the basic essence and the root of the Southern White Crane styles. Here, I will summarize the key training theories and points of the Ancestral Crane Fist.

The first concept that you should understand is that **most of the basic movements in the White Crane styles are manifestations of *Jin* (martial power). From this *Jin* manifestation, many options for techniques can be derived**. Therefore, when you see a performance of the White Crane styles, **you should not analyze the movements for the action of a technique**. If you do so, you have limited all possible applications to only a single one. In fact, it is possible that each *Jin* pattern includes the four categories of fighting techniques: kicking, striking, wrestling, and *Qin Na*.

The most basic and important *Jin* of White Crane, which marks the major difference of this style from others, is called Ancestral *Jin* (*Zong Jin*, 宗勁) or Trembling *Jin* (*Zhan Jin*, 顫勁). This *Jin* covers the three moving *Jin* patterns: Shaking (*Dou*, 抖), Rebounding/Springing/Whipping (*Tan*, 彈), and Bumping (*Zhuang*, 撞).

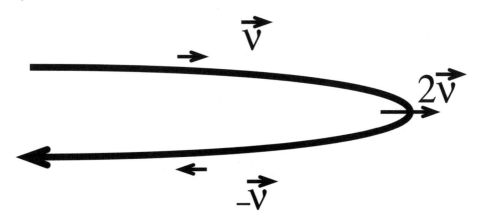

Figure 3–1. Whipping Speed

Shaking *Jin* is manifested like a dog or a bird which has just come out from the water and shakes the water away from its body. The standing root is firm and the power is generated and directed from the waist. In order to reach this goal, the spine must be strong yet relaxed. In addition, the waist area is utilized like the steering wheel of a car, directing the power in different directions. In order to operate this steering wheel (i.e., waist) comfortably, the waist must be soft and relaxed, otherwise, the power generated will be stiff. Shaking *Jin* is emphasized in all the Crane styles. It is believed that if Shaking *Jin* can be manifested correctly, the power generated is invincible. It is said:

十抖九虛搖，眞搖千軍擋不了。

Ten shaking, nine are false. A real shaking, (even) a thousand-man army cannot impede.

If there are ten martial artists manifesting Shaking *Jin,* nine will not catch the secret essence of the *Jin,* and the power manifested will be false and weak. If the Shaking *Jin* is the real one, then its power is so strong that even an army of a thousand cannot neutralize it. This implies the importance of the Shaking *Jin* training in White Crane styles.

Rebounding (Spring, or Whipping) *Jin* is just like the whipping of a whip forward and then rebounding it back. If the whipping velocity is v, and the rebounding velocity is another V, then at the instant of contact with the target, the velocity is 2v (Figure 3-1). The power can then be penetrating.

Bumping *Jin* relies on a firm stance, and uses the torso, hips, elbows, shoulders, knees, or any other part of the body to bump the opponent off balance. Because Southern White Crane is a southern style in which the hand techniques are heavily emphasized over kicking, in order to have strong power in the hands, the stances are firmly rooted. In addition, because hand techniques are trained more than kicking techniques, the fighting range between you and your opponent is usually kept short. In this case, often you can use any part of your body to bump the opponent off balance. This will provide a chance for further attack. It is said:

頭撞，肩撞，肘撞，胯撞，膝撞。善於聽勁，順勢撞抖。

The head bumps, the shoulders bump, the elbows bump, the hips bump, and the knees bump; all are good at Listening *Jin*, following the coming posture and bump-shaking (the opponent away).

There are five places which the White Crane style commonly uses to bump the opponent away. These five places are the head, the shoulders, the elbows, the hips (side of the hips), and the knees. In order to make bumping techniques effective, you must be good at feeling (i.e., skin listening) the opponent's incoming power and use the bumping and shaking power to redirect this force away.

When this situation occurs, even though your stances are firm, they must move swiftly and agilely. This will allow you to enter from long and middle ranges to short range fighting distance. This can also allow you to retreat rapidly when an urgent situation develops. It is said:

兩手如竹繩，兩腳似車輪，進如猛虎出林，退似老貓伺鼠。

Two arms are like bamboo being bound by rope, two feet (move) like a cart's wheels. Enter like a fiery tiger exits from the woods, and retreat like an old (i.e., experienced) cat waiting for a mouse.

When you fight, in order to protect your center efficiently, and in order to manifest power strongly, your two arms should be held in front of you with the elbows downward. This is as if the two arms have been bound at the elbows by a rope. In order to move in and out rapidly and agilely, the two feet are like the wheels of a cart, or more contemporarily, a car. When you enter from long range into middle or short range fighting distance, you are like a tiger exiting from the woods, unstoppable. When you retreat from a short distance into middle and or range fighting distances, be very careful, like an experienced old cat patiently waiting for the opportunity to pounce.

White Crane also places great emphasis on using the spine and the chest area to store *Jin*. Therefore, the strength of the torso and the chest is heavily trained. This can be seen in White Crane *Qigong*. Through White Crane *Qigong*, you will be able to strengthen your spine and chest to a higher level, which allows you to manifest *Jin* powerfully. It is said:

龜背鶴身，嚇退狗宗身。

Turtle back and Crane body. The (most) scary (power) is the dog's body shaking (*Jin*).

When you practice White Crane, you should emphasize body movement in which the back is like a turtle' shell (i.e., arced back with flattened scapula) and the chest is like a White Crane's body (i.e., chest sunk inward, shoulders down). If you can use the spine and chest skillfully, the shaking power generated (i.e., dog's shaking power) will be so strong that you can scare your opponent.

There are many sequences which exist in the Ancestral Crane style. However, the most basic ones are: Seven Stars (*Qi Xing*, 七星), Fan Crane (*Shan He*, 扇鶴), Five Plum Flower (*Wu Mei Hua*, 五梅花) and Five Steppings (*Wu Bu*, 五步).

B. Shi He Quan (食鶴拳) (or Zhao He Quan, 朝鶴拳)[2 & 4]

Shi He Quan means "Eating Crane Fist." From this meaning, you can see that this style specializes in using the beak to peck the opponent. *Zhao He Quan* means "Morning Crane Fist." The reason for this name is that Cranes look for food at dawn. This style has been popularly practiced in southern Taiwan, especially in Qikan (七坎), Xiluo (西螺), Anping (安平), Budai (布袋), and Dongshi (東石). According to legend, there were four Crane masters who went to Taiwan around the year 1922 A.D. and passed the art down to the southern Taiwanese people. One of them was Master Lin, De-Shun (林德順). His successor was Master Liu Gu (劉故), who wrote a book about this style.[5]

The basic theory of Eating Crane Fist is described in the following passage:

勾手喻鶴嘴，多用勾啄、指戮，手腳兼施。外動內靜，以靜養氣。以
靜為主，靜以養神守氣。

Hooking hands are like the Crane's beak, use the hooking (hands) to peck, fingers to poke, hands and legs are used in coordination. External is active and internal is calm; calm to nourish the *Qi*. Calmness is the major concern (in Crane) and when calm, (one is) able to cultivate the Spirit (*Shen*) and conserve the *Qi*.

When Eating Crane style uses a beak to attack the opponent, the fingers are bent in like a hook. The fingers are also commonly used to poke. In a fight, the hands and legs coordinate with each other. Although it is active externally, internally you remain calm. Only then will you be able to conserve your *Qi* and raise up your spirit of vitality.

In training, the Eating Crane style emphasizes the following key points:

身正步穩，穩靜內在，兩足為根，力由根起，勁在腰頭。

The body is upright and the steppings are steady (i.e., firm). Steadiness and calmness are held internally. Two feet are the root, the *Li* (i.e., muscular power) is originated from the root, and the *Jin* is (controlled) by the waist.

In fact, these key training points are used in every Southern White Crane style. The body should be upright and the head suspended. The stances and steppings are firm. In order to keep the body upright and the stepping firm, first you must be calm and firm internally. The common stepping used in the Eating Crane style is called "Three Points Five Plum Flower" (*San Dian Wu Mei Hua,* 三點五梅花). It is also called "Tri-Angle Horse" (*San Jiao Ma,* 三角馬). When you manifest *Jin,* the power is generated from the bottoms of the feet and directed by the waist.

There is another passage which describes the characteristics of this style:

四平八正，多用指法，猶為鶴啄食狀，敏捷多變。

(Train) four horizontals and eight directions, specialized in using finger techniques. The shape is like a Crane pecking food. (The techniques are) fast, agile, and variable.

Eating Crane emphasizes four horizontal and tri-angle horse stances (四平三角馬). The four horizontals are also called "four point gold" (四點金). This implies four importances (i.e., gold is precious). The four horizontals are: the head is horizontal (i.e., upright), the shoulders are horizontal (i.e., both sides are even and the body is neither leaning nor tilting), the legs are horizontal (i.e., the weight on both legs is equal), and the heart is horizontal (i.e., the mind is calm and is not disturbed).

The eight directions include forward, backward, two sideways, and four diagonal directions. When a Crane stylist fights, he or she should be able to take care of all eight directions in either offensive or defensive situations. Eating Crane Fist specializes in using the beak (i.e., fingers) to attack the vital points such as the temples, sides of the neck, and the sides of the chest, groin, etc. In order to make all of the pecking techniques effective, the movements must be fast and the techniques must vary, like a Crane trying to catch a fish in the water with its beak.

The most common basic training sequences in Eating Crane are: Angle Battle (*Jiao Zhan,* 角戰) and Three Battles (*San Zhan,* 三戰).

C. Fei He Quan (飛鶴拳)[2 & 4]

Fei He Quan means "Flying Crane Fist." From the name, you can probably guess that this style specializes in using the wings to strike the opponent. It is said:

兩臂喻鶴雙翅，收兩腿喻鶴爪，多模仿鶴振翅、行步動作。

Two arms are like the two wings of a Crane. Lock both legs inward like the Crane's legs. (Techniques) specialize in imitating the flapping of the Crane's wings with (the coordination of) moving steppings and body action.

Flying Crane specializes in training the flapping of the two arms, like a Crane. Both knees are locked inward, and the stances are like the Crane's postures. From this, you can see that, in order to have strong whipping power, the stepping must be firm and the action must originate from the body. Otherwise, the power will be weak.

The common basic sequences of Flying Crane Fist are: Eight Step Linking (*Ba Bu Lian,* 八步連) and Twenty-Eight Sleeping (*Er Shi Ba Su,* 二十八宿).

D. Ming He Quan (鳴鶴拳)[2 & 4]

Ming He Quan means "Shouting Crane Fist." This style emphasizes breathing. From deep breathing and the sound of shouting, *Qi* is led to the muscles to manifest *Jin* to its maximum. It is said:

注重腹式呼吸，鼻吸口呼，發聲如鶴鳴。掌爲主。

Pay attention to the abdominal breathing, inhale with the nose and exhale with the mouth. Emit the sound like a Crane's shouting. The palm (techniques) are used greatly.

Typical Martial Arts *Qigong* uses Reverse Abdominal Breathing. When you inhale, the abdomen withdraws and the *Huiyin* (Co-1) cavity (or anus) is held upward, and when you exhale, the abdomen expands outward and the *Huiyin* is released downward (Figure 3-2). When you exhale, the *Qi* is led to the muscular body and the *Jin* is manifested. In Shouting Crane, the Crane sound is uttered when you exhale and power is manifested. Shouting Crane emphasizes palm techniques.

About Shouting Crane Style, it is also said:

以形爲拳，以意爲神，發聲助力。

Use the shape as the fist, and use the *Yi* as the spirit (*Shen*). Uttering the sound to assist the strength.

Shouting Crane style manifests power from the physical body (i.e., shape) and also uses the *Yi* to lead the *Qi* to nourish the brain, raising up the spirit of vitality. Often, the sound can help you release emotional energy. From this shouting, you can raise up your spirit to a higher level. Naturally, the *Jin* manifested will also be strong.

Shouting Crane uses common steppings, such as Parallel Stepping (*Ping Xing Bu,* 平行步), Tri-Angle Stepping (*San Jiao Bu,* 三角步), and Single Kneeling Stepping (*Dan Gui Bu,* 單跪步). The major techniques are Poking (*Cha,* 插), Pushing (*Ding,* 頂), Pressing (*An,* 按), Coiling (*Chan,* 纏), Chopping (*Pi,* 劈), and Scooping (*Liao,* 撩). The common training sequences are: **Three Battles** (*San Zhan,* 三戰), **Four Doors** (*Si Men,* 四門), **Twenty-Eight Steppings** (*Er Shi Ba Bu,* 二十八步), **Upper Trapping** (*Shang Kuang,* 上框), **Middle Trapping** (*Zhong Kuang,* 中框), **Lower Trapping** (*Xia Kuang,* 下框), **Soft Arrow** (*Rou Jian,* 柔箭), **Seven Brocades** (*Qi Jin,* 七錦), **Soft Crane** (*Rou*

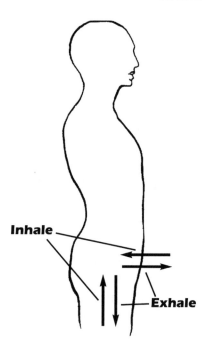

Figure 3-2. Reverse Abdominal Breathing

He, 柔鶴), and **Flowery Eight Steppings** (*Hua Ba Bu,* 花八步). Shouting Crane style has been popularly practiced in Fujian Province (福建), Hong Kong (香港), and Macao (澳門).

You should understand that even though the Southern Crane Styles have been classified into four types or styles, they all build upon the same theoretical root. Not only that, both the theory and techniques of each style have been somewhat mixed with those of the other three styles. For example, Flying Crane style also uses shouting in its movements and pecking in its techniques. In fact, a good Crane style should combine all of the good parts from each of the styles.

3. **Yongchun Quan** (*Wingchun*) 詠春拳 (永春拳)

Yongchun Quan was derived from Southern White Crane during the Qing Qian Long period (清乾隆, 1736-1796 A.D.). There is a saying that *Yongchun Quan* was started by the lady Yan, Yong-Chun (嚴永春) who learned Southern White Crane techniques from the Buddhist nun Wumei (五枚) in the mountains of Yunnan Province (雲南). Wumei's original name was Lu, Si-Niang (呂四娘). Later, Yong-Chun brought the techniques back to Canton, where they became *Yongchun Fist.*

It is also said that *Yongchun Quan* was created by the lady Yan, Yong-Chun (嚴永春) (also called Yan, San-Niang, 嚴三娘) in Fujian Yongchun County (福建，永春縣). Yet another saying is that *Yongchun Quan* was brought to Canton's Guang Xiao Temple (廣州，光孝寺) from Fujian Province (福建) by the *Shaolin* Head Monk, Zhi-Shan (至善). It is also said that *Yongchun* was created by Fang, Qi-Niang (Fang, Yongchun) (方七娘).[2 & 4]

Yongchun Quan has been popularly practiced in Guangzhou (廣州), Shunde (順德), Zhaoqing (肇慶), and Gaohe (高鶴). It has also spread to Hong Kong (香港), and Macao (澳門). Typical hand forms are Phoenix Eye Fist (*Feng Yan Quan,* 鳳眼拳) and *Willow Leaf Palm* (*Liu Ye Zhang,* 柳葉掌). Fundamental hand techniques are the Three Bridge Hands (*San Bang Shou,* 三榜手) together with File Hand (*Cuo Shou,* 挫手), Scoop Hand (*Liao Shou,* 撩手), Breaking Row Hand (*Po Pai Shou,* 破排手), Sunk Bridge (*Chen Qiao,* 沈橋), and Sticking Striking (*Nian Da,* 黏打) as supplements. The major stances include Four-Horizontal Horse (*Si Ping Ma,* 四平馬), Three Words Horse (*San Zi Ma,* 三字馬), Chasing Horse (*Zhui Ma,* 追馬), Kneeling Horse (*Gui Ma,* 跪馬), and Single Stance Stepping (*Du Li Bu,* 獨立步).

Its fundamental body requirements are: embracing the fist to protect the chest (抱拳護胸), sink the shoulder and drop the elbow (沈肩落膊), tighten the groin area (鉗襠), wrap the thigh (裹胯), and lock in the knees (扣膝). When they move, the two hands are no higher than the eyebrows and no lower than the groin, the left and right do not pass the shoulders, and they both attack the opponent's center while protecting the defender's. Kicks bring the upper body slightly forward to hide the attacking movements from the opponent. Speed is necessary for dodging, striking, and keeping close to the opponent in combat (i.e., short range). Traditional sequences are **Xiao Ren Tou** (小稔頭), *Biao Zi* (標子), and *Xun Qiao* (尋橋).

4. Five Ancestors' Fist (*Wuzuquan,* 五祖拳):

The full name of *Wuzuquan* is *Wuzu Heyang Quan* (五祖鶴陽拳). This fist was created by Cai, Yongming (蔡永明) (1853-1910 A.D. or 1849-1902 A.D.) in Jinjiang (晉江), Fujian Province (福建) during the Qing Dynasty (清咸豐).[4] Another saying is that *Wuzuquan* was created by Cai, Yu-Ming (蔡玉鳴) in Anhai Town, Jinjiang, Fujian Province (福建，晉江，安海鎮) during the Qing Xianfeng Period (清咸豐 1851-1862 A.D.).[2] I believe both persons to be the same individual. According to Chinese traditional custom, a person normally could have two or even three names.

It is said that Cai started learning White Crane Fist (白鶴拳), Monkey Fist (猴拳), *Luo Han* Fist (羅漢拳) (i.e., *Luo Han* means an *Arhan* in Buddhism; The *Arhan* are believed to be the perfect men of Hinayana, or the 500 disciples appointed to witness the Buddha-truth to save the world), *Da Zun* Fist (達尊拳), and *Taizuquan* (太祖拳). Later, he learned more martial arts from a martial artist named Heyang (鶴陽師), from Henan Province (河南). During the Qing Guangxu Period (清光緒, 1875-1908 A.D.) he combined all five styles together with his last master's techniques and called it *Wuzuquan* or *Wuzu Heyang Quan.* This style has been popularly practiced in Fujian Province (福建), Amoy (廈門), the Philippines, and Singapore.

Wuzuquan uses White Crane as its foundation. It is said: "White Crane's arms, monkey's fingers, *Taizu's* feet, *Da Zun's* body, and *Luo Han's* steppings" (白鶴手，齊天指，太祖足，達尊身，和羅漢步). This means that this style adopts the Crane's Trembling *Jin* (or Shaking *Jin*), generated from the waist and manifested in both arms and hands, the monkey's hand and finger techniques, which emphasize things such as first emitting before withdrawing, loose and then tight, exchanging actively and agilely, and *Taizu* Fist's leg kicking techniques which maintain below the waist kicking, fast and powerful. In addition, *Da Zun* Fist's body postures and techniques also adopt the head and body remaining upright, and the *Luo Han* Fist's firm stepping. The special characteristics of *Wuzuquan* focus on short range hand and leg fighting, fast and powerful. Consequently the kickings are low, and aim for the critical areas such as the groin, knees, shins and other targets below the waist. *Wuzuquan* has more than seventy sequences and is divided into two major categories. One is "Starting with Eight Steps" (*Ba Bu Tou,* 八步頭) in which the beginning section of the sequence is constructed from eight movements. This kind of sequence is known to be hard, strong, and powerful. The other is "Starting with Six Steps" (*Liu Bu Tou,* 六步頭), in which the beginning section is constructed from six movements. This kind of sequence is softer.

In addition to the above styles which are related to the Crane styles, there is a well-known sequence called **Tiger-Crane Double Shapes Fist** (*Hu He Shuang Xing Quan,* 虎鶴雙形拳) created by Master Lin, Shi-Rong (林世榮) of the Ping County, South Sea (南海平州) in the early 1900's. This sequence mixed the techniques and characteristics of the Tiger Claw, which is hard, and the techniques of the Crane, which are Soft-Hard, to become a very effective southern style practice sequence. However, there is only this single sequence, not a style. Master Lin wrote a book, ***Tiger Crane Double Shapes*** (*Hu He Shuang Xing*, 虎鶴雙形).

From the above informal information, we can conclude the following:

1. White Crane Styles and techniques have been practiced before the Chinese Song Dynasty (960-1278 A.D.).

2. There is a Northern Crane Style (*La Ma*) practiced in Tibet and its history is not known.

3. There are at least four existing Southern White Crane styles derived from Ancestral Crane Styles.

4. *Yongchun Quan* probably originated from the Southern White Crane style during the Chinese Qing Dynasty (1736-1796 A.D.).

5. White Crane martial techniques have been blended into other southern styles to develop into a new style or training sequence.

3-3. Training Theories of Southern White Crane Styles

Training theories are the root of every style. From understanding these theories, the actions or techniques are derived. If you train contrary to Crane style theories, then the techniques you are performing cannot be considered Crane style.

White Crane is considered a Soft-Hard Style, in which a beginner starts from hard and then gradually enters the soft. This also means that he or she will start with the external (i.e., more physical) and slowly enter into the internal (i.e., more emphasis on *Qi* cultivation). There are a few reasons that the training was set up this way.

1. **It is easier to be hard, and harder to be soft for a beginner.** This means it is easier to use muscular power and immediately adopt it into fighting. It was necessary in ancient times to learn how to defend yourself as soon as possible. Normally, three years of external training was enough to build good muscular techniques for defense in general.

2. **The theory of cultivating *Qi* is harder to understand for a beginner.** Not only that, since *Qi* cultivation is a high secret of *Jin*, often a master will not teach a student unless he or she has followed the master for a long period of time and has earned trust.

3. **The manifestation of Hard *Jin* is easier, and that of the Soft *Jin* is harder**. This is again related to the cultivation of *Qi*. However, another reason for this is that it is easier to injure the ligaments in the joints when the *Jin* manifestation becomes softer. Normally, in Hard *Jin* training, there is less problem with joint injury. We will discuss this subject in more detail in Part III of this book.

4. **The techniques based on the Soft *Jins* are much harder to perform.** For example, success in manifesting coiling *Jin*, controlling *Jin*, leading *Jin*, sticking *Jin*, and adhering *Jin* depends on a high level of comprehension and capability in performing listening *Jin* (i.e., feeling of the skin) and understanding *Jin*. In order to reach the high skill in these *Jins*, the body must be very soft, which allows the *Qi* circulation in the body smooth and free. This part of Crane training is exactly the same as that of *Taijiquan*.

From the above reasons, you can see that normally, when a master teaches a new student, he will **start with the Hard Crane *Qigong*,** which will help the beginning student build up physical strength in his legs, arms, fingers, and most importantly of all, his torso, including the spine and chest. From Hard Crane *Qigong* training, he or she will build a firm foundation for executing the hard techniques, which depend on strength and muscular power. Naturally, some of the Hard Crane Training sequences or routines will be taught, such as *San Zhan* or *Jiao Zhan,* mentioned in the last section.

Normally, **after a few years of training in Hard Crane *Qigong* and sequences, the practitioner will gradually enter the Soft Crane *Qigong*.** From Soft Crane *Qigong*, a practitioner will build up the strength and endurance of his ligaments. From the Soft Crane *Qigong*, he or she will also learn how to build up the *Qi* in the Lower *Dan Tian* and how to lead the *Qi* to the limbs with the mind. At this level, the *Jin* executed will be soft like a whip.

It is commonly known in Chinese external martial arts society that if a student practices the hard side of martial *Qigong*, and applies it into hard martial arts training for a time, then he or she must enter the Soft *Qigong* training in order to avoid the problem of **"Energy Dispersion"** (*San Gong*, 散功). Common symptoms of energy dispersion are rapid degeneration of the torso caused from over-training in tensing the physical body, joint pain, and high blood pressure. Lower back injury is also common. It is because of this that a White Crane practitioner, after practicing more than three years on the hard side of training, will slowly and gradually enter the soft side of training. The final goal of White Crane training is to manifest the Soft-Hard *Jin* more efficiently and effectively. That is, when it is necessary to be soft, he is soft and when it is necessary to be hard, he is hard. In addition, many White Crane *Jins* are first manifested as soft to lead the *Qi* to the limbs, and right before reaching the opponent, they tense up suddenly to protect the ligaments of the joints.

If you understand the above basic training theory, then you will be on the right course of training. Next, I would like to translate and make comments on some White Crane training secrets which have come down to us from the past.

In one of the documents, it is said:[4]

白鶴拳內重練意氣，講求以意行氣，意到氣到，以氣催力，吐氣生威
。外重練靈巧，其手法短，變化多。講求"運手柔，著手剛。"善發彈
抖勁，其步法多閃展，講求輕靈穩固。

Internally, White Crane Fist emphasizes the training of *Yi* and *Qi*. Demands using the *Yi* to transport (i.e., lead) the *Qi*. When *Yi* arrives, *Qi* also arrives. Use the *Qi* to urge the *Li*. From uttering (i.e., manifesting) the *Qi*, the awe-inspiring is generated. Externally, (it) specializes in the training of agility and skills. Its hand techniques are short and of many varieties. (It) particularly focuses (on the skills of) "moving the hands softly and landing the hands rigidly." (It) specializes in emitting the spring shaking (i.e., whipping and trembling) *Jin*. Most of its stepping techniques are dodging and evading, demanding lightness, agility, stability, and firmness.

In Chinese martial arts, all styles practice martial *Qigong*. Normally, the martial *Qigong* created in each style is used to cultivate the internal *Qi* to a stronger or more abundant level through breathing. It also trains the practitioner to use his mind to lead the *Qi* to the physical body and manifest martial power to its maximum efficiency.

It is the same in Southern White Crane style. Internally, White Crane trains the *Yi* and *Qi*. *Yi* (意) is the wisdom mind, which is clear, calm and firm. Through concentration and practice, this mind can reach a highly focused state. The other mind is called *Xin* (心)

which can be translated as "heart" or "emotional mind." The emotional mind is confused, irrational and often leads you to a state of excitement and wonder. In *Qigong* training, you are **training your *Yi* to govern the *Xin*.** From this control you will be able to **use your concentrated mind to lead the *Qi* in the muscular body to focus it to a higher, more powerful state**. The final goal of the training is that when the *Yi* is on target, the *Qi* immediately arrives and *Li* (muscular power) is generated. In order to lead *Qi* to the desired area smoothly and strongly, the *Yi* must be highly concentrated and strong. When the *Yi* is strong, the spirit is high. When the spirit is high, it can awe the opponent and he may become intimidated or scared.

When the *Yi* and *Qi* are manifested externally, you are demanding **agility and speed**. If you are able to apply the techniques at good speed, the skills manifested will be effective. The Southern White Crane styles specialize in short range fighting, and the techniques vary according to situation and strategy. For *Jin* manifestation, it emits the attack softly at the beginning. However, when the power reaches the opponent, it immediately turns hard. When you manifest your *Jin* in this Soft-Hard way, it can be as soft as a whip yet can be as hard as a staff. This *Jin* imitates the shaking or trembling action of an animal when it shakes water off its body.

Because the White Crane is a weak animal, when it fights, it must know how to dodge and evade an incoming powerful attack. From dodging and evading, it can set up the fighting strategy which is most effective. Sometimes, Southern White Crane is also called *"Z'ong He Quan,"* which means "Jumping Crane Fist." Naturally, in order to be effective for dodging and evading, the jumping must be light, agile, stable, and firm.

There is another document which summarizes the training theory of the Southern White Crane this way:[2]

在發勁上，講求以意行氣、以氣催力、勁發于腰。在形體上，要求頭
頂、項穩、拔背、鬆肩、沈腰、鬆胯、提襠吊肚。在步法上，力求穩
固，必須落地生根、五點金落地(五指用力抓地)。在手法上，要求天
對地(手足相應)，以達兩臂能發出顫抖之勁。

Of the *Fa Jin* (i.e., *Jin* emitting), talk about using the *Yi* to transport (i.e., to lead) the *Qi*. Use the *Qi* to urge the *Li*. *Jin* is originated from the waist. Of the shape (i.e., externally), the head must press upward, the neck is firm, the back arched, the shoulders are loose, the waist is sunk, the hips are relaxed, the groin area is lifted and the stomach is hanging (i.e., the sacrum is firm and the abdomen is withdrawn). Of the stepping, request stability and firmness. Must be rooted when (the feet) reach the ground. Five points of gold reach the ground (i.e., five toes grab the ground firmly). Of the hands, ask for Heaven and earth to correspond (i.e., the hands and the feet mutually correspond). It is desired to reach the goal of emitting Shaking and Trembling *Jin* from both arms efficiently.

When you emit *Jin,* you must first use your concentrated and firm wisdom mind to lead the *Qi*. From this *Qi* flow, the muscular power (i.e., *Li*) can be manifested in a most efficient manner. One of the special characteristics of Southern White Crane style is that **the power is often generated from the waist.** This is very different from many other Chinese martial styles, in which the *Jin* is generated from the legs, directed by the waist, and finally manifested in the hands. The reason for this is that the Crane often lands on small tree branches or at the tip-top of a tall bamboo shoot. When it shakes the water off its body right after a rain, you can often see that the branch does not move, yet the shaking power is strong. This is because the White Crane uses its waist to generate power to shake off the water. When power is generated from the waist, it is fast and the *Jin* is shorter. This is suitable for a style like Crane which specializes in short and middle range fighting distances.

Externally, Crane style requires the head to be upright and the neck to remain firm. In this case, you will maintain your physical and mental centers. The back arcs to store the *Jin* and prepare for emitting. This is the same theory as in *Taijiquan.* The shoulders are dropped and relaxed, the waist (and center of gravity) is sunk. Then, you will be rooted. The tail bone is tucked under and the abdomen is withdrawn. When you step, it must be firm and stable. All of the steppings must be rooted and the five toes grab the ground. The coordination of the arms and the legs is very important. Without a firm root, the power generated will be weak. Only when you have a firm root can the Shaking and Trembling *Jins* be strong.

拳訣講"鶴法全靠搖宗(顫)手," 搖爲柔，爲勁根。宗(顫)爲硬，爲勁
現。搖爲柔，主化勁，宗(顫)爲剛，主彈勁。要求剛柔相濟，"收手
軟如綿，出手弓送矢。"拳理要求"見力生力，見力化力，見力得力，
見力棄力。"

The fist secret says "the Crane techniques all depend on the Shaking and the Trembling hands." Shaking is soft and is the root of *Jin*. Trembling is hard and is the manifestation of *Jin*. Shaking is soft and (also) used as a main neutralizing *Jin*. Trembling is hard and used as a spring (rebounding) *Jin*. Requesting the hard and the soft mutually supporting each other. Withdrawing the hands as soft as cotton and emitting the hands as the bow sending the arrow out. The theory of the fist is asking "seeing the power, generate the power," "seeing the power, neutralize the power," "seeing the power, gain the power," and "seeing the power, soften the power."

The secret to White Crane *Jin* lies in the ability to manifest Shaking and Trembling *Jins.* **Shaking is the action generated from the waist.** In order to make the shaking power strong, your waist and entire torso must be as soft as a whip. This soft shaking power is the origin of *Jin* manifestation. Once this *Jin* is manifested on the limbs, then the trembling power is manifested into the target. Right before reaching the target, the attacking limbs (arm or leg) become suddenly hard. This action will generate strong rebounding power. In addition, since the shaking *Jin* is soft and is generated and controlled by the waist, it can also be used for neutralizing incoming strong power. A proficient martial artist should be able to maneuver the soft and hard skillfully, and should know how to use them to support each other when necessary. When you are soft, you are soft as cotton, and when you emit power with trembling *Jin,* your limbs are like the arrow shot from a strong bow. In order to reach this goal, you must know how to handle an opponent's power. This is called "understanding *Jin,*" which allows you to understand the incoming power and deal with it. You should practice until you reach the stage in which when you sense your opponent's power, you automatically generate a corresponding power useful for either redirecting or neutralizing. You should also train until you are able to use an opponent's power against itself (i.e., borrowing *Jin*), or even to lead the incoming power into emptiness.

鶴拳注重內外合一，氣沈丹田，或明或暗，深長爲主。精，氣、神高
度統一，凝精鑄神，以意取氣。

Crane Fist emphasizes unification of internal and external. *Qi* is sunk to the (Lower) *Dan Tian*. Either obvious (i.e., external) or hidden (i.e., internal), deep and long are the main (concern). (Aim for) the highest stage of unification in Essence, *Qi*, and Spirit, (enabling) the condensation of the essence and the concentration of the spirit. Use the *Yi* to lead the *Qi*.

Like other Chinese martial arts, Crane emphasizes the unification of the internal (i.e., *Qi*, *Yin*) and external (i.e., shape, *Yang*). In order to have a significant manifestation of power, the *Qi* must be abundant and sunk in the Lower *Dan Tian*. It does not matter if you cultivate the *Qi* internally or manifest it externally, you should practice breathing deeply. This will lead your mind to a calm state and store the *Qi* deeply within. Learn how to refine your essence into the *Qi*, and lead the *Qi* to the brain to raise the spirit of vitality. When you have a high degree of refinement in your essence and spirit, the mind will be able to lead the *Qi* strongly.

From the above two documents, we can obtain a brief but clear idea of the Southern White Crane styles. The Crane is a weak animal without much strength to use in fighting. However, when necessary, it can defend itself very effectively. A Crane defending itself relies on only three things: **the ability to jump, the breaking power of its wings, and the pecking of the beak.** Jumping is used to dodge an attack and also to approach the opponent for its own attack. When a Crane uses its wings to strike, it can generate enough power to break a large branch. The key to this kind of power is speed. Remember that even though water is soft, when squirted out fast enough it can be used in place of a knife in surgical operations. Finally, the speed and accuracy with which a Crane can peck with its beak is very effective for attacking vital areas. This survival skill is useful in another way, because the Crane uses its beak to catch fish. Next, I would like to summarize some of the key points together with some of my past thirty-five years of White Crane experience.

1. **Southern White Crane is a Soft-Hard Style**. For a beginner, the training tends more toward the hard side. It is commonly known that **the external styles train from external to internal and from hard to soft.** The reason is that it is easier to be hard instead of soft. Not only that, in order to use the soft to defend yourself, you must understand the theory of Listening *Jin* (聽勁) (i.e., skin feeling and sensing), Understanding *Jin* (懂勁), Following *Jin* (隨勁), Sticking *Jin* (沾勁), Adhering *Jin* (黏勁), and Coiling *Jin* (纏勁). Then, you must know how to apply the theories of each into practice. However, the most critical aspect of using soft against the hard is that you must know how to cultivate the internal *Qi* to an abundant level and be able to lead the *Qi* to energize muscular power with your concentrated mind. In order to reach this goal, it will usually take more than ten years of pondering and practice. Naturally, it is not easy for a beginner to learn these highly secret levels of the art.

    Normally, in an external style, a master will teach a student how to use the concentrated mind to generate local *Qi*, such as in the arms, and use this local *Qi* to energize the muscular power to a high level. **This kind of *Qigong* is classified as External Elixir** (*Wai Dan*, 外丹). From this training, the martial techniques can be taught and immediately applied for both defense and offense. This procedure was necessary in ancient times, when self-defense techniques were critical for surviving in martial society. Only after an external martial arts beginner reached a high level of skill would the master slowly introduce him to the way of meditation. Through meditation, the *Qi* is built up to a more abundant level in the Lower *Dan Tian*. **This kind of training is classified as Internal Elixir** (*Nei Dan*, 內丹). Normally, the first step of Internal Elixir training is Small Circulation (*Xiao Zhou Tian*, 小周天). Through Small Circulation practice, not only can the *Qi* be stored in the Lower *Dan Tian* at a higher level, but it can also be circulated in the two most important *Qi* vessels, the Conception and Governing Vessels. For more information on the *Qi* vessels, please refer to Chapter 4.

Finally, Grand Circulation (*Da Zhou Tian*, 大周天) is taught to the student. Through Grand Circulation practice, a student will learn how to lead the *Qi* correctly to the limbs, or any part of the body, to energize it to the highest level of Jin manifestation. In order to mentally lead the *Qi* to circulate smoothly and freely in the body, the physical body must be relaxed. A tense body will make the *Qi* circulation stagnant. Because of this, the body must remain soft.

Therefore, when a high level White Crane practitioner manifests *Jin* in his practice or in battle, the physical body is very soft at the beginning while the *Qi* is led to the limbs to energize the muscles for action. Once the power reaches the opponent, then the physical body is tensed suddenly. Again, this is why White Crane is called a Soft-Hard Style.

From this, you can see that the internal or the soft side of White Crane training, both in theory and practice, is the same as that of other internal Chinese martial styles. The reason for this is that it does not matter how a style was developed, it must follow the *"Dao"* (道) (Natural Way). I will explain the *Dao* of *Qigong* theory later.

In the past, it was commonly known that if a martial artist practiced the external styles and another practiced the internal styles for three years and then they fought, the external stylist would always win. The reason for this is that the external styles teach a practitioner how to use local *Qi* to energize the muscles and apply it to fighting immediately. This is not the same case for the internal stylist, who will still be learning how to be soft and searching for the ways to cultivate the *Qi* internally. However, after ten years of training, the external stylist will train toward the soft while the internal stylist moves toward the hard and martial applications. If they fight again, most likely they will balance each other easily. If you would like to know about these subjects, you should refer to the books: ***Tai Chi Theory & Martial Power, The Essence of Tai Chi Chi Kung, and The Root of Chinese Chi Kung***, by YMAA.

The beginning sequences of White Crane training, such as *Jiao Zhan Quan* (Angle Battle Fist, 角戰拳), *San Zhan Quan* (Three Battle Fist, 三戰拳), and *Qi Xing Quan* (Seven Star Fist, 七星拳), are harder in their training. While the very soft ones, such as *Shan He Quan* (Fan Crane Fist, 扇鶴拳) and *Hu Die Zhang* (Butterfly Palm, 蝴蝶掌), are extremely soft like *Taijiquan*. Many other sequences are a combination of soft and hard, and are trained for actual battles, such as *Ba Mei Shou* (Eight Plum Hands, 八梅手), *Z'ong He Quan* (Jumping Crane Fist, 縱鶴拳), and *Shi Ba Luo Han Shou* (Eighteen Luo Han Hands, 十八羅漢手).

2. **The Crane Sequences are constructed from different *Jins* instead of from individual techniques.** If you have learned different Chinese martial styles, you will have realized that the construction of most White Crane sequences, especially the beginning ones, are constructed from several *Jin* patterns. Normally, **the beginning sequences are short and only about five to ten *Jin* patterns are included**. The learning process is short and easy. However, the training process is very long and difficult. This is very different from many other Chinese martial styles such as Long Fist (*Changquan*, 長拳), Praying Mantis (*Tang*

Lang, 螳螂), or Eagle Claw (*Ying Zhua,* 鷹爪), in which the sequences are constructed from the techniques. Normally, these sequences are hard to learn and easier to train.

In the White Crane sequence training, **a firm root is the first requirement**. How to generate the different *Jin* patterns from the waist with the coordination of the breathing is the most critical aspect of the training. Normally, it will take many years for a beginner to grasp the essence of *Jin* manifestation. It is only after a *Jin* is manifested correctly and powerfully that the techniques derived from each *Jin* pattern are explained by the master. Generally, each *Jin* pattern includes four possible categories of martial arts applications: **Kicking**, **Striking**, **Wrestling**, and *Qin Na*. Again, there are several possible techniques in each of these categories.

In addition, speed training is heavily emphasized because it is believed that, without good speed and power in the Jin manifestations, even if you know many techniques, they will be useless. Therefore, **speed and power have become the most important parts of training at the beginning levels**.

3. **The spine and chest movements are the most important.** It is believed that the reason that long-distance flying birds, like migratory birds such as the White Crane or sea fowl, can fly long distances is because when they fly, they move their chest in coordination with their wings. Because of this, they use their body to execute the majority of their flying. This is different from local birds, such as the sparrow, who use their wings alone to carry their body and therefore cannot fly long distances. Naturally, when long range flying birds are fighting, they generate power from the center of their body and from their chest.

However, let us analyze *Jin* generation from the martial point of view. Theoretically, as long as there is a joint which allows you to bend and then straighten, then it is considered a bow. These bows are constructed from the muscles and tendons in the joints. Through contraction and extension, the bow is able to generate power. In our body, there are two large bows which are constructed from the two biggest muscle and tendon groups. These two bows are the torso and the chest. If you look at the body's structure, you will realize that through the contraction of the torso and chest muscles, you are able to pull, push, lift or do heavy work. Once you have injured these two bows, your power will be significantly reduced. Again, if you look at Olympic athletes who throw the javelin or discus, in order to generate great throwing power, the torso and chest must be skillfully applied to the movements.

In order to generate strong *Jin* for fighting, these two bows are emphasized in all Chinese martial styles. This is the same in Southern White Crane. **Southern White Crane specializes in the training of the torso and the chest.** We can see this from the White Crane *Qigong* training, in which the spine and the chest movements are the main focus. Through White Crane *Qigong* training, a practitioner will learn how to rebuild his spine and chest from weakness to a stronger level. This includes the muscles, tendons, and also the ligaments. Only after a practitioner has mastered the *Qigong* movements and coordinated it with his breathing, *Yi,* and *Qi*, can the *Jin* be manifested with the coordination of other, smaller bows such as the shoulders, elbows, and wrists to manifest the *Jin* to its maximum potential.

You should understand that in order to have strong Jin, you must have a strong physical body (*Yang*) and an abundant level of *Qi* (*Yin*). The physical body is like a machine and the *Qi* is like electricity. If either one is missing, the power will not be strong. Therefore, in White Crane you are training to generate power from the waist's jerking or shaking, and from this shaking, through the spine and chest, the power trembles outward and becomes the *Jin.*

Often, a White Crane beginner or a practitioner from another style only knows how to tense the muscles and tendons of the spine and chest without knowing how to relax them. It is common in this situation that the spine ligaments, the joints, or the muscles are damaged. This is commonly seen in *Karate* styles in which the tension of the torso is heavily emphasized.

4. **Southern White Crane specializes in short and middle range fighting.** As we have already seen, Southern White Crane developed in the south of China. Due to the background explained earlier, its hand techniques are highly developed. Normally, in northern styles, it is said: "Hands are like two door fans, raise the leg to kick the opponent."[6] This means that the two hands are like two pieces of a Chinese door which is used mainly to close for blocking. The key attack originates from kicking. However, in southern styles it is said: "Feet not higher than knees" (足不過膝). This means that when the southern styles are initiating a kick, the target is usually no higher than the opponent's knee. This implies that **Southern Styles emphasize low kicks instead of high kicking techniques.**

Because of the above reasons, normally when a White Crane martial artist fights, he or she will stay at long range from the opponent. When the timing is right and the situation allows, he or she will move rapidly into the middle and short ranges and take the advantage of skillful hand techniques to fight. Right after the attack, he or she will jump back to the long range immediately to avoid being grabbed. Since the Crane is a weak animal, once it is grabbed it will have little chance to escape. In order to fill this void, **Crane stylists specialize in wrestling and *Qin Na* (seizing and control) techniques to deal with the problems of being grabbed.** In fact, White Crane is considered one of the most well known styles which has expertise in *Qin Na.*

When White Crane training has reached a high level, the techniques of listening, following, sticking, adhering, coiling, and controlling become important. It is no different from *Taijiquan,* which emphasizes the same criteria and expertise in short and middle range fighting.

5. **Defense is used as offense.** Because the Crane is a weak animal without the advantage of strength, it has to use defense as its offense. It must be calm, quiet, and steady, but also alert and ready to attack. When the opportunity comes and the timing is right, an attack is executed in the blink of an eye. The strategy of the Crane is therefore to protect itself and wait for the opportunity to attack.

To conclude, Crane training focuses on keeping the proper distance, with jumping or moving, and speed and accuracy in attacks to vital areas.

3-4. Contents of Ancestral White Crane Styles

As mentioned earlier, there are many different styles of White Crane. Naturally, there are also many sequences that have been created to preserve the art. Sequences are called *"Quan Tao"* (拳套) or *"Tang"* (趟), and are constructed from many different techniques or *Jin* patterns. From repeated practice of the sequences, a practitioner is able to master the techniques and the methods of *Jin* manifestation. Sequences have also become a way of preserving the techniques understood by each master of the past. Some sequences were created for emphasis on speed, rooting and endurance, some for power, and some others for strategic movements. Although many sequences have been created, only those which were considered valuable and worthy of preservation were passed down generation to generation.

The contents listed in this section are those of only one White Crane style among many, and are only a portion of what my master passed down to me. In fact, it is my understanding that, even after thirteen years of learning from my White Crane master, I have probably learned only half of what he knew.

A. Barehand (Kong Shou) 空手

1. Seven Stars (*Qi Xing*) 七星
2. Great Shaking (*Da Yao*) 大搖
3. Little Shaking (*Xiao Yao*) 小搖
4. Shaking Drum (*Yao Gu*) 搖鼓
5. Eight Directions (*Ba Mei*) 八枚
6. Kicking Trigrams (*Ti Gua*) 踢卦
7. Jumping Crane (*Z'ong He*) 縱鶴
8. Fan Crane (*Shan He*) 扇鶴
9. Arcing Crane (*Gong He*) (Hard) 拱鶴
10. Spreading Wings (*Zhan Chi*) (Hard) 展翅
11. Trembling Crane (*Zhan He*) 顫鶴
12. Threading Needles (*Chuan Zhen*) 穿針
13. Buddha Hands (*Fo Shou*) (Internal) 佛手
14. Butterfly Palm (*Hu Die Zhang*) (Internal) 蝴蝶掌
15. Eighteen *Luo Han* Hands (*Shi Ba Luo Han Shou*) 十八羅漢手

B. Staff (Gun) 棍

1. Equal Eye-Brow Staff (*Qi Mei Gun*) 齊眉棍
2. Shoulder Pole Techniques (*Bian Dan Fa*) 扁擔法

* *Bian Dan is a common carrying pole which is used to carry things on each end, supported in the middle by the shoulder.*

C. Two Short Rods (Shuang Jian) 雙鐧

1. Seven Star Jian (*Qi Xing Jian*) 七星鐧
2. Spearing Heart Jian (*Chuan Xin Jian*) 穿心鐧
3. Killing Hand Jian (*Sha Shou Jian*) 殺手鐧

* *Jian: Name of an ancient Chinese weapon*

D. Sai (Chai) 釵

1. Seven Star Sai (*Qi Xing Chai*) 七星釵
2. Back Rolling Sai (*Bei Gun Chai*) 背滾釵
3. Jumping Crane Sai (*Z'ong He Chai*) 縱鶴釵

E. Saber (Dao) 刀

    1. Seven Star (*Qi Xing*) 七星

E. Others

    I. Short Weapons

    1. Double Dagger (*Shuang Bi Shou*) 雙匕首

    2. Double Sword (*Shuang Jian*) 雙劍

    3. Hook and Shield (*Gou* and *Dun*) 鉤盾

    4. Wu's Hook Sword (*Wu Gou Jian*) 吳鉤劍

    5. Hard Whip (*Ying Bian*) 硬鞭

    II. Long Weapons

    1. Spear (*Qiang*) 槍

    2. Trident (*San Cha*) 三叉

    3. Guan's Long Handled Saber (*Guan Dao*) 關刀

    4. Kicking Long Handled Saber (*Ti Dao*) 踢刀

    5. Chopping Horse Legs Saber (*Kan Ma Dao*) 砍馬刀

    6. Sweeper (*Sao Zi*) 掃子

    7. Spade (*Chan*) 鏟

    8. Hook Spear (*Gou Lian Qiang*) 鉤鐮槍

3-5. About This Book

When you read this book, you should keep a few points in mind.

1. From this book, you may grasp a clear concept of how a White Crane style developed and of its training theory and principles. However, honestly speaking, it is very hard to grasp the correct **feeling** of an art from a book. For example, in each White Crane *Qigong* movement, it is possible to relax as into the joints and bone marrow. If you do not have a deep and profound understanding of the *Qigong*, it is very difficult for you to gain the actual feeling of the practice. Normally, a videotape is able to help you catch the continuous movement of the practice. However, you should recognize an important fact: videotapes cannot teach you the feeling. These deep profound feelings must come from constant practice, pondering, and comprehension. Naturally, with a qualified teacher, you may find the correct training path much more easily.

2. This book does not intend to teach the practice routines or sequences. This book intends only to introduce Crane *Qigong* for health and for *Jin* emission for White Crane styles. Only when the reader has grasped this essence will the forms or sequences performed have meaning and root.

3. The *Qigong* part of this book can be used to improve health effectively. For those readers who are interested in health, Crane *Qigong* is one of the best *Qigong* practices existing today. Crane *Qigong* is not only able to build up the strength in the spine and chest, but can also improve *Qi* storage and circulation in your body.

4. Because Crane is considered a Soft-Hard Style, the *Jin* training in the third part of this book can be very beneficial for both Hard Style and Soft Style martial arts practitioners. From this book, a martial artist can grasp the keys to the *Jin* training for both Hard and Soft Styles.

5. Finally, I would like to point out that this book is not a definitive text. It originated from my personal White Crane martial arts background and understanding. This book is written for your reference only. There are many other White Crane styles. You should continue searching for the foundation and theory of these styles. Only then will you have an open mind and be able to absorb the real essence of the art. Truly, I hope other White Crane specialists can also share their knowledge through writing or seminars.

References

1. ***The Complete Arts of Shaolin Wushu***, 少林武術大全，德虔編著。北京體育出版社, p. 11, 1991.

2. 中國武術大辭典，(***Chinese Wushu Great Dictionary***), 人民體育出版社 (People's Athletic Publications), Beijing, 1990.

3. *Gong* means *Gongfu*. *Gong* has been commonly used to imply some special power and *Qi* trainings in the martial styles of China. In fact, *Gong* can be called the martial *Qigong* training in each Chinese martial style. From this training, a practitioner learns how to build up *Qi* in the Lower *Dan Tian* and then how to lead it to the physical body in order to energize the body to a higher level of power.

4. 中國武術實用大全，(***Zhongguo Wushu***), 康戈武 (Kang, Ge-Wu), 今日中國出版社 (Today's China Publications), Beijing, 1990.

5. ***White Crane Fist***, 白鶴拳，劉故 (Liu, Gu), 光明出版社 (Guangming Publications), Hong Kong.

6. 手是兩扇門，抬腳就打人。

Part II

White Crane Qigong

(Bai He Qigong)

白鶴氣功

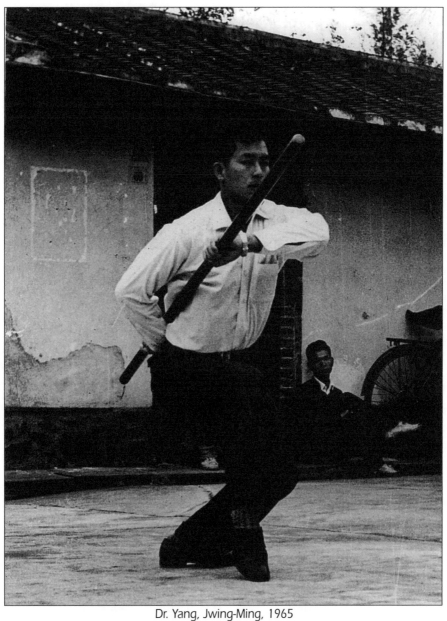

Dr. Yang, Jwing-Ming, 1965

Chapter 4

Theory

理論

4-1. Introduction

Before we discuss White Crane *Qigong*, I would like to remind you of a few things. First, Martial Arts *Qigong* is only one of four main *Qigong* schools in China, and it developed under the same theoretical root — the theory of *Yin* and *Yang*. Its development has always followed the same "path of nature," or **Dao**. Second, Martial Arts *Qigong* was originally created for martial arts purposes. All of its developmental influences were for fighting purposes. Therefore, some Martial Arts *Qigong*, especially **Hard *Qigong*, can be harmful to your health**. Third, no matter what kind of *Qigong* you practice, in order to have a long, healthy life, you must give equal emphasis to the *Yin* side of *Qigong* practice, which promotes smooth *Qi* circulation and a high level of *Qi* storage in the body, and the *Yang* side of physical training, which maintains physical strength and a healthy body condition. This is even more crucial in Martial Arts *Qigong*. In order to have great martial power (*Jin*), **you must develop not only the strength of your physical body (Yang) but also that of your *Qi* body (*Yin*)**. Only if you have trained both will you have the capability to manifest your power to its maximum.

Now, let us examine the White Crane *Qigong Yin-Yang* Chart (Table 4-1). This chart can be used for any style which trains both internal and external (i.e., soft and hard) techniques. In order to help you match the theoretical explanations with the chart, let us assume that whenever there is *Yang*, we represent it with "A," and whenever there is *Yin*, we will represent it with "B." First, White Crane *Qigong* can be divided into *Yang* (A) and *Yin* (B) training. Generally, *Yang* (A) training concentrates on developing the physical body's strength and endurance, while *Yin* (B) training focuses on *Qi* circulation, generation and storage.

Then, the *Yang* (A) side of physical practice can be sub-divided into *Yang* (AA) and *Yin* (AB). The *Yang* (AA) side is the shape of the movements in which *Jin* (i.e., martial power) is manifested; the *Yin* (AB) side is the applications which have been hidden inside the movements or the *Jin* patterns. The *Yang* (AA) side of *Jin* manifestation can yet again be divided into *Yang* (AAA) and *Yin* (AAB). The *Yang* (AAA) represents the expanding action with the coordination of the exhalation, and the *Yin* (AAB) represents the withdrawing action with the coordination of the inhalation. The *Yang* (AAA) expanding action, in turn, divides into *Yang* (AAAA) offensive expanding (which is the action of punching, bumping, etc.) and *Yin* (AAAB) defensive expanding (such as forward coiling or joint adhering movements). The *Yin* (AAB) withdrawing action, in turn divides into *Yang* (AABA), which is withdrawing but offensive (such as offensive rollback or leading action) and also *Yin* (AABB), which is withdrawing and purely defensive (such as yielding and retreating).

The *Yin* (AB) applications side divides into *Yang* (ABA), which is the action of the offensive applications, and *Yin* (ABB), which is the action of the defensive applications. The offensive *Yang* (ABA) can again be divided into straight forward offensive *Yang* (ABAA) and sideways offensive *Yin* (ABAB). In the same way the *Yin* (ABB) neutralizing defensive applications can again be divided into *Yang* (ABBA) offensive which is defensive but aggressive (such as wrestling or *Qin Na*) and *Yin* (ABBB) defensive which are purely retreating techniques (such as escape or hopping backward).

On the *Yin* (B) side of Crane *Qigong* training, the *Qi* practice is itself divided into *Yang* (BA), which is involved in the physical body's movements, and *Yin* (BB), in which the physical body remains at rest. The *Yang* (BA) side of physical movement again divides into two kinds of training: the *Yang* (BAA) side (which practices Hard *Qigong*) and the *Yin* (BAB) side (which practices Soft *Qigong*). The *Yang* (BAA) side of Hard *Qigong* training focuses on the drills of the skin and muscles, while the *Yin* (BAB) side emphasizes the physical condition of the tendons, ligaments, and marrow (i.e., joints and the interior of the bones). The *Yang* (BAA) Hard *Qigong* practice again divides into *Yang* (BAAA), in which the muscles are tensed while exhaling, and the *Yin* (BAAB), in which the muscles are relaxed while inhaling. In the same way, the *Yin* (BAB) Soft *Qigong* practice divides into *Yang* (BABA), in which the movements are on a large scale and the action is more tensed on the joints while the muscles remain relaxed, and *Yin* (BABB), in which the movements are very small and the relaxation of the joints is maximized.

The *Yin* (BB) still physical body practice, is divided into *Yang* (BBA), in which the *Yi* (i.e., wisdom mind) is actively leading the *Qi*, and *Yin* (BBB), in which the physical body remains still and calm. The *Yang* (BBA) side is again divided into *Yang* (BBAA), in which the *Qi* is led to circulate in the Small Circulation and also to the muscles and skin, and the *Yin* (BBAB), which uses the mind to lead the *Qi* up the Thrusting Vessel (i.e., spinal cord) to nourish the brain and raise the spirit. At this point, the *Yin* (B) side of White Crane training is manifested into the *Yang* (A) of physical action (i.e., Jin manifestation). The *Yin* (BBB) of physical stillness is divided into the *Yang* (BBBA), in which the physical body is tensed, such as Horse Stance training for endurance, and the *Yin* (BBBB), in which the body is very relaxed, such as in sitting meditation.

Naturally, if we went further, we could divide each *Yin* and *Yang* again and continue into very fine degrees of discrimination. This is the universal theory of *Yin* and *Yang*. *Yin* and *Yang* derive from *Wuji* (no extremity), and variegate into the Four Phases. Division is made from the Four Phases into the Eight Trigrams, and so on (Figure 4-1). From these derivations, tens of thousands of lives are generated. Therefore, any art created under the *Yin* and *Yang* theory is a living art, creative, dynamic and always growing.

In the second part of this book, we will discuss the theory of *Qigong* practice, which is the *Yin* (B) side of White Crane, to help you build your *Qi* internally. This shares the same root and theory as all other styles of Martial Arts *Qigong*. If you are able to grasp the essence of this part, you will understand one of the complete concepts of Chinese martial arts training.

In this part, we will include the *Yang* (BA) side of physical *Qigong* practice, which includes the *Yang* (BAA) Hard *Qigong* physical training mainly derived from Da Mo's **Muscle/Tendon Changing Classic.** Also included will be Flying Crane *Gong*, which is a unique part of *Yin* (BAB) soft White Crane *Qigong* and emphasizes the tendons, ligaments, and marrow. To my knowledge, there are only a few Soft-Hard Styles or even purely Soft Styles that practice this soft side of Martial Arts *Qigong*. If you wish to know more theory about Hard *Qigong*, you may read the book,

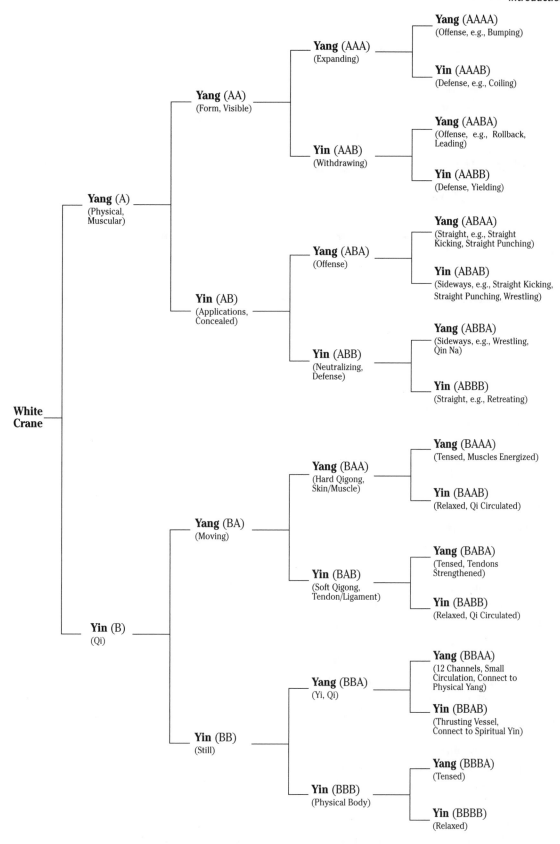

Table 4.1 White Crane Yin-Yang Chart

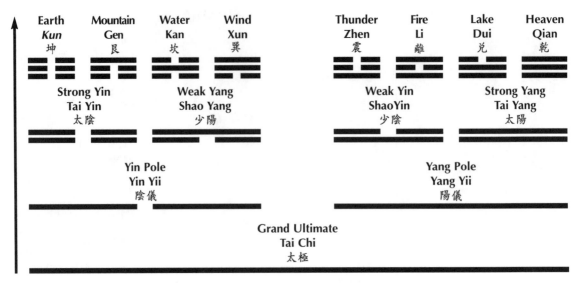

Figure 4–1. The Eight Trigrams are Derived From Taiji

Muscle/Tendon Changing and Marrow/Brain Washing Chi Kung, available through YMAA. This book will provide a clear idea of Hard *Qigong* training as derived from Da Mo's ***Yi Jin Jing.***

In addition, this second part will briefly discuss the *Yin* (BB) side of *Qigong* training, and how to coordinate the breathing to build up the *Qi* in the Lower *Dan Tian,* and how to lead it to the limbs for power manifestation. However, due to page limitations, Small Circulation theory and practice methods will not be discussed in detail in this book. For this knowledge, you should refer to the book, ***Yang's Small Circulation and Grand Circulation Meditation***, which is scheduled for publication in 1997.

4-2. General Theory of Martial Arts Qigong

As explained in the first part of this book, it is very likely that the Chinese martial arts did not incorporate internal *Qigong* training until 527 A.D., when Da Mo came to China to preach. Da Mo passed down the two *Qigong* classics, ***Yi Jin Jing*** (*Muscle/Tendon Changing*) and ***Xi Sui Jing*** (***Marrow/Brain Washing***). Since then, Chinese martial arts society has divided into external styles and internal styles. External styles train from external to internal and internal styles are from internal to external.

External styles normally start with the *Wai Dan* (external elixir) *Qigong* practices based on the *Yi Jin Jing* theory and training routines. At the beginning, a practitioner will learn how to use his concentrated mind to excite the local *Qi* in the limbs (for example the arms), to energize the muscles and tendons to a more powerful level. After a period of training, the muscles and tendons will be strengthened and built up. Endurance and a higher level of power manifestation are the goals of this kind of training. After practice, the *Qi* built up in the local areas will flow inward to the center of the body to nourish the internal organs. However, it was discovered over time that when the local physical body is over-trained in a short period of time, the *Qi* level can become overly abundant, and make the physical body too *Yang*. When this hyper-*Yang Qi* flows into the organs, it can make the *Qi* level circulating in the internal organs too *Yang* and therefore bring harm to the physical body. In addition, due to over training and stimulation of the physical body, when a practitioner stops training or gets old, the muscles and tendons can degenerate very quickly. The consequence of this over-development can be swift degeneration of the physical body, high blood pressure, or injury to the joint areas. In Chinese martial arts society, this phenomenon is called *San Gong* (energy dispersion, 散功).

The theory behind the problem of *San Gong* is very simple. When you keep training your body physically, you are building the size of your body machine (*Yang* side). Naturally, it requires an increased supply of *Qi* or energy to function. Normally, when you are still young, you will not encounter any serious problems. However, as you age and the *Qi* level decreases, the physical machine will not function as efficiently. The body becomes withered and weakened.

San Gong can also be seen in people who train very hard and then suddenly stop training, especially body builders who use steroid hormones to enhance their muscle growth. Theoretically, relying on outside sources such as steroids or electricity to build your physical body is not wise. It can only damage the balance of your *Qi* body and physical body. Generally, in order to prevent the problem of suddenly quitting after a period of heavy training, you must reduce your training gradually and allow your body to adapt to the new situation slowly. For example, if you jog five miles every day and then quit suddenly, your lungs will wither, shrink and possibly even collapse after experiencing pneumonia. Therefore, if you decide to stop jogging, you should reduce the distance from five miles slowly down to zero.

In Chinese external martial arts society, in order to remedy this problem a practitioner will slowly change from hard training into softer *Qigong* practice, and at the same time enter the practice of *Nei Dan* (internal elixir) Small Circulation. There are two goals in Small Circulation practice. The first is learning how to **build up an abundant *Qi* supply in the Lower *Dan Tian*** and the second is learning **how to use the mind to lead the *Qi* circulation in the two major vessels**, the Conception and Governing Vessels (Figures 4-2 and 4-3). According to Chinese medicine, it is known that these two vessels regulate the *Qi* level of the 12 primary *Qi* channels. Through practice, the problem of energy dispersion can be avoided. Moreover, since the amount of *Qi* which can be built up and stored in the Lower *Dan Tian* is much more significant than that of local *Qi*, leading the *Qi* from the Lower *Dan Tian* to the limbs to energize the muscles and tendons results in a higher level of power. This is the Grand Circulation. In order to make the *Qi* circulate smoothly and freely in the body, the body must be relaxed. All of the movements become soft and the training changes from hard to soft and from external into internal.

Then, **the internal styles started *Nei Dan* training**, which concentrates on building up the *Qi* to an abundant level in the Lower *Dan Tian*. Practitioners learn how to breathe correctly and use the mind to lead the *Qi* to the Lower *Dan Tian*, protecting and storing it there. At the same time, they also learn Soft *Qigong* movements to loosen the joints and condition the ligaments and tendons. Relaxation becomes the most important physical training. The reason for this is that in order to lead the *Qi* to the limbs for fighting, the joints must be relaxed and loose. This will result in relaxation of the muscles, allowing the *Qi* to circulate smoothly and freely. The first stage of this training is Small Circulation, in which a practitioner learns how to build up the *Qi* in the Lower *Dan Tian* and to circulate it in the Conception and Governing Vessels. Only after a long period of cultivation will they learn how to lead the *Qi* to the limbs to energize the muscular power to its maximum. Again, this is the Grand Circulation. Therefore, internal styles are from internal to external.

In *Nei Dan* training, practitioners also learn how to expand the *Qi* outward along the Girdle Vessel (Figure 4-4). The Girdle Vessel is the *Qi* vessel which encircles the waist area. This vessel is the only vessel in the body which is horizontal and parallel to the ground; all seven of the other vessels are perpendicular to the ground. The purpose of the Girdle Vessel is to help your balance.

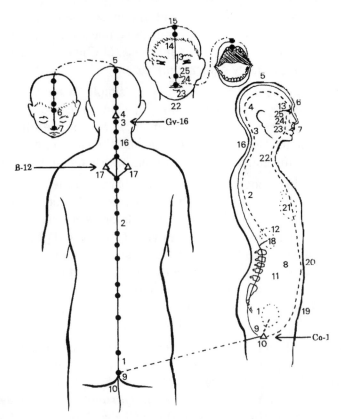

Figure 4–2. The Governing Vessel (Du Mai)

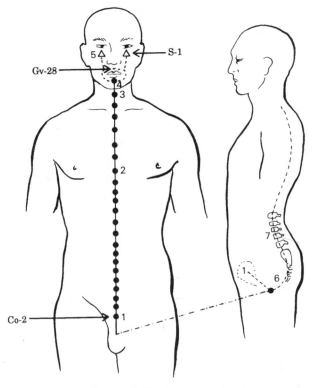

Figure 4–3. The Conception Vessel (Ren Mai)

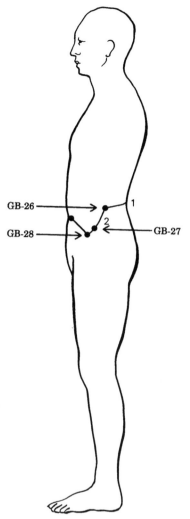

Figure 4–4. The Girdle Vessel (Dai Mai)

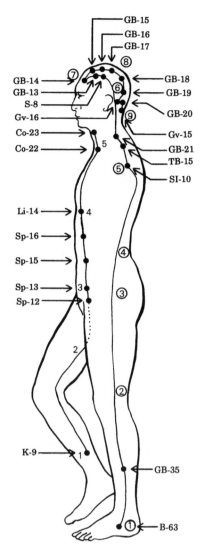

Figure 4–5. The Yang Linking Vessel (Yangwei Mai)
and The Yin Linking Vessel (Yinwei Mai)

If the *Qi* on the Girdle Vessel is strong, the feeling of balance will be stronger. This balance training is very important for a martial artist. **When there is balance, there is a center; when there is a center, there is a root; when there is a root, the fighting spirit can be strong.**

In addition, in order to develop a firm root, the *Qi* level in the *Yang* and *Yin* Heel Vessels and Linking Vessels on the legs must also be built up (Figures 4-5 and 4-6). Therefore, the sexual energy which supports the *Qi* in the legs must be stimulated, and the Horse Stance must be trained. Through a long period of correct training, the root can then be built up and made firm.

If a martial arts practitioner is able to reach a high level of *Qigong* training, then the last stage is the cultivation of the spirit. A practitioner must learn how to lead the *Qi* from the Lower *Dan Tian* through the Thrusting Vessel (i.e., spinal cord) to the brain in order to nourish and bring the brain cells to a more energized state (Figure 4-7). This can result in the raising of the spirit and hopefully a greater understanding of the meaning of life. If you are interested in any of the above subjects,

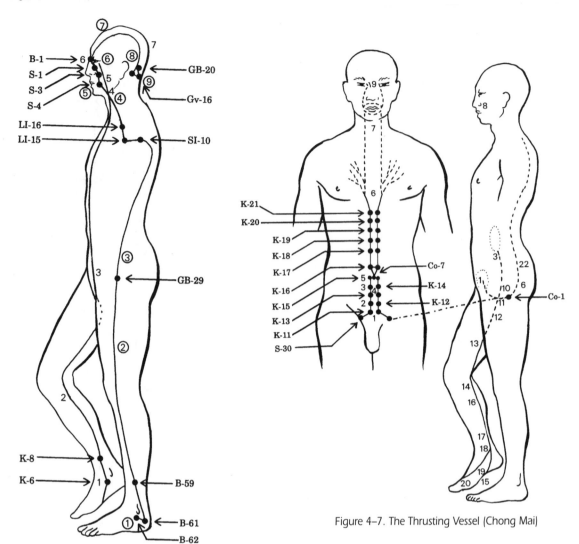

Figure 4–6. The Yang Heel Vessel (Yangjiao Mai)
and The Yin Heel Vessel (Yinjiao Mai)

Figure 4–7. The Thrusting Vessel (Chong Mai)

you should refer to the book: ***Muscle/Tendon Changing and Marrow/Brain Washing Chi Kung.***

Next, I would like to summarize the theory related to the training of Martial Arts *Qigong*. Before we discuss this training theory, again I would like to remind you that it does not matter which style of *Qigong* you practice, they all follow the same five training procedures as explained in Chapter 2. These procedures are: **regulating the body, regulating the breathing, regulating the mind, regulating the *Qi*,** and then finally **regulating the spirit**. You should also understand that even though there are five training processes in *Qigong* practice, it does not mean you can separate all the five processes independently. They are mutually related and cannot be separated. For example, in order to relax your body to a deeper level, you must first learn how to relax your mind and slow down your breathing. Conversely, in order to have a peaceful mind and comfortable breathing, you must first have a relaxed body. Even when you have reached the final stages of regulating the spirit, often you must still go back to regulate your body and breathing again in order to reach to a deeper and more profound level of relaxation, which then allows your spirit to reach a higher level of enlightenment.

When you practice coordinating both breathing and mind, you must first regulate your body until it is comfortable. However, this does not mean you have already regulated your body to the most desired state. You then enter the stage of regulating the breathing until the breath is smooth and comfortable. Regulate your mind until it is concentrated but still relaxed. This will provide optimal conditions for you to sense *Qi* flow. Then, again return to the first step of regulating your body, breath, and mind, and so on repeatedly. The more you repeat the entire process, the more profound a level of practice you will achieve. Naturally, this could take more than twenty years of pondering and practice. This repetitive process continues until someday you reach the stage of no doubts about your life, understanding the meaning of your life, and combining your energy and spirit with nature. This is the stage of enlightenment or Buddhahood.

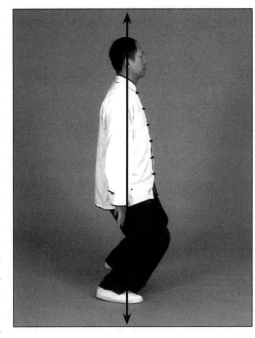

4–8

Finally, as explained in Chapter 2, when you regulate, you must reach the stage of **regulating without regulating**. This regulating is the real regulating. When you reach this level, each regulation will automatically happen without too much of your attention and effort. That means every regulating process has become second nature, and your mind does not have to be there all the time to make it happen.

1. Regulating the Body

Different types of *Qigong* training have different goals for regulating the body. Some Hard *Qigong* training focuses on muscular strength, while others place the primary emphasis on building endurance in the joints. Some Soft *Qigong* emphasizes simple relaxation of the joints, and others demand the most comfortable position or posture possible for meditation. We will discuss this subject by dividing it into Hard *Qigong* and Soft *Qigong*, and again divide each of these categories into Still and Moving.

Hard Qigong — Yang

The main goal for regulating the body in Hard *Qigong* is to regulate the still postures or the movements until they are accurate. Naturally, the first step is learning these correct postures for the movements. Then, through practice you learn how to maintain them correctly throughout the course of your training.

A. Regulating the Body for Still Hard Qigong

In Still Hard *Qigong*, correct posture is most important. Wrong postures can cause serious problems, such as joint injury or muscle/tendon damage. For example, in Horse Stance (*Ma Bu*, 馬步) training, you must first learn how to keep your spine straight and your head upright (Figure 4-8). This will provide you with a firm physical center, and will also avoid possible injury to the torso caused by incorrect posture. In addition, you must also be aware of the condition of the hip, knee, and ankle joints. You must build up the strength of your muscles, tendons, and liga-

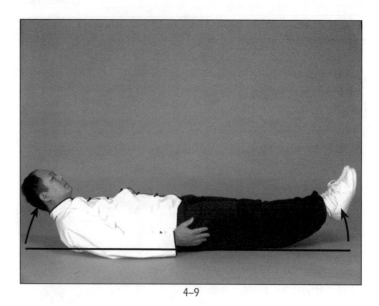

4-9

ments slowly. From Horse Stance training, you gradually make your bones more compact and strong. Only when your physical body is strong can you use your mind to lead the *Qi* downward to the ground and establish a firm root. We will discuss Horse Stance training in detail later.

Another typical example of Still Hard *Qigong* training is Iron Board Bridge. The purpose of this training is to build up endurance and strength in the torso. It is understood that power is directed or generated from the waist area and through the torso, manifesting itself in the limbs. The torso is considered one of the two major bows which can manifest your *Jin* powerfully. A weak torso is like a weak bow, and the power generated will not be significant. However, the most important reason for strengthening the torso is to avoid injury. A weak torso gets injured much more easily than a strong torso. The first stage of Iron Board Bridge training is to lift your head and heels a few inches from the floor, then hold that position for one minute (Figure 4-9). Later, when you feel stronger, increase to two minutes and then three minutes and so on. If you assume the wrong posture in this training, you can cause lower spine injury. Again, if you do not know how to regulate your body smoothly and correctly, you may gain more injury than benefit. We will further discuss this training later.

Normally, the regulating process for the body is easier in Still Hard *Qigong* than in Moving Hard *Qigong*. However, because most Still Hard *Qigong* trains the endurance of the muscles and tendons, often after some time a practitioner will change his or her postures without noticing it. Therefore, the mind has to be aware of the postures from the beginning until the end. At the higher levels of Still Hard *Qigong*, after you have built up the strength of the muscles and tendons, you learn to use your mind to relax your joints, and start to train the strength and endurance of your ligaments.

B. Regulating the Body for Moving Hard Qigong

Normally, Moving Hard *Qigong* is a simple movement or a sequence of movements which help a practitioner tense up the muscles and tendons in the right order. **The purpose of Moving Hard *Qigong*, other than building up strength and endurance, is to build up specific, smooth and strong patterns of movement for *Jin* manifestation**. Therefore, coordination of the breathing and concentration of the mind are very important. The key to success in emitting *Jin* is correct breathing, matched with techniques and a sense of enemy. After all, it is the mind and the spirit which direct the *Qi* through the muscular body for maximum power manifestation.

Naturally, the first step in Moving Hard *Qigong* is to learn the correct moving patterns, which were designed by masters in the past. These moving patterns have been studied, pondered, and experienced through many generations to bring you to the correct path of *Jin* manifestation. Some of them even have histories going back thousands of years. For example, Da Mo's *Yi Jin Jing* moving patterns have been trained for more than fourteen hundred years. In fact, based upon the same theory, many other sets of moving patterns have been created or discovered by many masters after Da Mo.

Some Moving Hard *Qigong* uses only arms, others move both arms and legs, and yet others move the entire body. Almost all Moving Hard *Qigong* training developed after Da Mo's time follows the requirements of the styles. For example, in order to manifest *Jin* strongly in the arms and hands/fingers, Tiger Claw martial styles created many Moving Hard *Qigong* patterns for strengthening the arms and fingers.

Soft Qigong — Yin

The purpose of regulating the body in Soft *Qigong* is to provide optimal conditions for the *Qi* to move freely and comfortably. For this reason, physical relaxation has become the highest training priority. Naturally, in order to relax your physical body, you must first relax your joints.

A. Regulating the Body for Still Soft Qigong

In Still Soft *Qigong*, the use of the muscles and tendons has been reduced to a minimum. The main purpose of Still Soft *Qigong* training is to build up internal *Qi* through coordination of the mind and the breath. The only part of the physical body in motion is the abdominal area (Lower *Dan Tian*). From the up and down abdominal movements, *Qi* is built up to an abundant level in the Lower *Dan Tian*.

At the next stage, the mind leads the *Qi* to circulate in the two major vessels, the Conception and Governing Vessels. This training is known as the **Small or Microcosmic Circulation**. In Small Circulation meditation, while you are leading the *Qi* to circulate, you may have a slight movement in the spine. Once you have completed Small Circulation practice over a long period of time, you learn how to lead the *Qi* from the Lower *Dan Tian,* following the spine upward and reaching outward to the arms. You must also learn how to lead the *Qi* from the Lower *Dan Tian* to the limbs. This practice is known as Four Gates Breathing, leading the *Qi* through the *Laogong* cavity in center of the palms and the *Yongquan* cavity on the soles of the feet.

From the above discussion, it may seem that the problems encountered in regulating the body are not as difficult as others. However, this is not true. In fact, regulating the body in Still Soft *Qigong* training is more important and significant than in other forms of *Qigong*. The reason is very simple. When you are in Still Soft *Qigong* meditation practice, in order to lead your mind into the most profound meditative state, your breathing must be very relaxed, soft and slender, and your body must be in the most relaxed and comfortable state possible.

In this practice, first look for an extremely **deep degree of relaxation**. At this level of relaxation, your *Qi* **will be able to move freely** and without stagnation. Once your *Qi* is able to move freely, then you can **feel and sense your body's balance**. Only when you have gained your balance can you **locate both your physical and mental centers**. Only after you have located these centers can you **be rooted**. Finally, once you have a firm root, you can **raise your spirit**. These are the required steps for regulating your body in Still Soft *Qigong* training. If you are able to

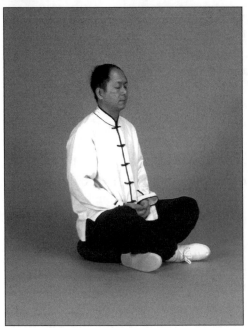 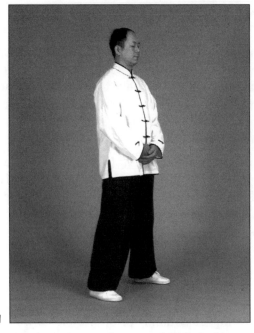

4-10   4-11

achieve these requirements, you will have provided the best conditions for your Still Soft *Qigong* practice.

Common examples of Still Soft *Qigong* practice are sitting meditation (Figure 4-10) and standing meditation. Standing meditation can be done while standing straight up (Figure 4-11) or while squatting down (Figure 4-12). Whatever method is trained, although the legs may be tensed, the torso and the neck should be as relaxed and comfortable as possible.

In this book, we will briefly discuss the training methods of Still Soft *Qigong*. The reason for this is simply that Soft *Qigong* training is a *Nei Dan* practice. In theory, it is much harder to understand and practice. It is also more difficult to train. In Soft *Qigong* meditation practice, you are dealing with your own mind and trying to promote your spirit to an enlightened level. Regulating the mind is the most difficult part of the training. For this reason, it is not easy for a beginner to grasp the essence of the training.

B. Regulating the Body for Moving Soft Qigong

In Moving Soft *Qigong*, the use of muscles and tendons is again reduced to a minimum while keeping your body in motion. You must move in a manner that allows your muscles and tendons to be in their most relaxed state. **The purpose of Moving Soft *Qigong* is the conditioning of your joints, including the ligaments and tendons**. Only when you are in this relaxed moving condition can you improve the *Qi* circulation through the joints to the bone marrow. This kind of **Moving Soft *Qigong* is the foundation of Soft Jin manifestation**. In Soft Jin manifestation, your entire body is treated like a soft whip. In order to reach this stage, the joints must be soft, loose, and relaxed. From this, you can see that Moving Hard *Qigong* emphasizes training the skin, muscles, and tendons, while Moving Soft *Qigong* focuses on training the tendons, ligaments, bones, and marrow.

From this, you can see that the first stage of regulating the body in Moving Soft *Qigong* is to learn the movements correctly. The movements can be a simple single motion, for instance the waving motion of a Crane wing, or a combination of many complex moving postures, such as a *Taijiquan* sequence. After you have learned the correct movements, then place your mind inside the joints to make the relaxation reach to a higher level, while coordinating your breathing with

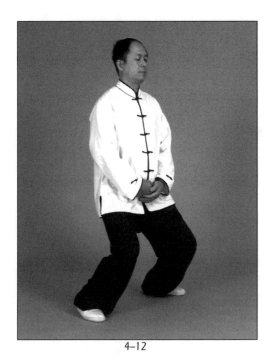

4–12

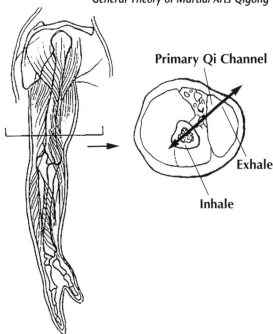

Primary Qi Channel

Exhale

Inhale

Figure 4–13. The Expansion and Condensing of Qi During Reverse Abdominal Breathing

the movements. Once your mind is able to feel deeply into the joints, you then learn how to fully loosen and relax these joints to a deep level. From this, you can see that in Moving Soft *Qigong*, coordination between mind and breath is crucial.

Generally speaking, the most difficult areas to regulate in Moving Soft *Qigong* are the spine and the chest. However, it is important to have these areas soft and relaxed. In Chapter 6, we will introduce White Crane style's Moving Soft *Qigong*, known as Flying Crane *Gong*. Hopefully, this book will enable you to make your spine and chest more healthy.

2. Regulating the Breathing

In *Qigong* practice, after you can remember the forms or patterns of movement, and have tuned your body the desired level of relaxation (Soft *Qigong*) or tension (Hard *Qigong*), you should start to pay attention to the process of regulating the breathing.

Breathing is considered to be the strategy of Chinese *Qigong*. Coordination of your breathing allows you to regulate your body and lead your *Qi* efficiently. There are two types of breathing which are commonly used in Martial Arts *Qigong*. The first is called "Normal Abdominal Breathing" (*Zheng Hu Xi*, 正呼吸) or "Buddhist breathing;" the other is called "Reverse Abdominal Breathing" (*Fan Hu Xi*, 反呼吸) or "Daoist breathing." **In Normal Abdominal Breathing, when you inhale the abdomen expands, and when you exhale the abdomen withdraws**. However, **in Reverse Abdominal Breathing, the abdomen withdraws when you inhale, and expands when you exhale**. It is usually easier to keep your body relaxed and comfortable with Normal Abdominal Breathing. This is why it is commonly used by *Qigong* practitioners who practice mainly for relaxation. According to past experience, when you use normal breathing, the major *Qi* flow circulates following the primary *Qi* channels (i.e., along the limbs), while a small amount of *Qi* expands both outward to the skin surface and inward to the bone marrow. However, if you use reverse breathing, the situation is completely reversed. The major *Qi* flow is directed to the skin surface and the marrow, while the secondary *Qi* flow goes to the limbs, the fingers and the toes. This implies that normal breathing enhances relaxation, while reverse breathing can make you more tense and excited, since the *Qi* is lead to the muscles to energize them (Figure 4-13).

To learn to regulate the breathing, the first step is to breathe from the abdomen. Physiologically, it is not possible to take air into the abdomen. The place into which air can be taken is the lungs. However, the air's intake and expulsion is controlled by the diaphragm, which acts like a pump and is controlled by the muscles attached to the abdominal area. If you wish to take in more air, the pump (i.e., diaphragm) must move down and up as much as possible. Moreover, the lungs and diaphragm areas must be as relaxed as deeply as possible. The reason for this is that the more these areas are tensed, the more oxygen they will consume. Furthermore, tension in the diaphragm area can only affect the smooth intake of air. In order to make the diaphragm and lungs relaxed, the muscles controlling the diaphragm should be used as little as possible. Through deep, slow, slender and relaxed abdominal breathing, oxygen and carbon dioxide exchange in the lungs will be more efficient. Abdominal breathing (*Fu Shi Hu Xi,* 腹式呼吸) is also commonly called "deep breathing" (*Shen Hu Xi,* 深呼吸).

Many people today falsely believe that the reverse breathing technique is against the *Dao,* or nature's path. This is not true. It is simply used for different purposes. If you observe your breathing carefully, you will realize that we use reverse breathing in two types of situations.

First, when we have an emotional disturbance, we often use reverse breathing. For example, when you are happy and laugh with the sound "Ha, Ha, Ha,....," you are using reverse breathing. While you are making this sound, your stomach or abdominal area is expanding. When this happens, your exhalation is longer than your inhalation, your Guardian *Qi* expands from the skin, and you become hot and sweaty. This is the natural way of releasing the excess energy in your body caused from excitement or happiness.

Also, when you are sad and you cry, making a sound of *"Hen"* while inhaling, your abdominal area is withdrawn. When this happens, your inhalation is longer than your exhalation, your Guardian *Qi* shrinks, and you feel cold and chilly. This is the natural way of preventing energy loss from inside your body. When you are sad, your spirit and your body's energy are low.

The second occasion in which we use reverse breathing is when we intend to energize our physical body, for example when pushing a car or lifting some heavy weight. When this happens, you realize that in order to do this heavy job, you first must inhale deeply and then exhale while pushing the object. If you pay attention, you will again see that you are using reverse breathing.

From the above discussion, we can generally conclude that **when we are disturbed emotionally, or when we have an aggressive intention in our mind, we use reverse breathing**. As you know, the final goal of Martial Arts *Qigong* training is power manifestation for fighting. That means that there is an intention. Often, Normal Abdominal Breathing is used in the beginning, and when the practitioner reaches the final stages of training, he will switch to using Reverse Abdominal Breathing since the mental intention is critical for leading the *Qi*.

Hard Qigong — Yang

The purpose of Hard *Qigong* is to lead the *Qi* to the muscles/tendons and skin forcibly in order to energize them to their maximum level, so that the Guardian *Qi* is mightily enhanced and strengthened. Normally, when the *Qi* is led to the skin surface and the muscles, blood is also led to these areas in order to nourish the cells for activity. Therefore, the cells multiply and the muscles and tendons grow bigger. Consequently, a typical byproduct of Hard *Qigong* practice is a bigger, more muscular body.

In order to lead the *Qi* strongly to the skin and muscles, **Reverse Abdominal Breathing is necessary**. Often, in order to energize the cells to a more excited state, fast and heavy breathing is commonly used. This kind of breathing is able to excite the body to a more highly energized state. Therefore, this kind of practice is called the "martial fire" (*Wu Huo,* 武火). Often (not always), holding the breath after the final exhalation is used to trap *Qi* in a particular area for longer-lasting stimulation. This can be seen in weight training, in which a practitioner will first inhale deeply and heavily, then lift up the weight to the shoulder area. Next, he will lift the weight upward with an exhalation to energize the muscles to their maximum. Finally, he will hold his breath in order to maintain the energization of his muscles. It is the same when you are pushing a car stuck in the mud — you will first inhale deeply and exhale when you push. At the end point, you will hold your breath in order to maintain the longer energization of the muscles

Furthermore, as mentioned earlier, in order to strengthen the Guardian *Qi* more efficiently, you must exhale longer than inhaling with reverse breathing. Normally, from the heavy martial fire breathing, the emotional mind can be excited and the spirit can be raised in a short time. Therefore, using this kind of breathing technique in coordination with the sound *"Ha,"* soldiers could be excited to a higher spiritual and courageous level before a battle in ancient times. Next, we will discuss the breathing techniques normally used in Still and Moving Hard *Qigong* sets.

A. Regulating the Breathing for Still Hard Qigong

The main purpose of Still Hard *Qigong* is to build up the strength and endurance of the muscles/tendons and ligaments with some specific postures, as explained earlier. Therefore, at the beginning, you should simply breathe naturally and pay more attention to the correct postures. After you feel comfortable in the postures and have built up your endurance, start to bring your mind to the area being trained with the coordination of your breathing.

Since you now have an intention in leading the *Qi* to the training area, you must use Reverse Abdominal Breathing. For example, in Iron Board Bridge training, at the beginning, you simply pay attention and avoid holding your breath. After a period of training, when your endurance and strength are built up, use Reverse Abdominal Breathing and your mind to lead the *Qi* to the torso. After a long period of training, you will enter the final stage of Iron Board Bridge training, or Iron Shirt Beating practice. In this training, you will need a partner who uses his hand, some short sticks, and eventually a rubber hammer to pound the front side of your body from the chest to the abdomen. During this training, whenever the pounding lands on the body, you should hold your breath for an instant in order to build up resistant strength in the muscles, and then relax.

Another example of Still Hard *Qigong* is Horse Stance training. Again, do not worry about your breathing at first, but use your mind in the coordination with Reverse Abdominal Breathing to lead the *Qi* to the joints, such as the ankles, knees, or hips to generate joint breathing. This helps you build up strength and endurance in these joints.

B. Regulating the Breathing for Moving Hard Qigong

In Moving Hard *Qigong* practice, Reverse Abdominal Breathing is adopted immediately to coordinate your movements. In the beginning, local *Qi* is used to energize the muscles and tendons. Normally, Reverse Abdominal Breathing is necessary to make progress. When you practice this, first inhale deeply and then exhale. When you exhale, concentrate your mind on the movement while tensing up your muscles and tendons. In this way, the muscles and tendons which support the movements will be built up. This is a typical *Wai Dan* training.

Later, if you have learned Small Circulation and Grand Circulation training, the *Qi* is led to the training area from the Lower *Dan Tian* by the mind to stimulate and energize the muscles and tendons. From this training, physical strength can be enhanced to a higher and more significant level.

The final stage is learning how to build up resistance to an enemy's attack through Grand Circulation. In other words, Iron Shirt Training.

SOFT QIGONG — YIN

A. Regulating the Breathing for Still Soft Qigong

Of all the *Qigong* practices that exist, Still Soft *Qigong* is probably the most difficult. In Still Soft *Qigong* practice, there is very little movement. However, it can be very challenging to manage the process of regulating the breathing, mind, *Qi*, and spirit.

In Still Soft *Qigong* training, the first task is to use the abdominal area to breathe, thereby allowing you to inhale the oxygen and expel carbon dioxide smoothly and comfortably. To became an expert in Martial Arts *Qigong*, you must first master both Normal Abdominal Breathing and Reverse Abdominal Breathing.

After you practice these two breathing methods for a long time and they feel natural, you should practice Embryo Breathing (*Tai Xi,* 胎息). From Embryo Breathing, you learn how to build up your *Qi* to an abundant level, and to use your mind to lead the *Qi* to the Lower *Dan Tian* for storage. In addition, you also learn Five Gates Breathing (*Wu Xin Hu Xi,* 五心呼吸), which allows you to lead the *Qi* to the five gates - the two *Laogong* cavities on the palms, the two Yongquan cavities on the soles of the feet, and the *Baihui* (Gv-20) cavity on the head or the Upper *Dan Tian* in the center of the forehead (also called the third eye).

Finally, you will also need to train Skin and Marrow/Brain Breathing (*Ti Xi* and *Sui Xi,* 體息、髓息). From this training, you learn how to lead the *Qi* to the surface of the skin in order to strengthen the Guardian *Qi*, and also to the marrow to keep it clean. In addition, you learn how to lead the *Qi* to nourish the brain and raise the spirit of vitality.

All of the above training is difficult both in theory and practice. This is in fact the path for reaching enlightenment or Buddhahood. Therefore, it is not an easy subject to cover in just one section of this book. If you are interested in these subjects, please refer to the books ***The Root of Chinese Chi Kung and Muscle/Tendon Changing and Marrow/Brain Washing Chi Kung***, by YMAA.

B. Regulating the Breathing for Moving Soft Qigong

In Soft *Qigong*, after you have regulated your body, then you must apply the abdominal breathing (either normal or reverse) into the movements. After you have practiced for some time, and have reached a good level of the Embryo Breathing in the Still Soft *Qigong* practice, then you should apply the Embryo Breathing into the soft movements of the forms.

Later, you will apply the Five Gates Breathing. This will allow you to use your mind to lead the *Qi* to the extremities easily, and train the brain to raise your spirit of vitality. Naturally, as with any other *Qigong* practice, the final goal is to build up an independence of the spirit.

3. Regulating the Mind

As explained in Chapter 2, we each have two minds. One is called *"Xin"* (心), which means "heart," implying the mind which is generated from emotional disturbance. *Xin* can therefore be called the "emotional mind." For example, when you see something happening or encounter some occurrence which generates an emotional response, the thoughts or "mind" generated from this emotional disturbance are *Xin*. Even if nothing happens, the emotional mind can be generated from your own internal emotional conflicts. For example, laziness is generated from the *Xin*.

The other mind is called *"Yi"* (意). If we analyze the construction of this Chinese word, we can see that it is a combination of three words: *"Li"* (立), *"Yue"* (曰), and *"Xin"* (心). *Li* means "to establish," "to create," or "to begin." *Yue* means "speaking," "saying," or "talking." Naturally, *"Xin"* is the "heart" or "emotional mind." From the structure of the entire word, notice that Xin is on the bottom, which implies that the emotional mind is under control. Under these conditions only is talking possible. Therefore, reason is generated from careful pondering of the thoughts originated in the emotional mind. *Yi* can thus be translated as "wisdom mind," or the mind which originates from wise judgment. For example, you may be agitated emotionally, yet before the emotional mind manifests itself as action, the wise clear mind steps in to analyze the situation. The action taken by this wise judgment is said to originate from the *Yi*. *Yi* is calm, clear, wise and is classified as *Yin*, while *Xin* is disturbed, agitated, emotional and is classified as *Yang*. In Chinese *Qigong*, *Xin* is analogous to a monkey, always moving and jumping around; it cannot be calm and steady. However, *Yi* is looked upon as a horse, calm and powerful. *"Xin Yuan Yi Ma"* (心猿意馬) means *"Xin* is monkey and *Yi* is horse."

As with all *Qigong* practice, the first step for regulating the mind in Martial Arts *Qigong* training is learning how to use the wisdom mind to govern the emotional mind. This is not an easy process. Simply speaking, much of the time most people are controlled by their emotional mind. On one hand they know that they should not do some act or another, while on the other their selfish desires tempt them to ruin. In martial arts, if you are completely controlled by your emotional mind, then your reactions in combat will be irrational, wild and animalistic, as though your mind has been lost. This kind of mind will make you enter an opponent's traps easily. However, if the emotional mind can be filtered first through the wisdom mind and tempered, then your fighting will be confident and courageous. The best mind in a fight is the emotional mind under the direction of the wisdom mind. The emotional mind is the source of motivation, spirit, and aggression, but the rational mind is necessary to direct the emotional mind to the right place, and to manifest your intentions effectively and logically. Without this tempering, the emotional mind is unfocused and violent. There must be a moral goal to your conflict, or you will become destructive and evil. If the emotional mind (*Yang*) and wisdom mind (*Yin*) can coordinate harmoniously, then you will fight rationally with a high spirit. The outcome of this mental battle, which your opponent must also wage, is the true source of all victory and defeat. Its result can have consequences long after the last blows are struck.

Therefore, in Martial Arts *Qigong* training, even though you need to build up your emotional strength, you must also exercise your calmness of mind and always remain in control of your actions. When you are calm, you are like an eagle calmly surveying a landscape for the slightest signs of movement, or like a cat carefully stalking its prey's every movement, despite burning hunger. When you act, you are strong and powerful both physically and spiritually, like a fierce tiger.

In order to reach this goal, you must use your *Yi* to lead the *Qi* efficiently. Your emotional mind makes the *Qi* excited and out of control, while your wisdom mind leads this strong *Qi* down the correct path. Your *Yi* is very important at the beginning of Martial Arts *Qigong* training. It is said: "Use your *Yi* to lead your *Qi*" (*Yi Yi Yin Qi*, 以意引氣). This refers to leading the *Qi* in the Small and Grand Circulations.

In addition, you must also understand the meaning of the saying: "The *Yi* keeps in *Dan Tian*" (*Yi Shou Dan Tian*, 意守丹田). No matter how you lead the *Qi*, the Lower *Dan Tian* remains the headquarters or the central residence of your *Qi*. The *Qi* begins here and returns here. Therefore, the wisdom mind should always recognize this center. Your *Qi* will then have a root and a firm source. When your *Yi* is kept in the Lower *Dan Tian*, your *Qi* can be sunken and abundant. When your *Yi* wanders away from the Lower *Dan Tian,* this root will be lost, and the *Qi* will float and become over-excited. Next, we will discuss how the mind can affect different Martial Arts *Qigong* practice.

HARD QIGONG — YANG

A. Regulating the Mind for Still Hard Qigong

At the beginning of your Still Hard *Qigong*, your emotional mind might be distracted. You should take at least five minutes to calm yourself down. At the end of this time you will have to decide whether to continue or give up until you feel more focused. The struggle at this stage is between your emotional mind and your wisdom mind, and it is very important. If your emotional mind is stronger, then you will not be able to continue to the end of your session. However, if your wisdom mind is in control and you finish your set, then you will have already completed the first step of Still Hard *Qigong* training. Even after you have built up a strong will from your wisdom mind for the training, you still must be careful. You must listen to your emotional mind, as it reflects the impressions and desires of your physical body. If you are over-exerting yourself out of a sense of stubbornness, then you have made the mistake of the minds, and have confused the one with the other. It will not, in truth, be the wisdom mind that controls you in your over-training, but your emotional mind.

Remember that to all things there is a balance. Remember that the strength of your physical body cannot be built in one day. The general rule is that if the emotional mind is caused from laziness, then it should be conquered. This is relatively easy to recognize in yourself. But there is another aspect of the emotional mind which fears above all your own human frailty and weakness, and which can drive you to train at the expense of other valuable parts of your life. This is more difficult by far to recognize in yourself. You must always be vigilant and recognize why it is you are training, whether out of strength or out of fear. This is not an easy task, and it is a constant threat no matter what your level of training or expertise.

After you have completed the first phase of endurance training in Still Hard *Qigong*, then you must learn how to use your mind to raise the local *Qi* to a higher level. From this training, you will experience increased will power and a raising of the spirit.

The final phase of Still Hard *Qigong* training is using your mind to lead the *Qi* from the Lower *Dan Tian* to the training area in order to build up strength or endurance to the highest possible level. Notice that the training has changed from external to internal.

B. Regulating the Mind for Moving Hard Qigong

In Moving Hard *Qigong*, you are not only building up your physical body but are also training a sense of enemy. One of the main reasons behind Moving Hard *Qigong* is to build up the foundation for *Jin* manifestation. However, how the *Jin* is directed and manifested depends on your mind and spirit. Therefore, in each movement of Moving Hard *Qigong*, the mind assumes different attributes depending on the purpose of the movement.

For example, the arcing chest and back Moving Hard *Qigong* is mainly used to build up the strength of the bow formed by the chest. Therefore, the beginning purpose of this *Qigong* is to strengthen muscles/tendons, bones structure, and firm the root in coordination with the breathing. The mind should be focused on the physical body. Later, after training for a period of time, you should place your mind on leading the *Qi* from the Lower *Dan Tian* to the upper torso and then outward. This expanding outward *Qi* training is a crucial part of both Iron Shirt Training and Wardoff *Jin*.

Another example is Iron Arm *Gong,* in which the strength of the arms is considered most important. The reason for creating strong arms is to develop a capability for blocking and intercepting an opponent's attacks. Strong arms also provide you with a foundation for more powerful Jin manifestation through the arms. Therefore, the mind for this training can be different than in others. In order to regulate the mind in Moving Hard *Qigong*, you must first understand the purpose and the motivation of the movement.

SOFT QIGONG — YIN

A. Regulating the Mind for Still Soft Qigong

Regulating the mind in Still Soft *Qigong* is probably the most difficult task in all *Qigong* training. Once your physical body has calmed down through meditation, your emotional mind starts to be more active. The conflict between your emotional and wisdom minds becomes stronger. Generally, your emotional mind will bring forth images of past events, forcing your wisdom mind to deal with feelings of guilt or regret which have been hidden beneath the surface of your consciousness. It acts as a mirror, reflecting the things behind the masks we all wear. Your emotional mind can also generate many fantasies beyond reality, and lead you into a deep, dreaming state.

Therefore, the first phase of regulating the mind is removing your mask and facing yourself. If you do not know yourself, how do you expect to know others, or to know nature? Normally, if you succeed in calming your emotional mind and remain in position for more than half an hour without disturbing thoughts, then you will be able to place your mind on your breathing, build up the *Qi* in the Lower *Dan Tian* to an abundant level, and lead the *Qi* for Grand Circulation. This is the second phase of regulating the mind, and is the key to success in Embryo Breathing, Five Gates Breathing, Skin and Marrow Breathing, and Spiritual Breathing. Without the correct mind, all your efforts to so regulate your breathing will fail.

B. Regulating the Mind for Moving Soft Qigong

As mentioned earlier, the purpose of Moving Soft *Qigong* is to relax the joints and build up the strength of the tendons and ligaments. In addition, from Moving Soft *Qigong*, the foundation for manifesting Soft *Jin* can be established. In Soft *Jin,* the entire body acts like a silken whip. In order to reach this goal, the joints must be very relaxed and coordinate the movements.

Therefore, at the beginning of Moving Soft *Qigong* training, the mind is on the joints to regulate the body until the movements are correct, and the joints are at their most relaxed. Next, you must learn how to lead the *Qi* from Lower *Dan Tian* to the area being trained in order to support the motions. This is again Grand Circulation. If you are practicing Moving Soft *Qigong* for health purposes, then you have reached your goal.

However, if you practice Moving Soft *Qigong* for martial arts, then your final goal is a sense of enemy. With this sense, you can lead your *Qi* to an area which allows you to manifest your *Jin* power into the opponent's body. It is like learning how to use a silken whip against a target. Your mind must focus on the target. Otherwise, the whipping power will not be manifested efficiently.

4. Regulating the Qi

Regulating the *Qi* is actually the result of regulating the body, the breathing, and the mind. This means that, in order to regulate the *Qi*, you must first provide the proper conditions for the *Qi* to be regulated. Therefore, regulating the *Qi* cannot be separated from the other three regulations.

Moreover, you should also consider the quality of your *Qi*. The kind of food you eat and the cleanliness of the air you breathe can significantly affect your *Qi*. Often, herbs are used to regulate the *Qi* in Chinese *Qigong* society. For example, Ginseng can enhance *Qi* circulation in the winter (when *Qi* can be deficient), but should be avoided in the summer (when *Qi* can be abundant). Likewise, when you are young, you should avoid taking Ginseng. When you are young, you already have an abundance of *Qi* in your body; if you take Ginseng, it can make your body too *Yang*. Furthermore, once your body has gotten used to the Ginseng, when you need it later, it will not be as effective. Another example is that you should eat more meat products in winter, and more vegetables and fruits in summer. But again remember that such foods should be eaten in moderation, and that in general grains, fruits and vegetables are better for you than meats and dairy products.

In addition, you should also consider your sexual activity. If you are male, too much sex is harmful for your *Qigong* practice. Moderation of your sexual activity and conservation of ejaculation can stimulate your balance both physically and mentally.

Under all these prior conditions, when you regulate your *Qi*, you can decide how strongly it should be regulated. If the *Qi* is built up to an abundant level in a short time, it can make your body *Yang*. This can be done through heavy and short abdominal breathing with the mind's concentration. As explained earlier, this manner of building up the *Qi* is called "martial fire" (*Wu Huo*, 武火). Martial fire *Qi* training is commonly used in external Martial Arts *Qigong*.

However, if you wish to build the *Qi* up slowly and smoothly, the mind must be calm and the breathing must be slender and slow. Holding the breath is not encouraged, especially for beginners. In this kind of Qigong training, through slow abdominal breathing and relaxation, a calm mind is generated. This is called the "scholar fire" (*Wen Huo*, 文火). This practice can cool down the body's *Yang* and make the mind enter a profound meditative state. Scholar fire practice is commonly used in still meditation or Soft *Qigong* movements like *Taijiquan*. Next, we will summarize *Qi* status in Martial Arts *Qigong* training.

HARD QIGONG — YANG

A. Regulating the Qi for Still Hard Qigong

The goal of Still Hard *Qigong* is the conditioning of the tendons and ligaments. Therefore, the joint areas receive special attention in this training. In order to condition the joints as deeply as possible, your breathing should be as slow as is comfortable. The *Qi* is then led to the joints by the mind. Sometimes, after you have led the *Qi* to the joints being trained, in order to trap it there for conditioning, you will hold your breath for a few seconds. However, usually the *Qi* is merely led into the deep joints and then led out. These are joint breathing exercises in which the joints are tensed due to the postures.

For example, in order to build up strength in the knees, use the Horse Stance (*Ma Bu*) posture, then inhale deeply while leading the *Qi* inward to the center of the joints. Next, exhale and use the mind to lead the *Qi* to the outside of the knees (i.e., joint breathing). Through practice, the knees can be strengthened.

B. Regulating the Qi for Moving Hard Qigong

As mentioned earlier, Moving Hard *Qigong* strengthens the muscles and tendons for manifestation of Hard *Jin*. Naturally, through Moving Hard *Qigong*, you can condition your physical body from weak to strong.

In order to reach this goal, you first inhale deeply and then exhale strongly while using your mind to either excite the local *Qi* or lead the *Dan Tian Qi* to the trained area and energize it to a higher state. In order to quickly energize the muscular body, the exhalation should be both strong and short. That means that "martial fire" should be used. This will make your body *Yang*, and result in the conditioning of your physical body. Often, once the *Qi* is led to the areas being trained, you hold the breath to trap the *Qi* there for stronger energization of the muscles. It is just like when you push a car — first you inhale deeply and then exhale while pushing. In order to energize your muscular power to a higher level, you hold the breath during the initial push.

SOFT QIGONG — YIN

A. Regulating the Qi for Still Soft Qigong

In Still Soft *Qigong*, since there is no significant physical movement involved, the mind can be very calm and the physical body can be very soft and relaxed. Therefore, the breathing can be very slow, slender, smooth, soft, and relaxed. The first goal of Still Soft *Qigong* is to build up an abundant supply of *Qi* in the Lower *Dan Tian* with the "scholar fire" technique. Next, the *Qi* stored in the Lower *Dan Tian* is led by the mind to circulate in the two most important vessels, the Conception and Governing Vessels, thereby completing the Small Circulation. This training theory is harder to understand and the practice is much more challenging than that of Hard *Qigong*. Normally, in order to avoid danger and injury, Small Circulation should only be taught and supervised by a qualified teacher.

After Small Circulation training, you should begin training the Grand Circulation. In this training, first you learn how to use your mind to lead the *Qi* from Lower *Dan Tian* to the limbs and back again. Next, you learn how to lead the *Qi* to some specific area in the body for special training — or example, as in Iron Shirt training.

You then learn how to lead the *Qi* from the Lower *Dan Tian* to the skin surface and beyond in order to strengthen the Guardian *Qi* and bone marrow. This is the skin-marrow breathing *Qigong* training. From this training, the *Qi* can circulate freely to any part of your body. Health and longevity can then be maintained more naturally. Moreover, through this training, a Sense of Enemy (i.e., alertness) can be significantly developed.

At an advanced level of Still Soft *Qigong* training, the mind leads the *Qi* up the spinal cord (i.e., Thrusting Vessel) to the brain in order to nourish the brain cells and energize their functioning to a higher level. Consequently, the spirit can be raised. This is the path of enlightenment or Buddhahood as practiced in Chinese monasteries.

The final stage of Still Soft *Qigong* training is to blend your *Qi* with that of nature, and return your thinking to the natural way. In other words, the unification of Heaven and humanity.

All of the above training is not easy. Often more than one lifetime of pondering and practice can be expected. You should understand that the final goal of Chinese martial arts training is looking for the meaning of life. In order to reach this goal, you must find the origin of life, *Wuji* (no extremity). From *Yin* and *Yang* balance and harmonious interaction, you can lead yourself toward your own spiritual center, and finally reach the center of *Yin* and *Yang*, or *Wuji* (Figure 4-14).

B. Regulating the Qi for Moving Soft Qigong

The goal of Moving Soft *Qigong* is to loosen up the joints, muscles, and tendons. From repeating the soft movements, you can also strengthen the ligaments and tendons in the joint areas for the requirements of Soft *Jin* manifestation. In order to maintain the softness of the physical body, the breathing is soft and relaxed and the mind leads the *Qi* to the joints.

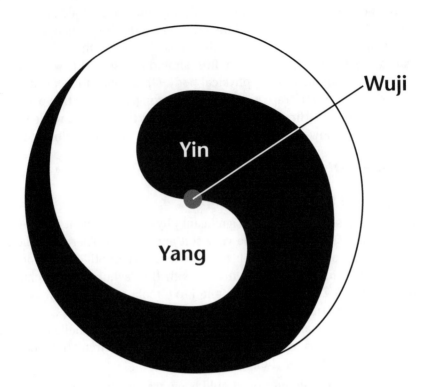

Figure 4–14. Yin and Yang Balance to Reach Wuji (No Extremity)

The Lower *Dan Tian Qi* is commonly used for Moving Soft *Qigong*. This means that Small and Grand Circulation training becomes critical in higher levels of Moving Soft *Qigong* training. *Taijiquan* and *Liu He Ba Fa* are both well known slow Moving Soft *Qigong*, while White Crane, Snake, and Dragon are well known faster Moving Soft *Qigong*.

5. Regulating the Spirit

Neutralization of the mental emotional mind (not becoming too excited or depressed) is the end result of regulating the spirit.

The first step in regulating the spirit is to understand the mutual relationships of human beings. From this understanding, morality is built up. In the first chapter we discussed some of the morality related to the martial arts. You should understand that the higher your morality is, the higher your *Qigong* practice can reach. Morality is the internal, invisible force driving you to a higher motivation for doing things. From this training, your spirit can then be raised.

When you have a high standard of morality, you will not have guilty feelings internally, and you need no thick mask on your face externally. You will then find that you have created a peaceful and calm feeling in your life.

For many martial artists of the past who trained in monasteries, the final goal of training was enlightenment. In order to reach this goal, the emotional mind was gradually neutralized toward the *Wuji* state. Then, nature and the human being can combine into one. This is called "the unification of Heaven and humanity" (*Tian Ren He Yi*, 天人合一). Next, we will discuss the goals of spiritual training in Hard and Soft *Qigong*.

HARD QIGONG — YANG

A. Regulating the Spirit for Still Hard Qigong

In Still Hard *Qigong*, in order to build up the tendons and ligaments to a stronger and more durable level, you first must conquer your laziness. The reason for this is that it is not an easy task to keep yourself on the correct training path. Often, most people are conquered by the laziness of their emotional mind.

Therefore, in order to reach your goal, you must build up a strong will, perseverance, patience, and endurance. Therefore, spiritually in Still Hard *Qigong*, you conduct a process of self-conquest. From this training, your spirit can be raised, and life's lessons can be understood more profoundly.

B. Regulating the Spirit for Moving Hard Qigong

In Moving Hard *Qigong*, you also look for methods of self-understanding and conquest. In addition, since you are moving for *Jin* manifestation, spiritually you must build up a **sense of enemy**. From the sense of enemy, the fighting spirit can be raised. From this high spiritual vantage, you can often convince your opponent to stop the fight. Remember, the best fight is no fight.

SOFT QIGONG — YIN

A. Regulating the Spirit for Still Soft Qigong and Moving Soft Qigong

The spiritual goal of both Still Soft *Qigong* and Moving Soft *Qigong* is to build a more peaceful and enlightened mind, which can lead to a deeper level of spiritual understanding. One of the *Taiji* songs says:

無形無象，全身透空。
忘物自然，西山懸磬。
虎吼猿鳴，泉清水靜。
翻江鬧海，盡性立命。

No shape, no shadow.

Entire body transparent and empty.

Forget your surroundings and be natural.

Like a stone chime suspended from the Western Mountain.

Tigers roaring, monkeys screeching.

Clear fountain, peaceful water.

Turbulent river, stormy ocean.

With your whole being, develop your life.

Ponder this song to discover the real meaning of Chinese martial arts.

4-3. Theory of White Crane Qigong

Since White Crane *Qigong* is a Martial Arts *Qigong*, it will naturally follow the same training procedures and theories discussed in the last section. In this section, we will summarize the points which most concern White Crane *Qigong*.

As explained in section 4-1, White Crane martial arts generally can be divided into the *Yang* side and the *Yin* side. The *Yang* side is related to the physical manifestations of the style. This again includes the *Yang* side, which is the actual movements of the forms, and the *Yin* side which involves the hidden applications of the forms. The *Yin* side of White Crane training is the *Qigong* practice related to *Qi* cultivation and circulation.

On the *Yin* side White Crane *Qigong* training, division can again be made into *Yang* side physical actions and *Yin* side stillness. On the *Yang* side physical actions are again divided into Hard *Qigong* and Soft *Qigong*. **Hard *Qigong* training is used to support the manifestation of Hard *Jin*, while Soft Qigong is used to support the manifestation of Soft *Jin*.**

HARD QIGONG (*Ying Qigong*, 硬氣功)

A. White Crane Theory for Still Hard Qigong

As mentioned earlier, Still Hard *Qigong* emphasizes building the endurance and strength of the muscles/tendons and ligaments rather than increasing their size. The quality of the muscles and tendons is emphasized instead of quantity.

In the beginning, local *Qi* is used to support the training. The training can be very simple, such as holding the push up position with the arms bent. From this training, the ligaments, tendons, and muscles will become more dense and durable. Naturally, the strength of the torso is also enhanced.

Later, after a practitioner has learned the Small and Grand Circulations, he will lead his *Qi* from the Lower *Dan Tian* to the local area, and then hold this position. Typical areas and joints for Still Hard *Qigong* training are the torso, fingers, wrists, elbows, and knees.

B. White Crane Theory for Moving Hard Qigong

In Moving Hard *Qigong*, first you place your attention on the local areas, such as the fingers, wrists, forearms or torso, and at the same time tense up the local tendons and muscles in coordination with the movements. This is a typical example of external elixir Martial Arts *Qigong* training. In this training, local *Qi* is used to support the tensed movements of the body. During this training, when you exhale the muscles and tendons will be tensed up, and when you inhale the muscles and tendons are relaxed and loose. Typically, when the body is expanding, such as when the arms are opened, you exhale, and when the body withdraws, you inhale.

Through repetition of this kind of practice, the muscles and tendons are slowly built up to a stronger and more durable level. This is no different from weight training. As mentioned earlier, this kind of Hard *Qigong* can build up the strength of the physical body in a short time. However, it can also over-stimulate the body, making it too *Yang*.

After you have learned how to build up the *Qi* in the Lower *Dan Tian* and know how to use the mind to lead the *Qi* from the Lower *Dan Tian* to circulate in your Conception and Governing Vessels for Small Circulation, then you should learn the Grand Circulation, which leads the *Qi* from the Lower *Dan Tian* to any part of the body. For a martial artist, the arms and legs are the two most important places. When you reach this level, you will again return to Moving Hard

Qigong. However, you will learn to **use the Lower *Dan Tian Qi*, rather than Local *Qi*, to energize the muscles and tendons**. In order to make this happen, you must be relaxed while your mind leads the *Qi* to the local area. Once the *Qi* has reached the area, you tense up the moving muscles and tendons to manifest the physical power to its maximum. A typical martial style which heavily follows this training is Tiger Claw style.

SOFT QIGONG (*Ruan Qigong,* 軟氣功)

A. White Crane Theory for Still Soft Qigong

The first step for training Still Soft *Qigong* in White Crane is learning to relax. You may simply lie down on your back or sit comfortably on a couch. Then, inhale deeply to the Lower *Dan Tian* and exhale while relaxing your entire body through the joints. This is called "self-relaxation hypnosis." From this training, you will be able to feel or even sense the *Qi* in your body. This practice is especially important right after Hard *Qigong* training.

You should then learn Small Circulation, which teaches you how to build up the *Qi* in the Lower *Dan Tian* to an abundant level, and also learn how to lead the *Qi* from the Lower *Dan Tian* to the limbs for Grand Circulation. In order to reach this goal, first both normal and Reverse Abdominal Breathing should be practiced. Then Embryo Breathing should be trained.

Next, you will learn the Four Gates Breathing (i.e., *Laogong* and *Yongquan* cavities) and also skin/marrow breathing. In addition, you must become familiar with Grand Circulation, which teaches you how to lead the *Qi* to the limbs for *Jin* manifestation.

Since Still Soft *Qigong* is such a big subject, it is impossible to include anything but its broadest outlines in this book. In the future YMAA will publish a comprehensive volume detailing this training.

B. White Crane Theory for Moving Soft Qigong

In the beginning of White Crane Moving Soft *Qigong* practice, you will focus your mind on keeping the muscles and tendons in the most relaxed and loose state. From this relaxed state, the joints are then moved. Through this movement, the ligaments and tendons are exercised. Keeping the muscles and tendons relaxed in order to exercise the ligaments is the major goal of the practice.

After a period of practice, when you can move your joints in a soft and relaxed manner, place your mind on the local joint areas to feel the *Qi* build up, and use the **local *Qi*** to support the movements. In order to keep the body in the most relaxed state, the movements are normally slow and they generally originate from the legs to be directed by the waist. In order to perform the movements softly, the spine and chest are usually very relaxed. From this kind of relaxed movement, joint injury caused from some forms of Moving Hard *Qigong* can be repaired.

After you have completed training the Small and Grand Circulations, you will learn how to lead the *Qi* to the local area in Moving Soft *Qigong* practice. This kind of *Qigong* is commonly used by internal or Soft Styles such as *Taijiquan*. From past experience, this kind of Moving Soft *Qigong* can not only repair physical damage and smooth the internal *Qi* circulation, but it can also bring the practitioner great health benefits.

SOUNDS

In White Crane *Qigong*, sounds are often used. The most common sounds are *Ha* (哈), *Hen* (哏), *He* (呵), *Sa* (煞), *Hei* (嘿), and *Hu* (呼). Naturally, there are more sounds which have been used in different White Crane Styles. Because the sounds are very important and closely related to the Crane *Qigong* and Emitting *Jin* (*Fa Jin*), one of the Crane styles is called "Shouting Crane," and places heavy emphasis on sound training (as explained in Chapter 1).

Ha is a well known *Yang* sound. When you are happy or excited, your internal organs are excited (especially the heart) and this will put the body into a too-*Yang* condition. This too-*Yang* condition is harmful to your health. Therefore, we make a *Ha* sound to laugh and release the excess energy through the skin. Thus, when you laugh, your exhalation is longer than your inhalation, and you sweat and feel hot. This means that the Guardian *Qi* is expanding. This is a natural method of regulating excess *Qi* excitement in the body. It does not matter which race or nationality a person is, the *Ha* sound is a common language for expelling excess energy from the body. Because of this, **Ha has been used in Chinese martial arts to raise the spirit of fighting. Moreover, with Ha, the Qi can energize the physical body to a much higher level of power manifestation**. Normally, to manifest attacking Jin, you first inhale deeply, and then manifest the *Jin* with the sound of *Ha*. With a short exhalation, you can condense the power into a short, powerful pulse. This was considered the secret for Emitting *Jin* for a long period of time in Chinese martial arts society.

Hen is a *Yin* sound. When you are crying and sad, you will make the sound of *Hen* either when you inhale or exhale. In this case, your inhalation is longer than your exhalation. If you make the sound of *Hen* while inhaling, you lead the *Qi* inward, the Guardian *Qi* shrinks, and you will feel chilly. That means you are storing the *Qi* in the body to a higher level. However, if you make the *Hen* sound while you are exhaling for crying or sighing, then in one way you lead the *Qi* inward and the other way release stagnated *Qi* from inside your body. Therefore, in Chinese martial arts, if you inhale with the sound of *Hen*, then you are storing the *Qi* for *Jin* manifestation. However, if you exhale with the sound of *Hen*, you are manifesting your *Jin* but are holding some of the power back to prevent yourself from becoming too *Yang*, which might be used against you by your opponent.

The *He* sound, like *Ha*, is commonly used for attacking, but the power manifested is more round instead of the straight power generated by *Ha*. In Chinese *Qigong* and medical societies, *He* is known for regulating the heart. For example, it is very bad for your heart to remain in a very excited state. This excited state may be caused by exercise, excitement, fear, or nervousness. *He* can calm down the heart's excitement and regulate the *Qi* circulation more smoothly. *He* is also used in martial arts for regulating the heart's condition during a fight.

Sa is the sound of killing; it is violent, cruel, and cold blooded. This sound can often raise the spirit of killing and make an opponent scared. When power is manifested with the sound of *Sa*, it is sharp and penetrating and the spirit is high. *Sa* is considered unfriendly and evil, only to be used when necessary.

Hei is used in martial arts to regulate the lungs. This sound is used both during inhalation and exhalation. *Hei* is used heavily in Crane styles. *Hei* is a sound which can clear the lungs and increase the intake of air. For martial purposes, the short sound of *Hei* is used to generate power in the arms or body.

Finally, *Hu* is used to relax the body and the lungs after a heavy fight or exercises. *Hu* is known to regulate the spleen in Chinese *Qigong* and medical society.

Other than the above sounds, there are many other sounds used by different styles. Naturally, each sound has different, specific purposes.

4-4. Summary

From the above discussion, you can see that White Crane style is a Soft-Hard Style, and includes both the hard side and the soft side of *Qigong* practice. As explained earlier, normally the hard side emphasizes the strength of the physical body, while the soft side is used to loosen the body and strengthen the *Qi*. From the martial arts perspective, if you are a good martial artist, you should be an expert in both Hard and Soft *Jin*. Only then can you position your fighting strategy and techniques in the most effective and efficient way.

From the point of view of health, you must have a healthy strong physical body (*Yang*) as well as abundant and smooth *Qi* circulation in the body (*Yin*). Only by balancing this *Yin* and *Yang* can you maintain the healthy condition of your entire self. Again, White Crane *Qigong* covers both the *Yang* and *Yin* sides of this balance. Be aware that too much *Yang* training is not good for your health, as is an over-abundance *Qi* combined with a weak physical body.

Chapter 5

Crane Hard Qigong

(Crane Strength Gong)

鶴壯功

5-1. Introduction

In the last chapter, we discussed the **Dao** of martial arts *Qigong*. This *Dao* is a universal paradigm describing the natural ways we manifest and demonstrate our *Qi* (internal energy) into forms of strength and power. Therefore, no matter how a style of martial arts *Qigong* developed, it must follow this natural theory of *Dao*. It is from this *Dao* (i.e., root), that the many martial arts *Qigong* patterns or methods (i.e., branches) were derived.

Since there are so many different Chinese martial arts styles, and each of them has its own special characteristics of manifesting *Jin,* they all have different patterns of *Qigong* training. For example, by imitating the strength of the tiger, Tiger Claw styles will focus on how to lead the *Qi* to the arms and thereby build up the muscles in the arms, energizing them to manifest power. In order to anchor the power, the rooting must be firm and the waist and spine must be strong. Therefore, a firm root, strong waist and spine, and powerful arms have become the characteristics of Tiger Claw *Qigong*.

Often in the past, when you learned martial arts from a master, there was no set schedule which directed you systematically from the shallows to the depths of the art. A master would teach you whenever he or she pleased. It is the same for White Crane *Qigong*. My master would teach us only one movement and would leave us alone for a month or so. Only some days, if he desired, he would teach another form. In order to more easily preserve the secrets of White Crane, I compiled the White Crane *Qin Na* (*Chin Na*) together with other techniques that I learned from my Long Fist (*Changquan*) teacher. Here, I will also compile the *Qigong* from my White Crane master into a more organized whole. Naturally, after more than thirty years of experience, I have also contributed some of my personal understanding and modifications.

We know that Martial Arts *Qigong* can be categorized into Hard *Qigong* and Soft *Qigong*, and further divided into still and moving. In this chapter we will introduce the Hard *Qigong* training in the Crane style. The Soft *Qigong* training of the White Crane style will be introduced in the next chapter. Since the basic training foundation of all Chinese styles are the same, you can expect many of the training methods to be used in many other martial styles.

In this chapter, we will first introduce the Still Hard *Qigong*. Then, we will discuss the training methods of Moving Hard *Qigong* in section 5-3. You should always remember that **Hard**

Qigong training is the foundation of Hard *Jin*. Without this training, the manifestation of Hard *Jin* will be shallow and the power will be weak.

As explained before, Hard *Qigong* can be very harmful, since much of it was created for martial purposes. Some of the Hard *Qigong* training (*Ying Qigong*, 硬氣功) such as Iron Sand Palm (*Tie Sha Zhang*, 鐵砂掌), Iron Head Gong (*Tie Tou Gong*, 鐵頭功), Spear Against the Throat (*Jin Qiang Shuo Hou*, 金槍鎖喉), and Break the Cement Block on the Chest (*Xiong Shang Shui Shi*, 胸上碎石), etc., which are considered harmful training methods, will not be discussed in this book. It is strongly recommended that you do not practice these harmful *Qigong* forms, since they are no longer necessary in today's society.

5-2. Stationary Hard Qigong (*Ding Gong*, 定功)

There are many Still Hard *Qigong* training methods which exist in Chinese martial arts society. It is impossible to introduce all of them in such a small section. The purpose of this introduction is to offer you a guideline and some examples. If you understand the theory and the purpose of the training, you will be able to adapt the similar training techniques into your style without injuring yourself.

1. Crane Horse Stance (*He Ma Bu*, 鶴馬步)

The purposes of Crane Horse Stance are first to build up the endurance and strength of the legs, especially in the joint areas such as the ankles, knees, and hips. Second, from Crane Horse Stance training, you learn how to line up your torso correctly, and enhance the strength of your lower back. The third purpose is to build up a firm root, which is considered a crucial factor in martial arts training. With a firm root, the spirit can be raised to a higher level.

In fact, almost all of the fundamental stances can be used to train endurance in the ankles, knees, and hip joints. However, if you have trained well in any one of them, you have already grasped the trick of the others.

In Crane Horse Stance training, you start by squatting down, with the angle formed by your thigh and calf at about 90 degrees. To prevent injury, at the beginning you should line up your knees and your toes (Figure 5-1). This will prevent injury caused by the mis-alignment of the knees. Only after you can stand for five minutes easily should you start the second phase of the training.

In the second phase of the Crane Horse Stance training, you push both your knees inward (Figure 5-2). Naturally, the knees will not line up with the feet, and as a consequence the ligaments on both the inner and outer sides of the knees will be strained. Beginning with only a minute or so, gradually increase the time you stand like this to five minutes. Normally, this goal can be reached after about six months of training. The purpose is to train the tendons and ligaments in the knee area. If you speed up the training, you may cause serious knee injury.

Once you can stand in this second phase of the Crane Horse Stance correctly for five minutes, you should continue your training by standing on bricks; the brick should be lying down with the spine upright (Figure 5-3). In this training, you should coordinate your breathing and mind. First inhale deeply, and then exhale while using your mind to lead the *Qi* downward until it reaches underneath the bricks. This will become rooting training as you progress. Occasionally, you may inhale and lead the *Qi* to the deep places of the joints, such as the ankles, knees, or hips, and then exhale and lead the *Qi* outward in these same areas. This kind of practice is called "Joint Breathing" (*Guan Jie Hu Xi*, 關節呼吸). This kind of training is commonly used to strengthen the

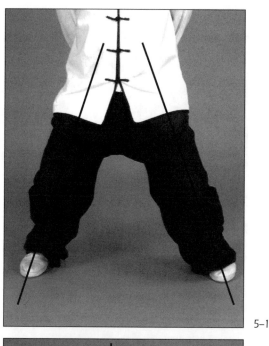
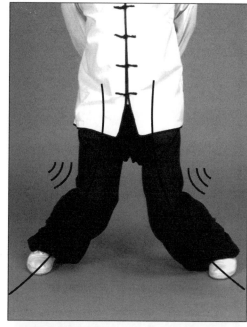

5–1   5–2

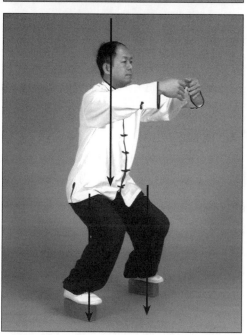
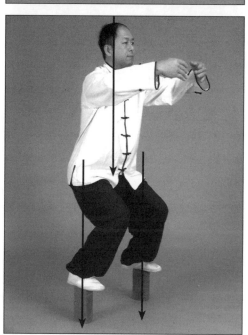

5–3   5–4

joint areas, or can be used to heal joint injuries with the mind and breathing. Often, when it is used for healing, the joints are relaxed instead of being tensed.

If you can stand on the spines of the bricks and feel the root underneath them, then stand on the sides of the bricks while they are standing upward (Figure 5-4). Again, repeat the entire training process for rooting. Normally, this will take one to two years of training. Then, place another brick on top of the first brick and repeat the same training process (Figure 5-5). Finally, stand on top of three bricks for five minutes. **This is an extremely difficult training routine at first, and there is an element of danger to it no matter what your level. When you train, you should always be very cautious.** If you can reach this goal, you have built up a firm center and root like the ancient Chinese martial artists were able to reach. Naturally, the entire training process can take five to ten years, depending on your *Qigong* foundation.

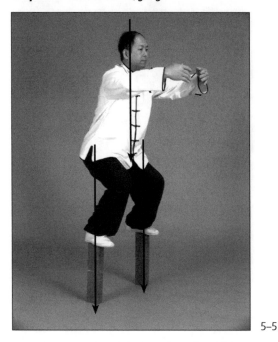

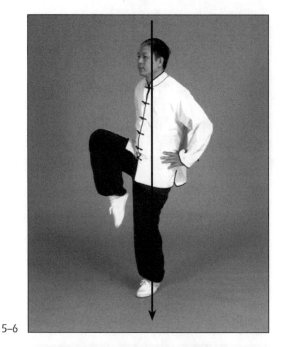

5–5   5–6

2. White Crane Stands with Single Leg

(*Bai He Du Li Shi,* 白鶴獨立勢)

White Crane stands with single leg is important for training stability and rooting in the Crane style. From this, you can build up the sensitivity of the soles of your feet. This training also develops the endurance of your legs.

At the beginning, place your hands beside your waist while standing on a single leg (Figure 5-6). Start at one minute on each leg. After you have practiced for a long time and feel that it is too easy for you, then start for two minutes on each leg, building up to five minutes per leg. In order to prevent injury, the standing leg should be bent slightly. Otherwise, the long period with locked knees can make the *Qi* and blood circulation stagnant.

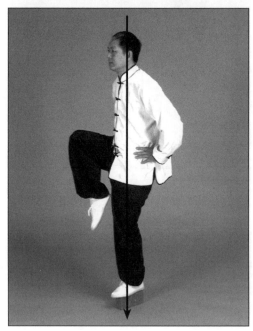

5–7

Once you can stand easily for five minutes on each leg, lay a brick on its narrow side and stand on its spine (Figure 5-7). If this is too easy, lay the brick on its small side and stand on its crown. (Figure 5-8). The final point is standing on two or three bricks (Figure 5-9).

Standing on a single leg training has been popularly trained in both external and internal styles. Popular postures are Child Worships the Buddha Posture (*Tong Zi Bai Fo Shi,* 童子拜佛勢) (Figure 5-10) and White Crane Soaring Posture (*Bai He Ao Siang Shih,* 白鶴翱翔勢) (Figure 5-11).

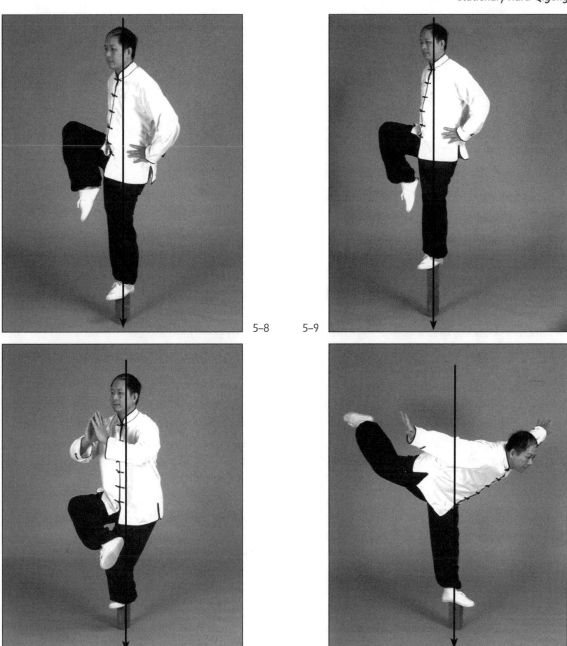

5–8 5–9

5–10 5–11

In this kind of training, the coordination of the mental center and the physical center is very important. This training can not only build up stability and a firm root, it can also help you establish a strong upright spirit, which is an essential factor for raising the spirit. At the beginning, train with your eyes open. From the eye contact with your environment, you can maintain your balance relatively easily. Later, you should train to stand with your eyes closed, and use your other senses to feel your center and root. This will lead you to a very deep level of stability in your training.

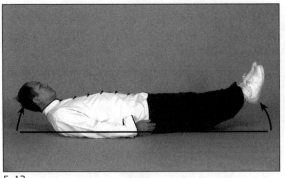

5-12

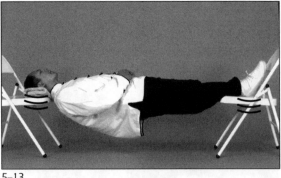

5-13

3. Iron Board Bridge Gong (*Tie Ban Qiao Gong*, 鐵板橋功)

Iron Board Bridge *Gong* is well known in Chinese martial arts society, and almost every traditional style trains it. The main purpose of the training is to build up a stronger and more durable torso. The torso is considered one of the two major bows in the body, and it can manifest *Jin* to a significant degree all by itself. Another bow is the chest. The training here is to build a strong bow for *Jin* manifestation.

In this training, at the beginning, simply lie down with your face looking upward and lift your head and heels a couple of inches off the ground (Figure 5-12). The entire leg should be straight. The distance from your head to the ground and also from the heels to the ground should not be too high. If they are too high, pressure will build up in the lower spine and generate injury. A proper height for the lifting of the head and the heels can keep the rear side of the torso stretched and the front side properly tensed.

You should start at only one minute. After you have trained for some time, if you feel comfortable, increase to two minutes and so on until you can hold it for five minutes. If you can reach this goal, you have built up the foundation for Iron Board Bridge training.

Next, place your head and heels on the edge of two chairs with nothing under the torso (Figure 5-13). Again, start with one minute and progress until you can stay for five minutes. Then, start to place some light weights on your abdominal area. Start with one pound and gradually increase to thirty pounds. If you can reach this final goal, then you have built up a very strong bow in your torso. Naturally, you have also established a firm foundation for Iron Shirt Training of the torso.

When you train, you should take your time. Do not hold your breath while training. Speedy training can only harm you. You should remember that **your body must be conditioned slowly and gradually**. If you have too much ego, once you have injured yourself, it will take a long time to heal, and once you have injured yourself once, you will never be quite the same. The results of mis-training can be devastating.

4. Crane Claw Push Up Gong (*He Zhua Ting Shen Gong*, 鶴爪挺身功)

Crane Claw Push Up *Gong* is used to build up the strength and endurance of your fingers and palms. To White Crane and Eagle Claw styles, the strength of the fingers is extremely important since grabbing is one of the main fighting techniques.

At the beginning of this training, hold yourself in a push-up position with your arms bent and the fingers spread (Figure 5-14). Do not use the finger tips to push up. If you do, you will not be training the tendons and ligaments in the fingers. Moreover, according to Chinese medicine, the six primary *Qi* channels at the end of the finger tips will be affected, and the *Qi* circulation from the fingers to the outside of your body will be diminished. That means that the *Qi* status of the

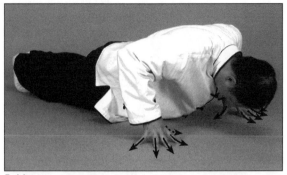

5-14

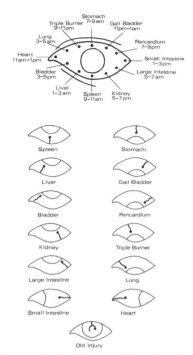

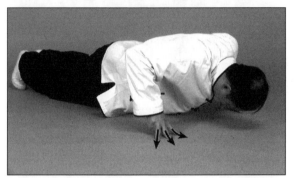

5-16

Figure 5-15. Eye Diagnosis of Injuries in the
Primary Qi Channels

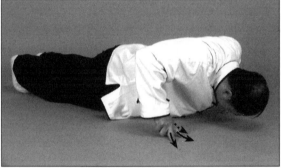

5-17

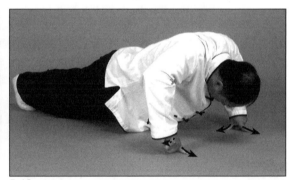

5-18

six internal organs will also be affected.
Furthermore, Chinese medicine also postulates that the *Qi* circuits from the fingers tips are connected to the eyes (Figure 5-15). Too much stimulation on the finger tips can therefore damage your eyes.

You should start with thirty seconds. After practicing for some time, you may increase the time in five second increments weekly. If you can hold the correct posture

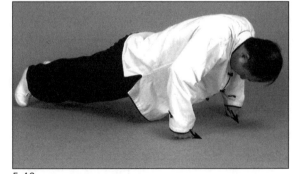

5-19

for five minutes, you have built up very strong finger power and endurance. Naturally, this training can also strengthen the torso from the push-up position.

If you can do this for five minutes, then you should start to lift the pinkie from the pushing (Figure 5-16), and later, also the ring finger (Figure 5-17), middle finger (Figure 5-18), and finally the index finger (Figure 5-19). That means you will be pushing up with only the thumbs.

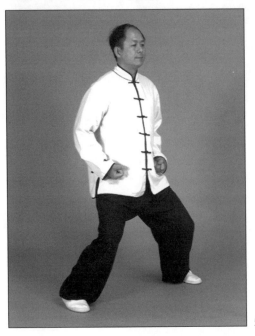 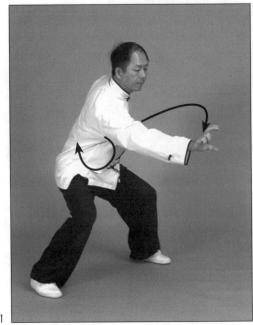

5-20   5-21

5-3. Moving Hard Qigong (*Dong Gong,* 動功)

In this section, I would like to introduce four simple Moving Hard *Qigong* exercises as examples. From these four examples, you can understand how the training is done. Then, I will introduce a training set for Moving Hard *Qigong*. Every piece of this set can also be practiced independently.

1. Crane Claw Gong (*He Zhua Gong,* 鶴爪功)

The purpose of Crane Claw Gong is to train the grabbing power of the fingers. In this training, stand in Horse Stance while placing both of your hands beside your waist (Figure 5-20). Next, twist your body to the left and inhale, while extending your right fist out and toward the left with the palm facing upward. Then, twist your body to the right and exhale while using the twisting power to circle your right arm and form your right hand into a Crane Craw, palm facing forward (Figure 5-21). Close the fingers knuckle by knuckle until the hand becomes a fist again and return it back to your waist with the palm facing upward, as in the beginning posture. Repeat the same process with your left hand.

When you practice this exercise, inhale deeply and withdraw your lower abdomen, then exhale strongly with the lower abdomen pushing out while placing your mind on the grabbing. You should imagine that you are crushing an object with your three fingers' grabbing power. You can also practice different angles of grabbing. For example, grabbing with the palm facing inward (Figure 5-22), or sideways (Figure 5-23).

If you have completed the Small Circulation and Grand Circulation training, then you may use your mind to lead the *Qi* to the fingers first (*Nei Dan*), and then grab with the fingers intensely. If you do not know Small and Grand Circulation, you should keep training using local *Qi* (*Wai Dan*). The use of *Nei Dan Qi* circulation techniques can do great harm if you have not been trained by a qualified master.

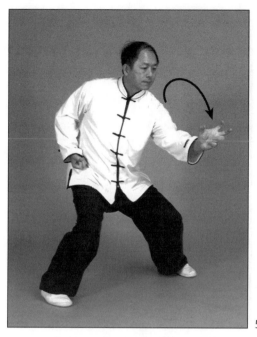
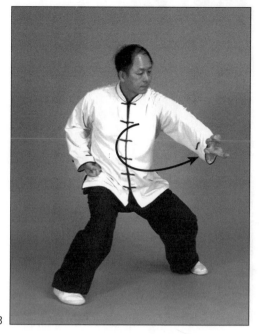

5-22   5-23

2. Turning the Wrist Gong (*Zhuan Wan Gong*, 轉腕功)

Turning the Wrist *Gong* can be used to strengthen the tendons in the wrist area. If you do not have wrist injuries or arthritis, you may practice this exercise the hard way. As explained earlier, Hard *Qigong* can build up physical strength. However, if you have already had problems and you practice Hard *Qigong*, the tension generated in the wrist area will compress the joints, which may cause more serious injury. In this case you should use the same movements, but with Soft *Qigong*. That means you simply do the movements without tensing the muscles and tendons. From the repeated relaxed circular movement, blood and *Qi* circulation can be improved and injury and arthritis can be healed. In fact, this is a simple way to treat arthritis in Chinese medicine. If you are interested in knowing more about how *Qigong* can aid in the treatment of arthritis, please refer to the book: ***Arthritis — The Chinese Way of Healing and Prevention*** (formerly *Qigong for Arthritis*), by YMAA.

In the Hard *Qigong* practice of this technique, first hold your right hand in a fist, bending it down and circling to the left, upward, and finally to the right (Figure 5-24). As you do this, hold the fists tightly and try to make the circle the wrists trace as large as possible. Start with only ten repetitions, then reverse the circling direction for another ten repetitions. After you have practiced for a while, you should increase to fifteen repetitions, and then to twenty. Remember, **if you over-practice this exercise, you may cause joint injuries which can trigger arthritis later in life.** Therefore, you should pay attention to the condition of your wrist while you are training.

After you have trained fist wrist turning for a period of time, you should open your palms and repeat the same exercises (Figure 5-25). When you open the palms for this training, the conditioning can more effectively reach the deeper tendons.

3. Contain in the Chest and Stretch the Back Gong (*Han Xiong Ba Bei Gong*, 含胸拔背功)

The main purpose of this training is first to stretch the upper torso and later to build up a stronger physical upper body, either for Hard *Jin* manifestation or for Iron Shirt training. Again, too much of this training can be harmful. You should be cautious and patient in your training. This training includes two parts. The first part is "Thrusting the Chest Forward" and the second part is "Arcing the Back." When you practice, you may combine the two parts into one. That means thrusting your chest first, followed by arcing the back, and so on.

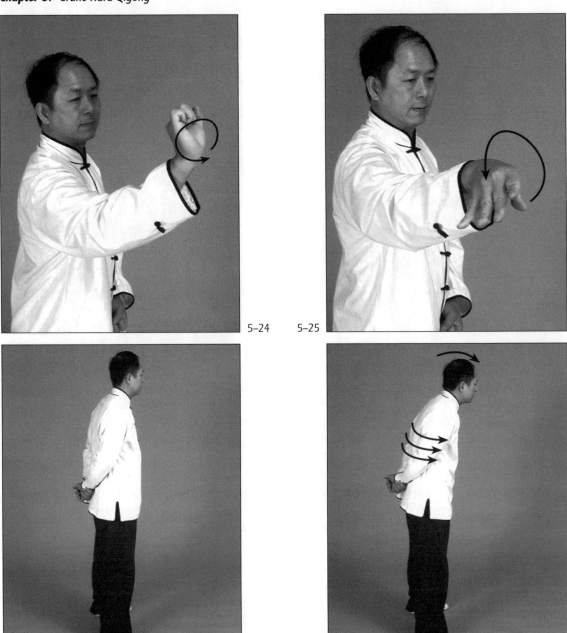

5–24   5–25

5–26   5–27

A. Thrusting the Chest Forward

In this training, first use one of your hands to hold the wrist of the other behind your back (Figure 5-26). Next, hold your chest inward to relax the upper chest while inhaling deeply (Figure 5-27). Then, thrust your upper chest forward and keep the spine upright while exhaling (Figure 5-28). While you are exhaling, gradually tense your upper body until it reaches its maximum limit. Hold the breath at this position for five seconds, and then hold your chest inward to relax the upper chest again and repeat the entire process. At the beginning, you should practice about ten times and gradually increase to twenty times.

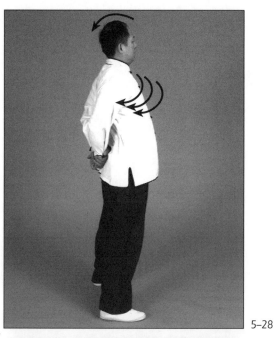

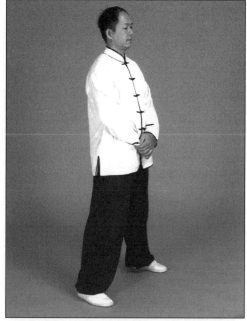

5-28   5-29

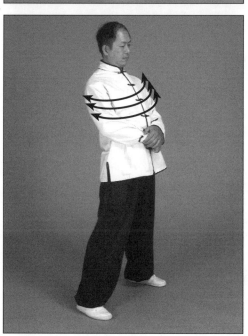

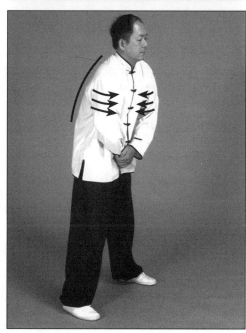

5-30   5-31

B. Arcing the Back

In this training, again use one of your hands to hold the wrist of the other in front of your abdomen area (Figure 5-29). Next, thrust your chest gently forward while inhaling deeply (Figure 5-30). Then, starting from your lower torso, arc backward, tensing upwards and gradually extending to the upper torso, until your entire spine and torso arcs backward (Figure 5-31). While you are doing this, you should also exhale in coordination with the movement. When you reach the maximum extension, you should hold your breath for five seconds. Again, repeat the same training. In the beginning, you should repeat about ten times and gradually increase to twenty times.

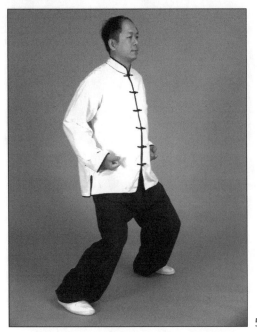
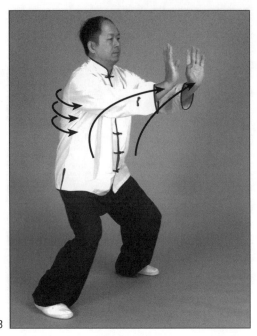

5-32   5-33

4. Iron Arm Gong (*Tie Bi Gong,* 鐵臂功)

There are two major purposes of Iron Arm *Gong* training. The first is to build up more phys-ical strength in the arms, which enables you to manifest Hard *Jin* from the arms more efficiently. The second purpose is to establish a higher, more durable resistance in the arms which allows you to intercept an opponent's attack without pain or injury. The second purpose is considered an important part of Iron Shirt Training.

A. Forward Pushing

First, hold your fists tightly, and place them beside your waist while inhaling deeply (Figure 5-32). Next, exhale and extend your arms forward with the palms facing forward, while drawing your chest in and arcing your back (Figure 5-33). You should keep extend-ing until your arms are slightly bent and all the fingers are pointing upward. Hold your breath for five seconds in this position.

Next, inhale deeply, relax your arms and torso, change your palms into fists, rotate your arms until the palm faces downward (Figure 5-34) and move the fists back to the sides of the waist with the palms facing upward (Figure 5-32). Then, exhale and extend your arms again to repeat the same training process. You should start with ten repetitions only. After you have trained for a period of time, you should gradually increase the number of repetitions.

When you train, due to the tension in the physical body, you may experience a headache. In this case, you should reduce the repetitions. If you have high blood pressure, you should not train this kind of heavy physical exercise.

B. Side Arm Forward Pushing

In this training, again inhale deeply while placing your fists beside your waist (Figure 5-35). Next, move your arm to the front of your solar plexus area while turning the fists until the palms are facing downward (Figure 5-36). As you are doing this, you should start to

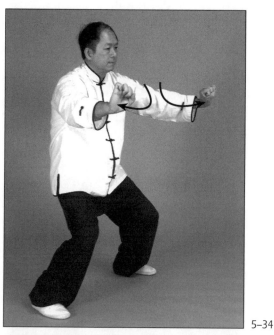

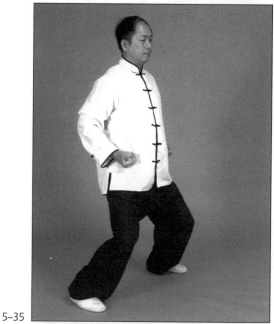

5–34   5–35

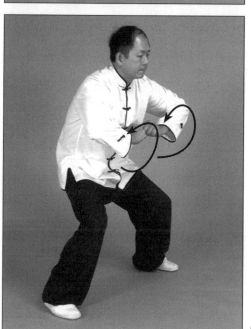

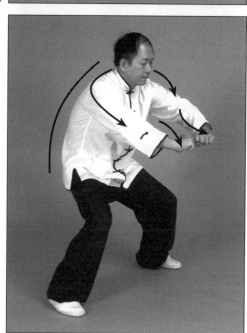

5–36   5–37

exhale. Continue your exhalation while using the sides of your forearm to push forward intensely while arcing your chest and back (Figure 5-37). You should push forward until both of your arms and your chest form a circle. Stay there and hold your breath for five seconds.

Next, relax your fists, arms, and torso while inhaling and turning your palms upward. Continue your inhalation and return your fists to the sides of your waist (Figure 5-35). Repeat the exercises ten times. Later, if you find this too easy, you should gradually increase the number of repetitions.

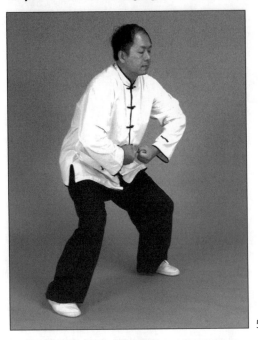
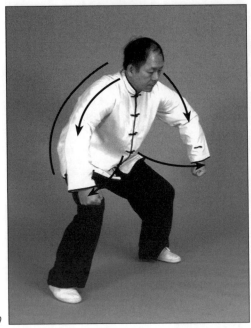

5-38   5-39

C. Sideways Arcing

In this training, first hold your fists right in front of your abdominal area, inhale deeply and tighten your fists and arms (Figure 5-38). Next, exhale and expand your arms sideways while arcing your chest and back (Figure 5-39). Stay at this position and hold your breath for five seconds.

Then inhale, relaxing your fists, arms, and torso while moving your arms back to the beginning position (Figure 5-38). Repeat the exercise ten times. Later, if you find this too easy, gradually increase the number of repetitions.

D. Upward Drilling

In this training, first inhale deeply while placing your arm right in front of your lower chest with both arms lined up (Figure 5-40). Next, tighten up your fists and arms, and arc your chest and back while drilling both of your arms forward until both palms face upward (Figure 5-41). You should continue this extension until both arms are slightly bent. Stay in this position and hold your breath for five seconds.

Then inhale, relaxing your fists, arms and torso while moving your arms to the sides with palms facing downward (Figure 5-42). Finally, return your arms back to the beginning position (Figure 5-40). Repeat the exercises ten times. Later, if you find this too easy, gradually increase the number of repetitions.

After you have practiced for some time, repeat the same process with the palms opened. Generally speaking, practice with the fists is easier than practice with the palms opened.

In the above training, and often in some of the moving training, weights are sometimes held in the hands. This is to train a practitioner's strength and weapons handling capability. You should understand that weapons were frequently used in most ancient battles. Strength and power with a weapon was a critical factor for victory and survival. Normally, a battle lasted for many hours. If you did not have the strength and endurance to last until the end of the battle, you would be the first one killed. Therefore, holding some weight in the hands while training Hard *Qigong* was very common.

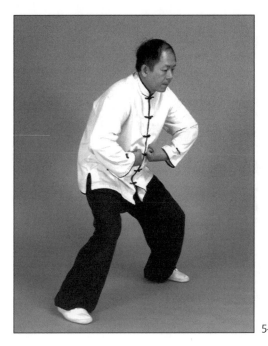

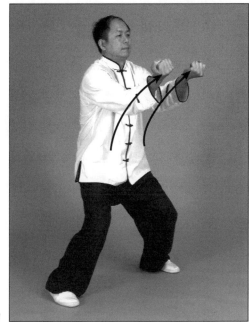

5-40   5-41

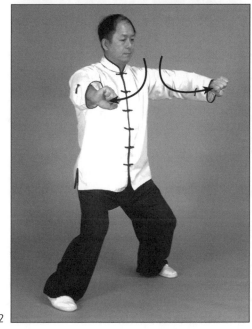

In addition, in order to lead the *Qi* strongly with the mind, and in coordination with the breath, "*Hen*" and "*Ha*" sounds were also commonly used. Whenever you inhale to lead the *Qi* inward, use the "*Hen*" sound, and when you exhale to lead the *Qi* to the skin surface, use the "*Ha*" sound.

From the last few exercises, you may have already figured out that most Hard *Qigong* practices can be used for Iron Shirt training. There are two main components of Iron Shirt training. One is to establish a stronger and more durable physical body, while the other is to build up abundant *Qi* in the Lower *Dan Tian* and lead it to the skin surface. Hard *Qigong* practice is a typical method of achieving the first goal of Iron Shirt training.

5-42

Before we introduce the moving sets for Hard *Qigong*, I would like to remind you again that too much tension can provide your body with too much energy and thereby make it too *Yang*. If you over-train, it can be harmful to you. In addition, if you have high blood pressure, heart problems, arthritis or joint injuries, you should not practice the training introduced in this chapter. Instead, you should practice Soft *Qigong*, which will be introduced in the next chapter.

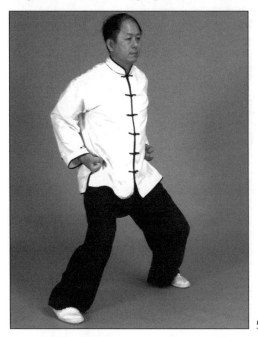

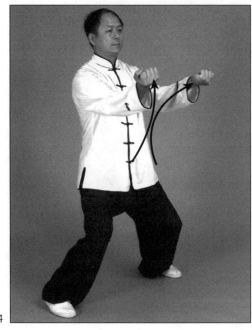

5-43   5-44

MOVING SETS:

Here, I would like to introduce two moving sets, the Fist Set and the Palm Set. In the Fist Set, both hands are held as fists. When the hands are formed as fists, because of the tightness of the wrists, the *Qi* will be trapped in the arms, especially in the forearm areas. From this, strength and endurance in the arms can be built to a higher level.

The second set, the Palm Set, is used to lead the *Qi* to the fingers or even beyond. Often, palms and fingers are used in a fight. The Palm Set can build up a firm physical foundation for this purpose.

When you practice, you should at first start with six repetitions until you feel the training has become easy and comfortable. Then, increase to eight repetitions and then ten. If you can do the entire set with twenty repetitions of each piece, you have built up firm physical strength for the manifestation of Hard *Jin*.

If you like, you may choose only a single piece and practice that piece independently. This will offer you more focus on the practice of a single piece while you have great energy. Of course, you may mix the order in any way you like. Remember, the art is alive and creative. If you find that it is difficult to catch the correct moving patterns, it may be a good idea to get the demonstration tapes from YMAA.

FIST SET:

1. Extend Both Arms Forward (*Shuang Bi Ping Zhang*, 雙臂平展)

In this piece, first place both of your fists beside your waist (Figure 5-43). Next, inhale deeply while holding in your chest, and arc your back backward. Then start to exhale, and at the same time extend both of your arms from the center of your chest outward (Figure 5-44). While you are exhaling, you should gradually tense up your fists, arms, and torso until the arms are extended but slightly bent. The distance between your elbows and chest should be about a palm's width.

Next, start to inhale and turn both of your fists until the palms are facing down, relax your arms and upper torso, and circle both of your fists to the side (Figure 5-45). Finally, return them

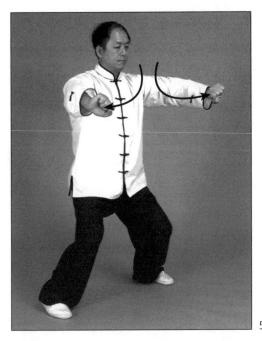

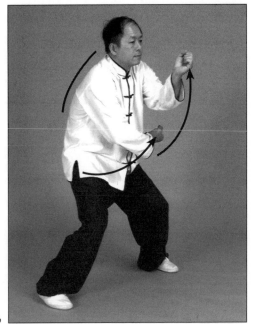

5–45   5–46

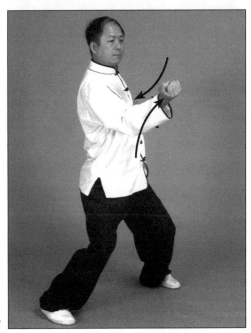

to the sides of your waist again with the palms facing upward (Figure 5-43). Repeat five more times.

The movements of this piece are very similar to those of the Upward Drilling training in the Iron Arm *Gong* introduced earlier. The difference is that, when you are extending both of your arms forward, the fists are also pushing sideways.

5–47

2. Left and Right Bending the Bow (*Zuo You Kai Gong,* 左右開弓)

From the last piece, start to inhale, and arc your spine and chest in, while crossing your forearms in front of your chest with the left arm on the top and the right arm on the bottom (Figure 5-46). Next, exhale and continue to extend your right arm forward while rotating your left arm until the palm is facing down, then pull it back to the left hand side of your upper chest (Figure 5-47), and straighten up your torso.

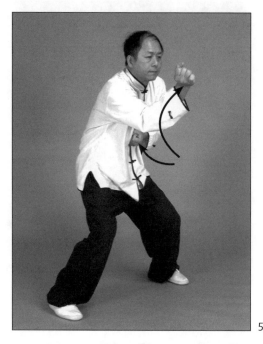
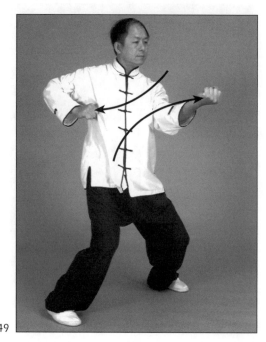

5–48   5–49

Inhale, cross both of your forearms with the right arm on the top and the left arm on the bottom, and rotate both of your fists until the right palm is facing down and the left palm is facing upward (Figure 5-48). Finally, exhale while extending your left arm forward and pulling your right fist back to the side of your left upper chest to complete a cycle of this piece (Figure 5-49). Repeat five more times for both sides.

3. Press Downward and Drill Forward (*Xia Ya Shang Zhuan,* 下壓上鑽)

Continuing from the last piece, inhale deeply while arcing your spine and chest inward, turn your left arm until the palm is facing down, and move your right fist to the side of your right waist (Figure 5-50). Next, exhale, straighten your torso and thrust your chest out while continuing to cover your left arm down and drilling your right fist over your left arm (Figure 5-51). In this position, your left fist should be extended forward while your right fist is under the left elbow.

Change sides by covering your right arm downward and rotating your left fist until the palm is facing upward (Figure 5-52). Finally, exhale and drill your left fist forward while continuing to cover your right arm downward (Figure 5-53). Repeat the entire process five more times.

In this practice, when you are inhaling, you are relaxed and when you are exhaling, you gradually tense up your torso and arms.

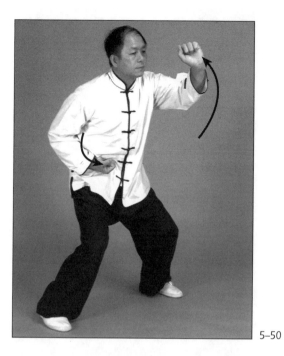

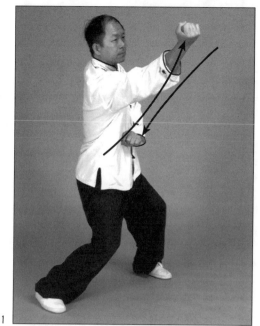

5–50   5–51

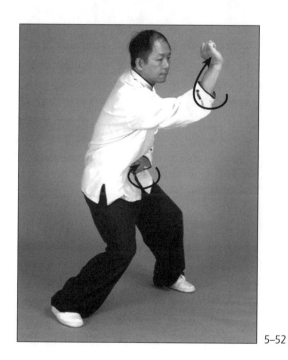

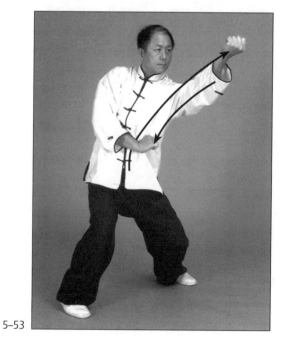

5–52   5–53

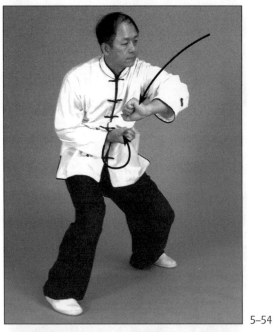

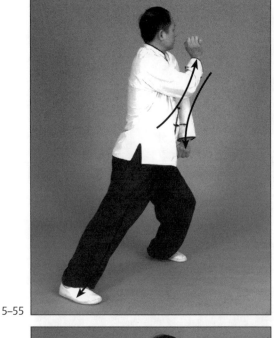

5–54   5–55

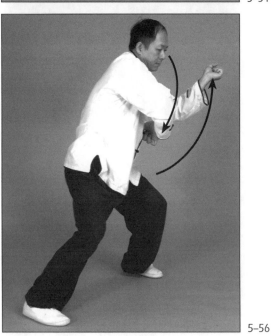

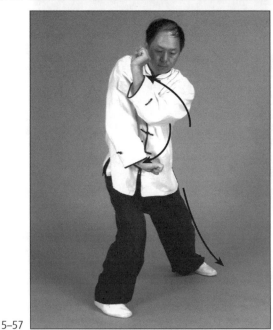

5–56   5–57

4. Left and Right Bump (*Zuo You Lan Kao,* 左右攬靠)

Continuing from the last piece, inhale deeply, arc your torso and chest, and cover your left arm down while rotating your right arm until the fist is facing upward (Figure 5-54). Next, exhale and gradually tense up your torso and arms while pushing both arms to your left with your right leg straightening up (Figure 5-55). Keep both arms slightly bent.

Inhale and rotate your right arm downward while moving your left arm upward (Figure 5-56). Finally, exhale while gradually tensing up your torso and arms and pushing both arms to your right (Figure 5-57). Again, keep both of your arms slightly bent and left leg straight. Repeat the entire process five more times.

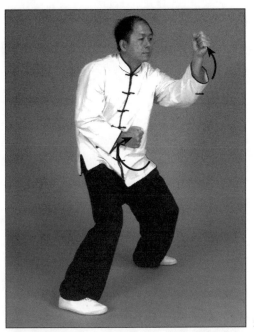

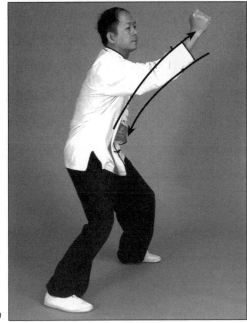

5–58   5–59

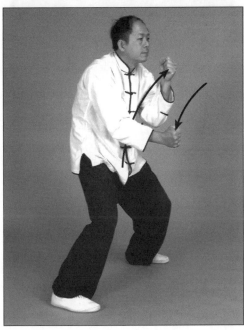

5–60

5. Linking Cannon Fist (*Lian Huan Pao Quan,* 連環砲拳)

After you have completed the last left push, turn your body to face forward, inhale and cover your left arm downward while moving your right fist to the front center of your lower body (Figure 5-58). While you are doing this, you should arc your torso backward and hold in the chest. Next, exhale and continue to cover your left arm downward while pushing your right fist forward (Figure 5-59). At this time you should straighten your torso and thrust your upper chest forward while gradually tensing it along with your arms.

Change sides by covering your right arm down while inhaling and arcing your torso and chest. Finally, continue your right hand's covering while pushing your left fist out (Figure 5-60). Repeat the entire process five more times.

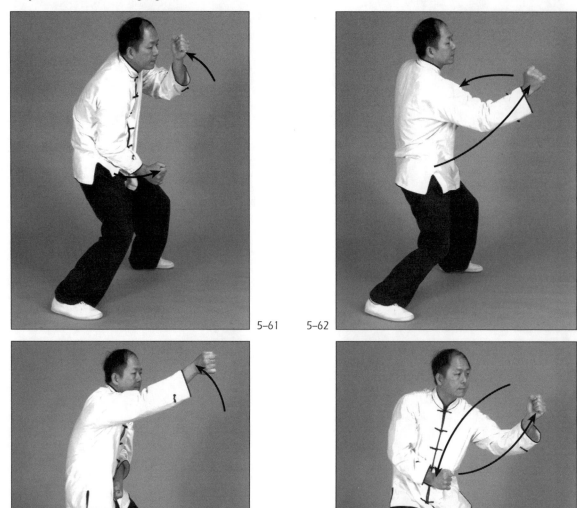

5–61   5–62

5–63   5–64

After you have finished six complete repetitions on both sides, reverse the rotation of the arms for another six times. The transition begins right after you push your left fist forward in the last movement. From there, inhale, rotate your left arm upward, and arc in your torso and chest (Figure 5-61). Next, exhale, pushing your right fist forward and upward while moving your left fist to the stomach area (Figure 5-62). Continue the left fist pushing by moving your right arm up and back to the stomach area while pushing your left fist out (Figures 5-63 and 5-64). Again, repeat the entire process five times.

6. Double Arms Arcing and Embracing (*Shuang Bi Gong Bao,* 雙臂拱抱)

After you finish the left push in the last section, inhale and move your left arm back to the

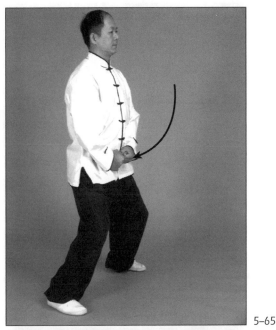

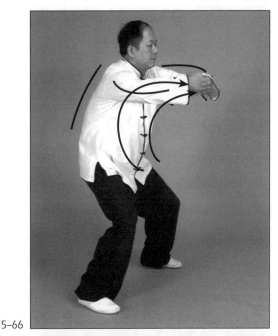

5-65   5-66

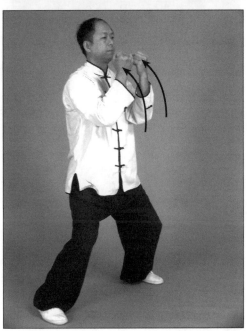

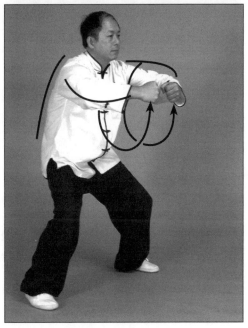

5-67   5-68

abdominal area (Figure 5-65). Next, exhale and circle both of your arms upward and then forward, gradually arcing your back and holding in your chest while tensing up (Figure 5-66). Your arms and back should form a circle and the expanding force should be like a fully inflated beach ball. Finally, inhale, relax your body and straighten up while thrusting your chest out and moving both of your arms to the abdominal area to repeat the movement (Figure 5-65). Repeat five more times.

Next, repeat the same training except this time the circle is reversed. First, inhale and relax your body while straightening up and thrusting your chest out as you move both of your arms to the upper chest area (Figure 5-67). Next, exhale and circle both of your arms downward and then forward while arcing your spine and chest (Figure 5-68). Repeat five more times.

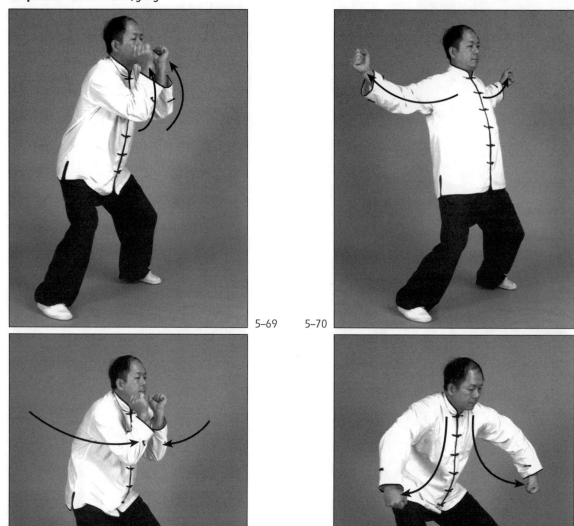

5–69   5–70

5–71   5–72

7. Feudal Lord Pulling the Bow (*Ba Wang La Gong,* 霸王拉弓)

Continuing from the last piece, first inhale and bring both of your arms to the front of your chest, and arc your back (Figure 5-69). Next, start to exhale and expand from the center of the chest outward to the shoulders and finally straighten out both arms as far as possible (Figure 5-70). Inhale again and bring both of your arms back to the chest and repeat five more times.

After you have completed six repetitions pulling, then keep the last expanding movement and inhale deeply. Exhale, arc your back and hold in your chest while squeezing both of your fore-arms inward until in front of your chest (Figure 5-71). Inhale, relax your torso and expand your chest and arms to repeat five more times.

8. Left and Right Arcing the Wings (*Zuo You Gong Chi,* 左右拱翅)

Once you complete the final squeezing movement in the last piece, stay in the same posture

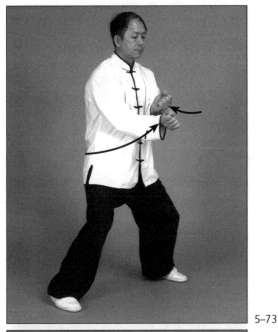

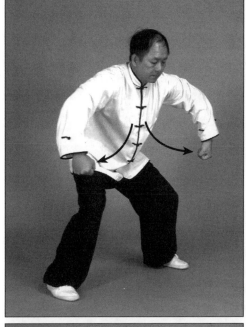

5-73 5-74

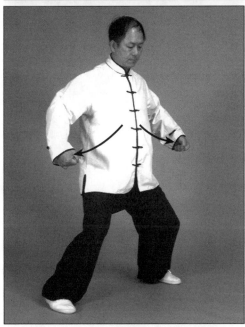

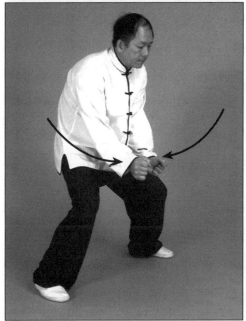

5-75 5-76

and inhale deeply. Next, exhale and circle both of your arms downward and then sideways (Figure 5-72). Both of your arms are arcing outward and your torso is arcing backward.

To repeat the movements, first, inhale, relax your torso, straighten your body and thrust your chest forward while bringing both of your arms to the front of your chest again to repeat five more times (Figures 5-73 and 5-74).

After you have completed six repetitions, inhale and bring both of your hands back to the front of your abdominal area, and then exhale while your entire body is relaxed. Next, inhale deeply, straighten your torso and thrust your chest out while expanding both of your arms to the sides of your body (Figure 5-75). Exhale, arc your back and hold in your chest while pushing both arms inward toward the abdominal area (Figure 5-76). While you are pushing both arms toward each other, imagine that you are using both of your arms to squeeze a ball right in front of your abdomen. Repeat five more times.

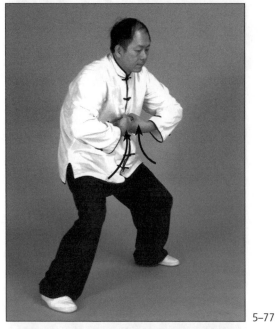
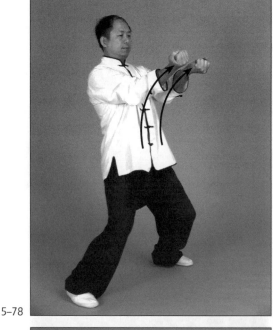

5–77   5–78

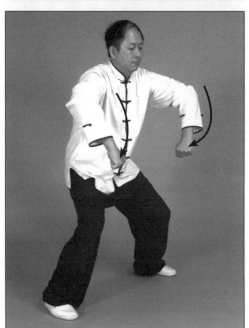
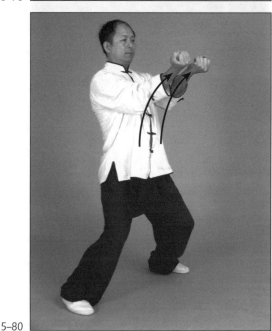

5–79   5–80

9. Up and Down Drilling Fist (*Shang Xia Zhuan Quan,* 上下鑽拳)

Right after you have completed the final squeezing in the last piece, rotate both of your fists inward and then upward while you are inhaling (Figure 5-77). Exhale, straighten your torso upward, and thrust your chest out while drilling both of your fists forward from your upper chest (Figure 5-78). Inhale again, rotate both of your fists downward toward the abdominal area, arc your back, and hold in your chest (Figure 5-79). Finally, exhale again while drilling both of your fists forward (Figure 5-80). Repeat the same practice four more times.

After you have completed the upward drilling, inhale, straighten your torso and thrust out your chest while rotating both of your fists upward and then downward in front of your face

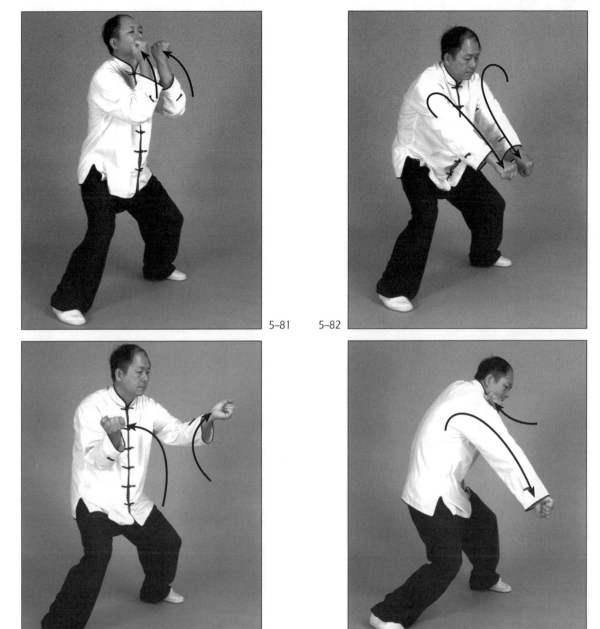

5–81   5–82

5–83   5–84

(Figure 5-81). Exhale, drill both of your fists forward and downward while arcing your back and holding in your chest (Figure 5-82). Repeat five more times.

10. Left and Right Downward Fist (*Zuo You Zai Quan,* 左右栽拳)

Continuing from the last piece, right after you completed the last downward drilling, inhale, rotate both of your fists upward and then toward your face (Figure 5-83). Next, exhale and twist your body to your left while pushing your right fist downward and forward (Figure 5-84). Inhale, straighten your torso, thrust your chest out, and circle your right fist upward while circling your

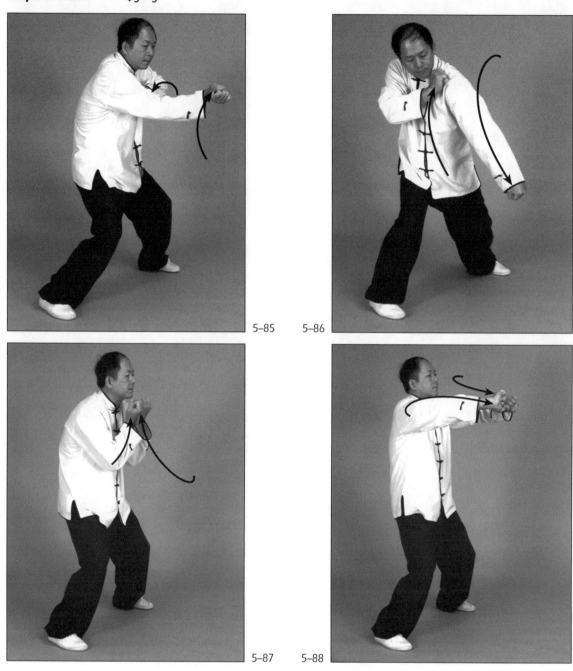

5–85   5–86

5–87   5–88

left fist downward (Figure 5-85). Finally, exhale, arc your torso and hold in your chest while push-ing your left fist downward and forward (Figure 5-86). Repeat five more times each side.

11. Forward Arcing and Backward Pushing (*Qian Gong Hou Tui,* 前拱後推)

From the final posture of the last piece, inhale, arc your torso, hold in your chest, and move both of your fists toward your face (Figure 5-87). Next, exhale, straighten your torso, thrust out your chest while continuing to rotate both of your fists until the palms face forward, then push out in front of your upper chest (Figure 5-88).

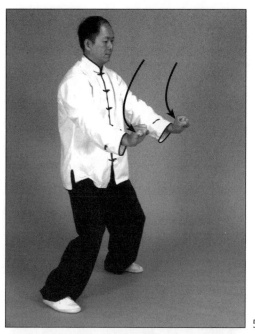

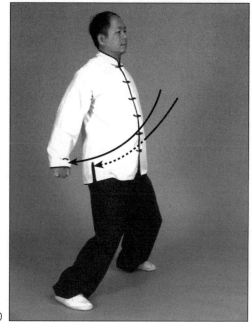

5-89   5-90

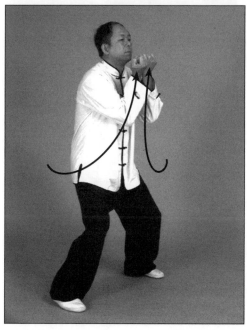

5-91

Inhale and relax your torso while moving both of your fists backward beside your waist (Figure 5-89). Finally, exhale, thrusting your chest forward while pushing both of your fists backward and downward (Figure 5-90).

To repeat, simply inhale deeply, relax your torso, and move both of your fists to the front of your upper chest (Figure 5-91). You should repeat five more times to make a total of six repetitions.

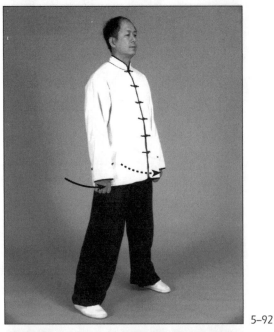
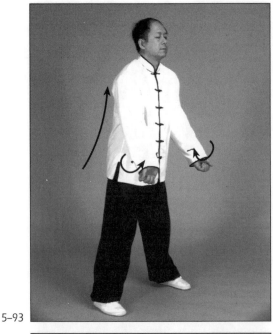

5-92   5-93

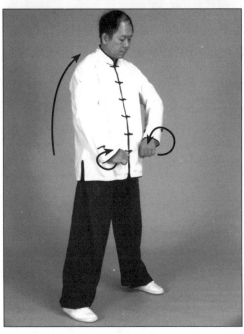
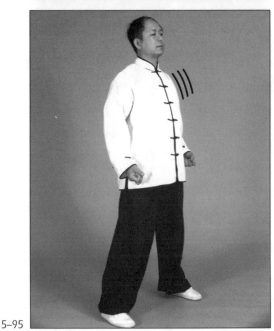

5-94   5-95

12. White Crane Softens Its Body (*Bai He Ruan Shen,* 白鶴軟身)

This last piece is very important, and is used to recover from the tension of the physical body caused by Hard *Qigong* training. Right after you have completed the last eleven pieces, breathe naturally and drop both of your fists naturally downward beside your waist while relaxing your torso (Figure 5-92). Next, move your spine like a wave upward from the sacrum area while rotating both of your fists following the wave movement of the spine (Figures 5-93 and 5-94).

If you would like to coordinate your breathing, inhale first, gently thrusting your chest out while keeping your palms facing forward (Figure 5-95). Next, exhale, and move your sacrum back to start the waving motion of the spine or torso again. When this wave reaches the shoulders and

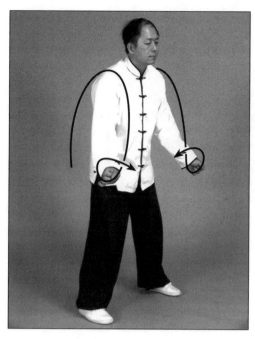

5-96

the arms, circle your fists naturally beside your waist area (Figure 5-96). You should keep practicing this Soft *Qigong* until the entire torso is relaxed.

From *Qigong* theoretical concepts, after you have practiced a Hard *Qigong* set, your physical body will have built up an excited level of *Qi*. If this energy stays trapped in your physical body, it can cause your body to become too *Yang*. Therefore, you should loosen your body, especially the joint areas, and lead the *Qi* out through the limbs.

After you have completed the entire set, you should walk for at least five minutes to loosen up your legs. While you are walking, continue to swing your arms forward and back, rotating your shoulders gently in both directions, and twisting your body gently from side to side. Naturally, if you have time, after you have recovered from Hard *Qigong* practice, you should begin the soft moving Crane practice explained in the next chapter. This specializes in helping you loosen up your torso and joints.

Before we finish this section, I would like to remind you of a few important points:

1. All of the above Hard *Qigong* practices are designed for Hard *Jin* manifestation. Hard *Jin* is then applied into the fighting techniques. Therefore, after you have mastered the above practice, you should coordinate it with stepping when you are practicing. The stepping in Chinese martial arts is used to coordinate the techniques. Therefore, you may simply imagine the stepping coordination with the upper body movements.

2. After you have practiced for a long time, you will feel that the number of repetitions cannot satisfy your need to build up strength. In this case, you should increase the number of repetitions.

3. You should always remember that Hard *Qigong*, though able to build up the strength of your physical body, can also be harmful if over trained. **Know how to build up the *Qi* through tension and also how to circulate and release the *Qi* through relaxation. One is *Yang* and the other is *Yin*.**

4. The final goal of the practice is reaching the "**unification of both internal and external.**" For a long term goal, you should also learn Small Circulation, which teaches you how to

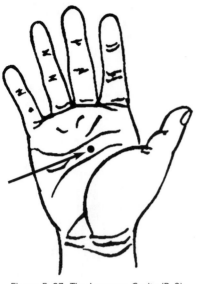

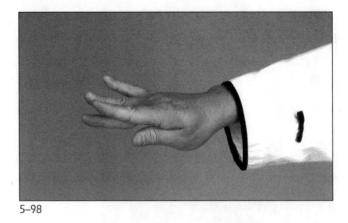

5–98

Figure 5–97. The Laogong Cavity (P–8)

build up the *Qi* in the Lower *Dan Tian* to a more abundant level and how to circulate the *Qi* in the Conception and Governing Vessels. In addition, you should also understand the practice of Grand Circulation. From Grand Circulation practice, you will lead the *Qi* from the Lower *Dan Tian* to the torso and limbs for *Qigong* practice.

Next, we will introduce the Palm Set of Hard *Qigong* training. Soon you will realize that many pieces of the Palm Set are similar to those of the Fist Set. The only difference is that one uses the fists and the other the palms. Actually, this should not be surprising, since the basic theory and training principles remain the same. The only difference between the Fist Set and Palm Set is that **in the Fist Set, the *Qi* is always trapped in the wrists and arms, which can help you build up the physical body easily, while in the Palm Set, the *Qi* will be emitted through the *Laogong* cavities (P-8) and finger tips** (Figure 5-97).

Before we start the Palm Set, you should first pay attention to the hand form. The thumb and the middle finger are pushed slightly forward, while the index finger is straightened and the ring finger and pinkie are pushed backward (Figure 5-98). This hand form imitates the wing of a crane. The reason for this hand form will be explained in the next chapter.

PALM SET:

1. Extend Both Arms Forward (*Shuang Bi Ping Zhang,* 雙臂平展)

This piece is very similar to the first piece of the Fist Set. First, place both of your palms beside your chest area (Figure 5-99). Next, inhale deeply while holding in your chest and arc your torso gently backward. Start to exhale and at the same time extend both of your arms from the center of your chest outward (Figure 5-100). While you are exhaling, you should gradually tense up your palms, arms, and torso until the arms are extended but slightly bent. The distance between your elbows and the chest should be about a palm's width. Your fingers are pointing slightly sideways.

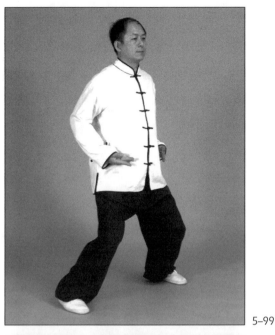
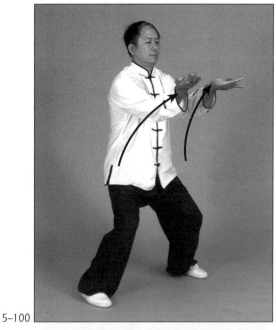

5-99   5-100

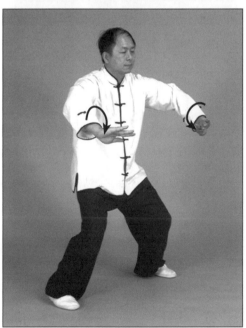
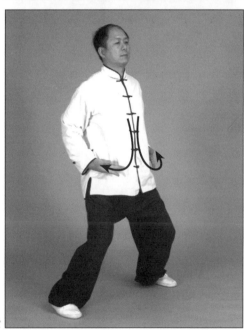

5-101   5-102

Next, start to inhale, relax your torso, and turn both of your palms until the palms are facing down (Figure 5-101), then pull them back to the sides of the upper chest area and turning the palms until they are facing upward again (Figure 5-102). Repeat five more times to make six repetitions total.

2. White Crane Expands Its Wings (*Bai He Zhan Chi,* 白鶴展翅)

From the last piece, start to inhale, arc your back and hold in your chest as the forearms cross each other with the left arm on the top and the right arm on the bottom (Figure 5-103). Next, exhale and continue to extend your right arm forward while rotating it until the palm is facing

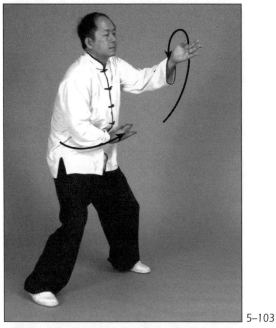
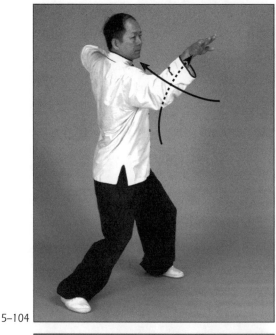

5–103   5–104

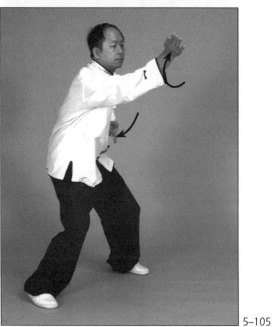
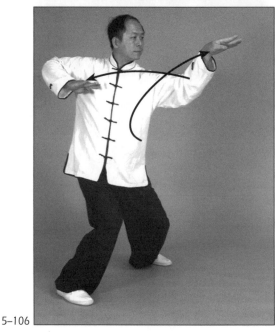

5–105   5–106

down, and pull your left hand back to the left hand side of your upper chest, palm facing downward (Figure 5-104). When you do this, you should straighten your torso and thrust your chest out.

Inhale, arc your back and hold in your chest again. Cross both of your forearms with the left arm on the bottom and the right arm on the top, rotating both of your hands until they face upward (Figure 5-105). Finally, exhale, straighten your torso and hold in your chest while extending your left arm forward and pulling your right hand back to the side of your right upper chest to complete a cycle of this piece (Figure 5-106). Both palms should face downward at this time. Repeat five more times.

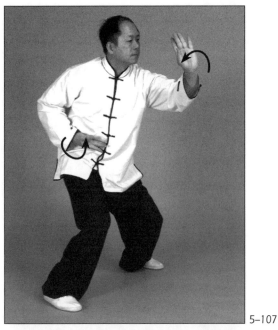
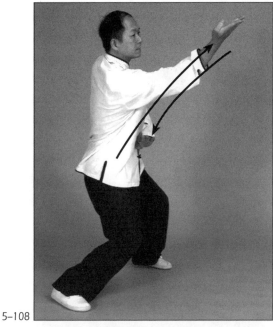

5–107   5–108

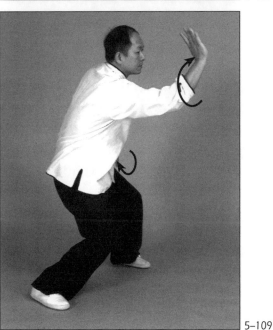
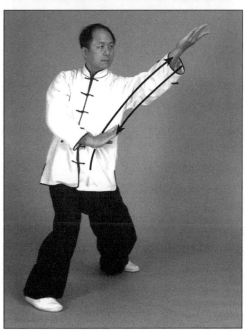

5–109   5–110

3. Press Downward and Drill Forward (*Xia Ya Shang Zhuan,* 下壓上鑽)

Continuing from the last piece, inhale deeply while arcing your spine and chest inward, cover your left palm downward and toward your right lower chest, and rotate your right arm until the palm is facing upward (Figure 5-107).

Next, exhale, straighten out your torso and thrust out your chest. Continue to cover your left hand down while extending your right hand forward over the left arm (Figure 5-108). At this position, your right hand should be extended forward while your left palm is under the right elbow.

Change sides by covering your right hand downward and rotating your left hand until the palm is facing upward (Figure 5-109). Finally, exhale and drill your left hand forward while continuing to cover your right hand downward (Figure 5-110). Repeat the entire process five more times.

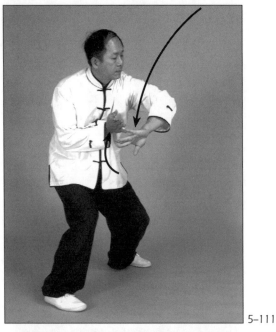
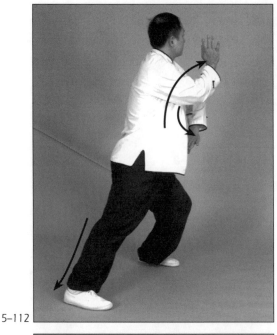

5–111   5–112

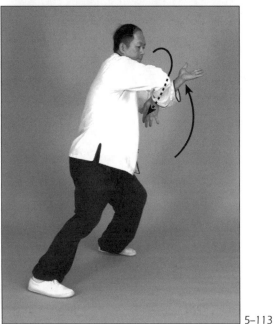
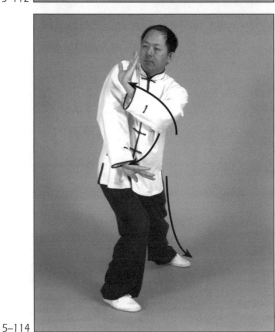

5–113   5–114

4. **Left and Right Bump** (*Zuo You Lan Kao,* 左右攬靠)

Continuing from the last piece, inhale deeply, arc in your torso and chest, and move your left hand down while starting to push your right palm to your left (Figure 5-111). Next, exhale and gradually tense up your torso and arms while pushing your right hand and your left arm to your left (Figure 5-112). Keep both arms bent.

Inhale, rotating your right hand downward while moving your left hand upward (Figure 5-113). Finally, exhale and gradually tense up your torso and arms while pushing your left hand and right arm to your right (Figure 5-114). Again, keep both of your arms bent. Repeat the entire process five more times.

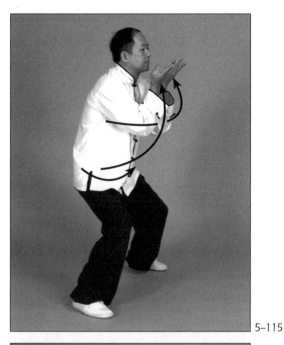
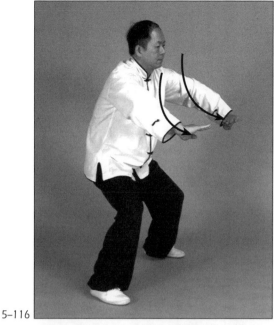

5-115   5-116

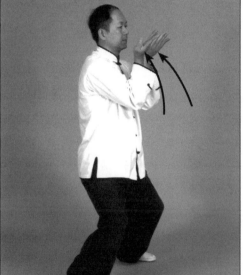
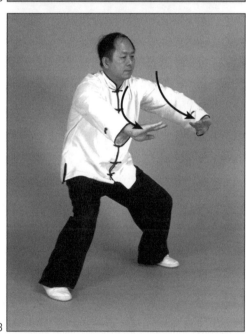

5-117   5-118

5. Double Hands Cut Forward (*Shuang Shou Ping Qie,* 雙手平切)

After you have completed the last right hand side pushing, inhale, face forward, and relax your torso while moving both of your hands toward your upper chest (Figure 5-115). Next, exhale, arc your back and hold in your chest, while using the sides of your palms to push and press forward and downward (Figure 5-116).

To repeat the form, simply inhale again and relax your torso while bringing both of your hands to your upper chest, then push and press your palms forward and downward again (Figures 5-117 and 5-118). You should continue the training until you have pushed and pressed six times.

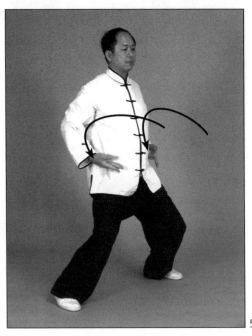

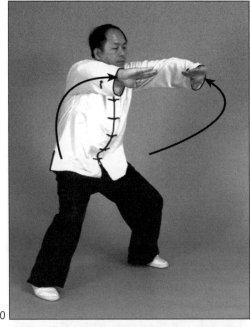

5-119   5-120

6. Double Arms Circular Embracing

(*Shuang Bi Huan Bao,* 雙臂環抱)

Continuing from the last piece, inhale deeply, straighten up and relax your torso while bringing both hands toward your waist area and start to form a circle (Figure 5-119). Next, exhale, arc your back, and extend the arcing circular motion into the arms until the finger tips on both hands almost reach each other (Figure 5-120).

To repeat the form, inhale, relax and straighten your torso, and bring both of your hands back to the waist area again. You should repeat the movement six times.

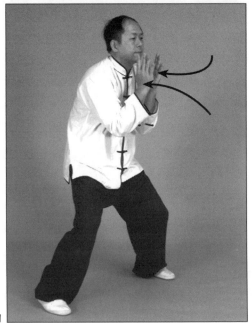

5-121

7. Left Right Pulling the Bow (*Zuo You Zhang Gong,* 左右張弓)

Continuing from the last piece, inhale and bring both of your arms to the front of your chest with the palms facing each other, and arc your back (Figure 5-121). Next, start to exhale and expand both arms from the center of the chest outward to the shoulders and finally straighten out both arms as far as possible (Figure 5-122). Inhale again and bring both of your arms back to the chest and repeat five more times.

After you have completed opening six times, hold the final expanding posture and inhale deeply. Next, exhale, arc your back and hold in your chest while squeezing both of your forearms inward until they are in front of your chest (Figure 5-123). Then inhale, relax your torso, and expand your chest and arms to repeat five more times.

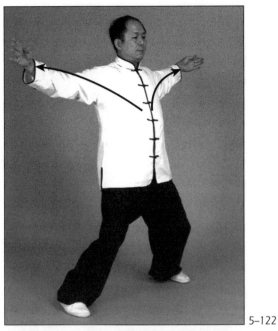
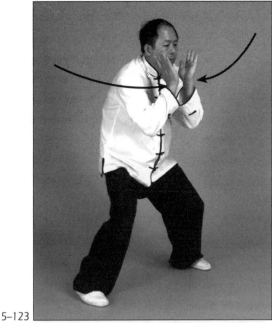

5-122   5-123

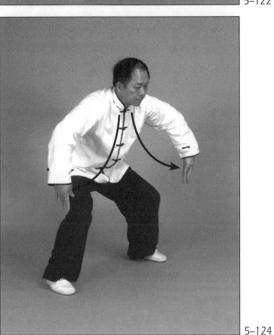
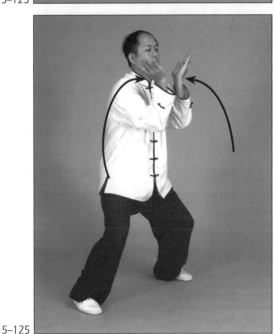

5-124   5-125

8. Left and Right Arcing the Wings (*Zuo You Gong Chi*, 左右拱翅)

When you complete the last squeezing movement in the previous piece, stay in the same posture and inhale deeply. Next, exhale and circle both of your arms downward and then sideways (Figure 5-124). Both of your arms are arcing outward and your torso is arcing backward. Your palms face each other.

Inhale, relax your torso, straighten your body and thrust out your chest while bringing both of your arms to the front of the chest to repeat five more times (Figure 5-125).

After you have completed six repetitions, inhale and bring both of your hands back to the front of your chest area. Exhale, again arc your back and hold in your chest while expanding both

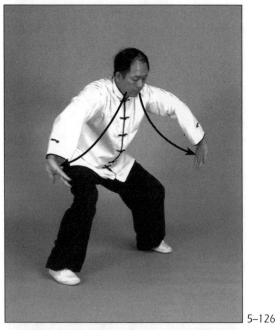 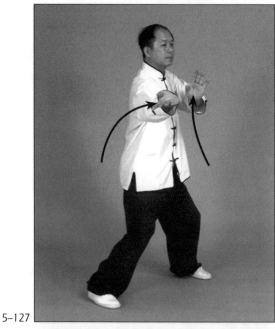

5-126   5-127

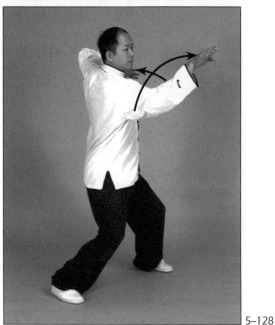 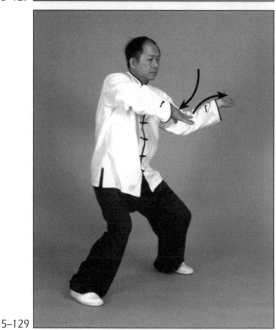

5-128   5-129

of your arms to the side (Figure 5-126). When you are doing so, you should rotate both of your wrists and push both of your hands outward. To repeat the training, inhale again and bring both hands to the chest area and then exhale to repeat the form. Repeat five more times.

9. White Crane Covers Its Wings (*Bai He Yan Chi*, 白鶴掩翅)

After your have completed the last piece, inhale and bring both of your hands up to your chest area (Figure 5-127). The torso and chest are relaxed. Next, exhale and pull your left hand to the left armpit with the palm facing downward while covering your right hand downward (Figure 5-128). When you do this, you should twist your body to your left.

Next, inhale, circle your right hand inward toward your upper chest while starting to cover your left hand (Figure 5-129). Again, the torso and chest should be relaxed. Exhale, pulling your

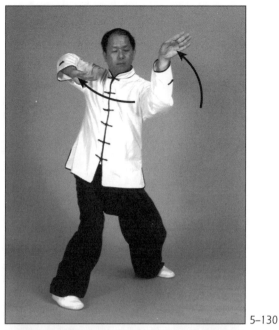
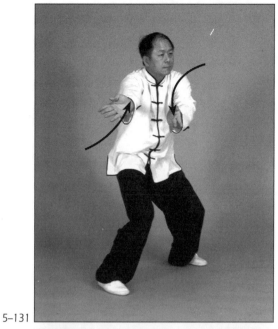

5-130 5-131

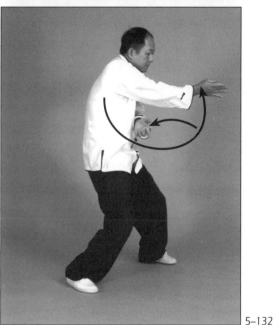
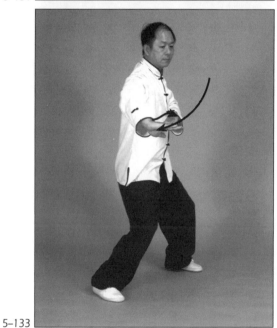

5-132 5-133

right hand to the right armpit area with the palm facing downward, while covering your left hand in front of your upper chest (Figure 5-130). The body should be twisted to the right and tensed at this point. You should repeat the entire process another five times.

10. Left and Right Cut Horizontally (Zuo You Pan Qie, 左右盤切)

After you have completed the left hand's covering in the last piece, inhale and pull both of your hands to the chest area (Figure 5-131). Next, circle your left hand counterclockwise horizontally in front of your stomach area, while circling your right hand counterclockwise to the right side of your chest (Figure 5-132). Your back should be arced and your chest held in. Exhale and continue circling both hands until your left hand is over your right lower rib area and your right hand is stretched out to the right side of your body (Figure 5-133). The torso is straight and the chest is thrust out.

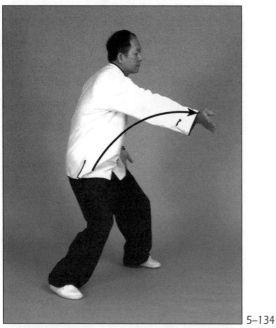
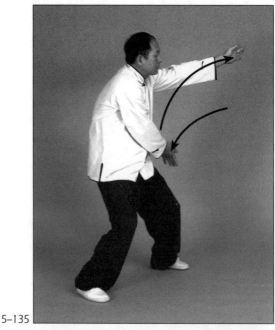

5-134   5-135

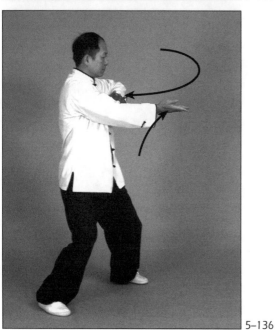
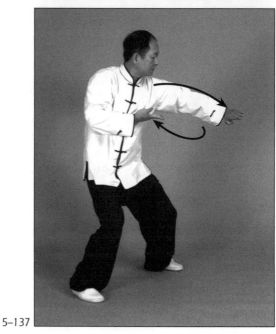

5-136   5-137

Inhale, twist your body to your left, and turn your right hand until the palm is facing upward, moving it to the left (Figure 5-134). Continue to move your right hand to your left lower rib area while circling your left hand up and forward clockwise (Figure 5-135). Next, circle your right hand and left hand clockwise with the left hand one-half circle behind (Figure 5-136). Finally, pull your right hand back to your chest area while pressing your left hand out to your left (Figure 5-137). You should train this left and right exercise another five times.

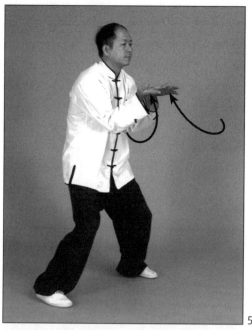

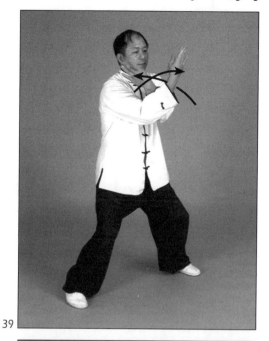

5-138   5-139

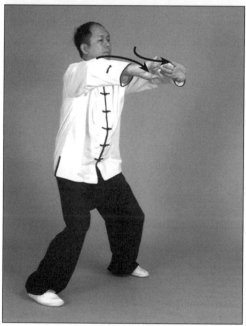

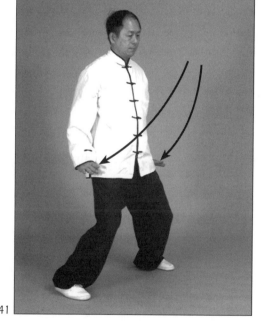

5-140   5-141

11. Forward Arcing and Backward Pushing (*Qian Gong Hou Tui*, 前拱後推)

From the final posture of the last piece, start to inhale and pull both of your hands back to your upper chest area (Figure 5-138). Continue your inhalation and thrust out your chest while rotating your wrist until both palms are facing outward (Figure 5-139). Next, exhale, arc your torso and hold in your chest while pushing both of your hands out in front of your upper chest (Figure 5-140).

Inhale and relax your torso while moving both of your hands backward beside your waist (Figure 5-141). Finally, exhale and thrust your chest forward while pushing both of your palms backward and downward (Figure 5-142).

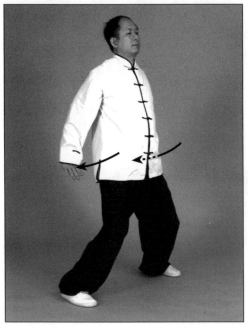
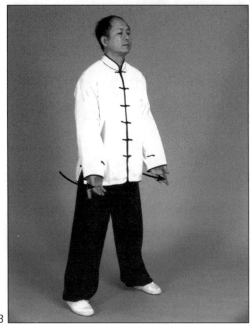

5-142   5-143

To repeat, simply inhale deeply, relax your torso, and move both of your hands to the front of your upper chest. Then, rotate both of your hands and push forward to repeat the practice. You should repeat five more times to make six repetitions.

12. White Crane Softens Its Body (*Bai He Ruan Shen,* 白鶴軟身)

This last piece is very important and is used to recover from the tension in the physical body caused by Hard *Qigong* training. Immediately after you have completed the last eleven pieces, breathe naturally, and drop both of your hands naturally downward beside your waist while relaxing your torso (Figure 5-143). Next, move your spine like a wave upward from the sacrum area while rotating both of your palms naturally, following the wave movement of the spine (Figure 5-144).

If you would like to coordinate your breathing, first inhale, gently thrusting your chest out while keeping your palms facing forward (Figure 5-145). Next, exhale and move your sacrum back to start the waving motion of the spine or torso. When this wave reaches the shoulders and the arms, circle your hands naturally beside your waist area (Figure 5-146). You should keep practicing this Soft *Qigong* until the entire torso is relaxed. Finally, stand still, relax and breathe deeply for a while to complete the entire palm set (Figure 5-147).

From *Qigong* theoretical concepts, after you have practiced a Hard *Qigong* set, your physical body will have built up an excited level of *Qi*. If this energy remains trapped in your physical body, it can cause your body to become too *Yang*. Therefore, you should loosen your body, especially the joint areas, and lead the *Qi* out through the limbs.

After you have completed the entire set, you should walk for at least five minutes to loosen up your legs. While you are walking, continue to swing your arms forward and back, rotate your shoulders in both directions gently, and twist your body gently from side to side. Naturally, if you have time, after you have recovered from Hard *Qigong* practice, you should enter the soft moving Crane practice explained in the next chapter, which specializes in helping you loosen up your torso and joints.

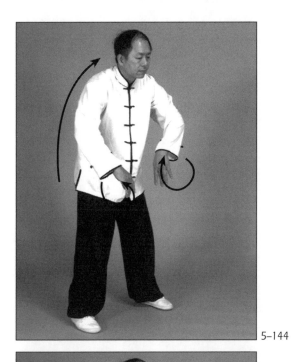

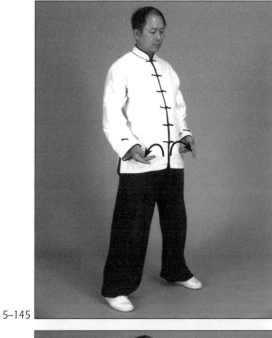

5-144   5-145

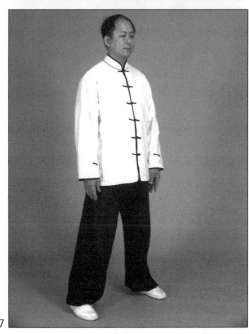

5-146   5-147

Again, when you practice this Palm Set, start with the use of local *Qi* to energize the physical body. Later, after you have completed Small Circulation and Grand Circulation practice, you should apply Lower *Dan Tian Qi* to the training.

Chapter 6

Crane Soft Qigong

(Flying Crane Gong)

飛鶴功

6-1. Introduction

The last chapter presented an idea of how Hard *Qigong* can be trained in White Crane style. You may apply the same theory and training principles into other styles. This can be done because no matter what style, the *Dao* of martial arts remains the same. From understanding and continued pondering, the arts can be promoted to a higher level.

It is not surprising that, in Chinese martial society, even in the same style there can be many different types of *Qigong* practice. These originated from different teachers' understandings about the styles, which were then applied into the training. From this, different *Qigong* training methods within the same styles were developed. For example, there are more than four crane styles existing today, and each one of them has its own special way of training *Qigong*. For instance, the Shouting Crane style emphasizes stillness and internal cultivation of the *Qi* in the Lower *Dan Tian*, applying this *Qi* to raise the spirit of a Crane practitioner with the sound of shouting. Jerking or Trembling Crane (also called Ancestral Crane) style focuses on the softness and the strength of the spine and the chest in order to manifest the *Jin* strongly from the torso. Another example of this is the many different styles of *Taiji Qigong* which are used in different *Taiji* styles today.

The main style of White Crane which I learned was the Jerking or Trembling Crane, which imitates the jerking or shaking power of a crane. In order to have a high level of Soft *Jin* manifestation, both Hard and Soft *Qigong* were heavily emphasized. Jerking *Jin* is a typical way of manifesting Soft *Jin*. The movement is just like a crane shaking the water off of its feathers after a rain. In order to generate strong jerking power, the torso and chest must be strong and soft. In addition, the motion of the jerking generated either from the legs or the waist must be able to be manifested from the fingers. Because of this the body, from the bottom of the legs to the finger-tips, must act like a soft whip. In order to reach this goal, **the joints must be very relaxed and the entire body connected and treated as one unit**. This soft side of White Crane training completely matches the training theory of *Taijiquan*. In fact, it was my White Crane background that led me to a deeper understanding of my *Taijiquan* practice.

In the next section of this chapter, I would like to briefly discuss the Still Soft *Qigong* training of White Crane. Due to the deep and profound theory of this *Qigong*, it is impossible to fully cover this subject in a short section. Here, I can only offer some theory and basic training.

In Section 6-3, Moving White Crane *Qigong* training will be introduced. In this section, first some important stretching methods, especially for the spine and the chest, will be introduced. Next, some warm up exercises which can be used to stimulate the torso's muscles, tendons and ligaments will be demonstrated. Through such preparation, you can produce an appropriate and beneficial condition for your White Crane *Qigong* and *Jin* practice. I will then introduce Flying Crane *Qigong*. Flying Crane *Qigong* can be considered the essence of the Jerking, Trembling or Shaking Crane style.

6-2. Stationary Soft Qigong (*Ding Gong,* 定功)

In Stationary Soft *Qigong* training, the body's condition is extremely relaxed and soft. In fact, there is only a limited physical movement generated from the abdominal area for breathing. Other than that, the entire physical body remains completely still. From this, it might seem that since there are no significant physical movements involved, the Stationary Soft *Qigong* should be very easy. As a matter of fact, as explained in Chapter 4, Stationary Soft *Qigong* (or Still Meditation) is the most difficult *Qigong* simply because in this practice, you must face your own mind and learn how to regulate it.

Generally speaking, in order to reach a profound level of Stationary Soft *Qigong* practice, you must first be able to reach a high level of regulating your body, breathing, and mind. Only then will you have provided a proper condition for your mind to lead the *Qi* to circulate in the body as you wish. The final goal of this practice is using your mind to lead the *Qi* upward following the spinal cord (i.e., Thrusting Vessel) to nourish your brain for enlightenment. If you are interested in knowing more about this theory and training, you may refer to the books: ***The Root of Chinese Chi Kung, Muscle/Tendon Changing and Marrow/Brain Washing Chi Kung,*** and ***The Essence of Tai Chi Chi Kung,*** by YMAA. In this section, I will first summarize the four most important Stationary Soft *Qigong* practices. These are Self-Hypnosis Relaxation Meditation, Small Circulation, Grand Circulation, and Spiritual Cultivation. Of these four, only Self-Hypnosis Relaxation Meditation will be explained in detail. The reason for this is that, unlike the other three, there is no danger involved in this training. In addition, this subject is not as complicated and difficult to understand as the other subjects, and is therefore possible to cover in one section. However, you should understand that although self-hypnosis relaxation meditation is simple, it is important in its fundamentals, and can provide you with a foundation for other practices.

Self-Hypnosis Relaxation Meditation

Self-Hypnosis Relaxation Meditation can be described as the first, most basic and important step in Still Soft *Qigong*. This practice can be done after a hard day of physical training or work. It does not matter if you are a martial artist or not, this practice can produce a deeply relaxed physical body.

You should understand that, in order to have smooth *Qi* circulation, you must learn how to relax your body. Every minute, thousands of body cells die. New cells must constantly be produced to replace the old ones.

As mentioned in Chapter 2, aging is a product of the degradation of health that occurs between cellular generations. For some reason, the newly formed cells are not as healthy as the earlier cells. One of the main purposes of *Qigong* practice is to produce healthier cells, and to learn how to make the cellular replacement process more efficient.

In order to have smooth cell replacement in your body, you must learn how to keep the blood and the *Qi* circulation smooth. The most important factor in reaching this goal is to maintain both a relaxed physical and mental body. Whenever your mental and physical bodies are tensed, your blood and *Qi* circulation will be stagnant. When you are relaxed, the blood and the *Qi* circulation can be smooth. This results in healthy cell replenishment.

From this, you can see that relaxation is one of the most important keys to maintaining health and slowing down the aging process. The relaxation that you practice must reach to the depths of your joints and to all the internal organs. Physical degeneration often starts in the joints, and sickness and disease often involve the failure of an internal organ. In order to achieve such deep relaxation, you must begin by relaxing your muscles and tendons. Only then can your mind reach into or feel the ligaments and the deep places of the joints. When the joints are relaxed, the *Qi* and blood circulating in the bone marrow will be smooth. Consequently, the bone marrow will function efficiently, creating more healthy blood cells. Remember, healthy blood cells will promote proper blood and *Qi* nutrition to all parts of your body.

You must also learn how to relax as deeply as possible, right into your internal organs. When you relax to these organs, not only does cell replacement increase, but the normal functioning of the internal organs can also be maintained.

The trick to relaxing the muscles and tendons is to treat the joints like the two ends of a rope. At the tips of your muscles are tendons, which attach the muscles to the bones. At the ends of the bones are the ligaments, which hold the joints together. When the two ends of the rope are relaxed, the entire section of that muscle can be relaxed. Only when the muscles and tendons are relaxed will you be able to feel the deep spaces in the joints. Then, through mental awareness and breathing techniques, you will be able to relax all your joints.

At this time, you must understand an important point. The key to successful *Qigong* practice is learning how to improve mental communication with your physical body, which is *Yang*, and also to the *Qi* body, which is *Yin*. Through this communication, your mind can bring both the physical and *Qi* bodies to a deeply harmonious state. When the *Yin* and *Yang* bodies are harmonious, the *Qi* and the blood will circulate smoothly in the body.

You can now see that the primary key to successful training is your mind. The deeper your mind can feel or communicate, the deeper you can relax your body. Therefore, you must learn how to meditate in stillness in order to reach the deepest parts of your mind. In order to achieve a deep meditative state, you must first learn to detach yourself from emotional disturbance, realizing fully that the problems of your past and future cannot touch you during meditation unless you allow them to. Your mind will then become neutral to the outside world, and as your mental body relaxes, you will be able to develop a deep sense of peace and well being. When you achieve this deep meditative mind, you can gradually begin to feel or sense your internal organs. This deep feeling, combined with correct breathing techniques, will help you to relax the internal organs.

We now know that one of the main keys to successful relaxation practice is to have a deep, meditative mind. But how does one achieve such a state? The task of controlling your own mind is one of the most difficult steps in *Qigong* practice. Like falling asleep, the harder you try, the less you will succeed. The trick to falling asleep is very similar to the trick to meditation. The main difference between sleep and meditation is that in meditation, your conscious mind is still functioning quietly in the background, but while you are sleeping your conscious mind is no longer in control. The tricks for reaching a deep meditative mind are: do not resist, do not concentrate, do not persist, and most importantly of all, do not be disturbed emotionally.

In meditation, the more you restrict your mind from wandering, the more it will try to escape your control. It is like trying to force yourself to sleep — it just cannot be done. The mind is very stubborn and cannot be pushed. It can, however, be led. Like water, the more you push, the more ways it will find to get around you. But if you lead it correctly, it will flow smoothly even into the deepest places.

Moreover, when you meditate in this way, you should not concentrate. Too much concentration will only generate greater resistance. Instead, simply pay attention. Concentration will make you tired and tense. This will worsen the situation. You should not allow your mind to dwell upon thoughts or problems occurring outside of your body. When you notice that your mind is constantly returning to the same thought patterns, bring it gently back to the center of your spirit. The center of your spirit is located at what is called the third eye, in the center of your forehead. Remember that deep, even breathing can help you to achieve and maintain this mental centering.

Above all, never become upset with yourself if you have difficulty leading your mind into a deep meditative state. Emotional disturbance will only create more tension in your mind, and further hamper your efforts.

Another important key to achieving deep meditation is learning how to breathe correctly. Observation of natural human behavior reveals that when we are happy and excited, our exhalation is longer than our inhalation. One example of this, as previously mentioned, is that when you are happy, you laugh. The sound of laughter is one of the natural sounds which can release over-accumulated fire or *Qi* in the body, bringing it to the surface of the skin. Consequently, the Guardian *Qi* is strengthened and the accumulated *Qi* is led outside of the body. This is one reason why you feel warm when you are happy.

Conversely, when you are sad, you make the sound of *"Hen"* while inhaling. Moreover, sadness produces an inhalation that is longer than the exhalation. Therefore, the *Qi* is led inward to the bone marrow, and the Guardian *Qi* is weakened. When this happens, you may feel cold.

This model also holds that, while awake, our exhalation is relatively longer than our inhalation, and that skin temperature is relatively higher. When we sleep, however, inhalation becomes longer than exhalation, the heart beat slows down, and the skin temperature is lower. The Guardian *Qi* is considerably weaker when you sleep. Consequently, you feel chilly when you first wake up.

From the above observations, you can see that in order to lead your mind into a deep meditative state, besides calming down your mind, you should also pay attention to your breathing. You should inhale calmly, gently and slowly. After this deep inhalation, relax and let the air out of your lungs smoothly and naturally. This will gradually slow down your heart beat, cool down your excited mind, and relax your physical body. Finally, you will find yourself slipping off to sleep, or entering a deep meditative state.

Normally in meditation practice, you should avoid falling asleep. Your mind should be in the state of sleepy wakefulness. In this state, you can still use your mind to lead or regulate the *Qi* in your body while you are in a deep and relaxed state. However, in self-relaxation hypnosis, you do not have to worry if you are falling sleep. The reason for this is simply that you are not using your mind to regulate the *Qi* circulating in the body. What you are doing is simply bringing your mind and your physical body to a deep, meditative state which allows the *Qi* to flow or re-distribute by itself to a more harmonious state in your body.

In fact, falling asleep in this practice can be beneficial. This is because when you are asleep, as long as you do not have a nightmare, both your mental and physical bodies are in an extremely relaxed state. Sleeping is the most natural method of re-balancing *Qi* which has become unbalanced during wakefulness. When you are awake, you are in *Yang* state, and when you are sleeping, you are in the *Yin* state. When you are in the *Yin* state, physical action ceases. During sleep, the physical body and the brain regain their *Qi* nourishment. Self-relaxation hypnosis can help you make this *Yin* recovery process more efficient. This is one of the keys to health and longevity.

Now, let us summarize the purposes of self-relaxation hypnosis.

1. For both mental and physical relaxation. From mental and physical relaxation, smooth *Qi* and blood circulation is produced. Most important of all is to relax the internal organs, which provides a healthy environment for their functioning. In addition, through relaxation, stress or strain in the internal organs can be reduced.

2. To improve the *Qi* and blood circulation. When the *Qi* and blood circulation is smooth, cellular replacement in the body can be enhanced. Physical degeneration or defects can be prevented.

3. To reduce mental pressure. From self-relaxation hypnosis, you will be able to bring your mind into a neutral state, and therefore reduce or even remove mental stress and depression.

4. To expedite the recovery of fatigue. Due to smooth *Qi* and blood circulation, the poisons produced by muscular fatigue can be removed quickly and smoothly.

5. To help sleep. Self-relaxation hypnosis is the best way to lead your mind to sleep without drugs. This has been practiced in China for thousands of years. If you ponder the theory and practice diligently, you will soon discover that the benefit it can bring you is beyond price.

Important Concerns for Self-Relaxation Hypnosis

Before you start your practice, there are a few important points which you should note.

1. Place:

The place you choose for your self-relaxation hypnosis practice should be quiet and comfortable, providing a peaceful feeling. In addition, the air should be fresh and circulating well.

2. Orientation:

If you can, before you lie down, you should face the south to match the orientation of the earth's magnetic field. Normally, this self-relaxation practice should take place inside of the house, avoiding direct sunlight.

3. Posture:

When you lie down, your posture should be the most comfortable possible. One of the best choices is lying down, facing upward and placing your arms beside your body. To prevent tension in your neck, you should place your head on a soft pillow.

4. Prevent Disturbance:

During meditation, the most serious interruption is to be suddenly startled by noise. The telephone should be unplugged. Place a "don't disturb" sign on the door. Any noise which can startle you should be avoided.

5. Keep Warm:

In self-relaxation practice, your heart beat slows down, your skin temperature drops and your Guardian *Qi* retreats. In this state, you can catch cold easily. Therefore, you should cover your body with a blanket to keep warm.

6. Falling Asleep:

As mentioned previously, normally when you meditate, if you are using your mind to lead the *Qi* for special *Qigong* practice, you should not fall asleep. However, in this self-relaxation practice, since you are not using your mind to lead the *Qi*, there is no danger to falling asleep. In fact, to lead your mind into a sleepy state is the main purpose of self-relaxation meditation. When you are in the sleeping state, your physical body is very relaxed and your mental body is neutral. This will provide the best conditions for *Qi* circulation. Therefore, if you feel sleepy, it is okay to let go. The more you resist, the more your mental mind and physical body will be tense.

Self-Relaxation Hypnosis Procedures

1. Bring your mind to your spiritual center.

First, bring your mind from outside of your body to inside your body. To do this, focus your mind on the area known as the third eye, located in the center of your forehead. Breathe deeply and slowly, and pay attention to this third eye. As you exhale, try to relax the third eye area. If you do this correctly, you will feel almost as if your third eye is breathing with you. Repeat this a total of five times.

2. Relax your solar plexus.

Next, bring your mind downward to your solar plexus area. Pay attention to the solar plexus and feel how tense or tight it is. Inhale deeply and slowly, and then exhale. While you are exhaling, use your mind to melt the tension from the solar plexus area. Again, inhale deeply and bring your mind deep inside your solar plexus, then exhale and lead any remaining tension out, and relax your solar plexus. Once the solar plexus is relaxed, the front side of your torso will be opened, and the *Qi* can circulate smoothly and freely. You should repeat the solar plexus relaxation a total of five times.

3. Center your mind on the Lower Dan Tian.

After you relax your solar plexus, bring your mind to your abdomen or Lower *Dan Tian*. Inhale deeply, expanding your abdomen slowly and comfortably, then release all the carbon dioxide naturally and easily. You should inhale longer than you exhale, as though you are sleeping. This will cool your physical body down. When you exhale, try to feel all the joints in your entire body and relax them. You feel like your body is collapsing, and every piece of bone is falling to the floor naturally. Not even the slightest tension exists in the muscles or tendons. Again, you should repeat this practice five times.

4. Relax your toes.

Next, bring your mind to your toes. Feel all the joints in your toes. Inhale deeply, and bring your mind to deep within these joints. Then exhale, relax these joints and lead out any *Qi* stagnation there. Again, inhale deeply, then exhale to relax the joints. Repeat five times.

5. Relax your feet.

Now bring your mind to your feet. Inhale deeply to the center of each foot, then exhale and relax both feet completely. The *Yongquan* (K-1) cavity area is more sensitive to sensation than any other place on the foot (Figure 6-1). *Yongquan* is a *Qi* gate which connects the kidneys to your environment. Relax these two gates, open them up, and allow the *Qi* to pass through naturally and easily. Repeat five times.

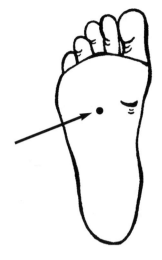

Figure 6–1. The Yongquan Cavity (K-1)

6. Relax your ankles.

Next, you should bring your mind deep into your ankles, inhale deeply and then exhale while relaxing the entire joints. Repeat five times.

7. Relax your calves.

Now bring your mind to your calves. In order to relax the calf muscles, you must first relax their ends, and the tendons that connect them to the bone at both the ankles and the knees. Inhale deeply into the joints, and then exhale while relaxing the entire calf muscle. Repeat five times.

8. Relax your knees.

Bring your mind to your knees. Inhale deeply into the knees and then exhale while relaxing the entire joints. Repeat five times.

9. Relax your thighs.

Next, bring your mind to your thighs. In order to relax the thigh muscles, first relax their ends at the waist and knees, and the tendons that connect them to the bones. Inhale deeply into the joints and then exhale while relaxing the entire thigh muscle. Repeat five times.

10. Relax your hips.

Bring your mind to your hips. Inhale deeply into the hips, and then exhale while relaxing the joints. Repeat five times. At this point, you should feel that your legs, from the hips down to the toes, are so relaxed and comfortable that they seem to be floating.

11. Relax your fingers.

Next, bring your mind to your fingers. Inhale deeply and bring your mind deep into the joints. Then, exhale and loosen every joint and relax them. Repeat five times.

12. Relax your hands.

Now bring your mind to the hands. Inhale deeply to the center of the hands and then exhale while relaxing all the joints. You will feel the *Laogong* (P-8) cavity area is more sensitive than any other place on the hand (Figure 6-2). *Laogong* is a *Qi* gate which connects the pericardium to your environment, and it is used to regulate the Heart Fire. Relax these two gates, open them up, and allow the *Qi* to pass through naturally and easily. Repeat five times.

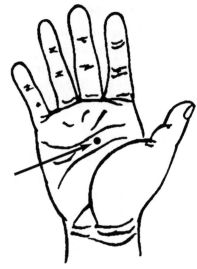

Figure 6–2. The Laogong Cavity (P-8)

13. Relax your wrists.

Next, bring your mind to your wrists. Inhale deeply into the wrists and then exhale while relaxing the joints. Repeat five times.

14. Relax your forearms.

Bring your mind to your forearms. In order to relax your forearms, first relax the muscles and tendons at their ends, near the wrists and the elbows. Inhale deeply into the joints and then exhale while relaxing all of the forearm muscles. Repeat five times.

15. Relax your elbows.

Next, bring your mind to your elbows. Inhale deeply into the joints and then exhale while relaxing deep into the joints. Repeat five times.

16. Relax your upper-arms.

Next, bring your mind to your upper-arms. In order to relax your upper-arms, first relax the muscles and tendons near the elbows and the shoulders. Inhale deeply into the joints and then exhale while relaxing the muscles. Repeat five times.

17. Relax your shoulders.

Next, bring your mind to your shoulders. Inhale deeply into the joints and then exhale while relaxing all the joints. Repeat five times.

18. Relax your abdomen and Lower Dan Tian.

After you loosen and relax your limbs, bring your mind to your abdomen. Inhale deeply and bring your mind to your body's center of gravity. Then, exhale slowly and relax the entire abdominal area. Repeat five times.

19. Relax your stomach area.

Now bring your mind to your stomach area. Inhale deeply and bring your mind deep into the stomach area. Then, exhale slowly and relax the entire area. Repeat five times.

20. Relax your chest.

Bring your mind to your chest. Inhale deeply and place your mind at the solar plexus. Exhale slowly and relax the solar plexus, easing the tension and leading the accumulated *Qi* to the lungs. Repeat five times.

21. Relax your neck.

After you loosen and relax your chest, bring your mind to your neck. Inhale deeply and focus on the neck, deep into the joints. Exhale slowly and relax the entire neck. Repeat five times.

22. Relax your mind.

Now that you have relaxed your entire physical body, it is time to relax your mental body. Inhale deeply and allow your mind to enter into a deeper meditative state. The trick for doing this is to inhale deeply and then exhale, letting all thoughts go and leading the physical body deeper into a relaxed state. Repeat as many times as you wish.

23. Recovery.

When you decide to wake up, stretch out your arms for several minutes. Then turn your body to the sides a few times to loosen up the torso. You have now completed the entire practice.

Small Circulation (Microcosmic Circulation)

Generally speaking, there are two main purposes of Small Circulation Meditation practice. The first purpose is learning to build up an abundant amount of *Qi* and store it in the Lower *Dan Tian*. The Lower *Dan Tian* is the battery which can store bioelectricity in your body. It is from this central battery that the *Qi* is distributed to the eight vessels (*Qi* reservoirs). From these eight *Qi* vessels, the *Qi* circulating in the twelve primary channels is regulated. When the *Qi* storage in the Lower *Dan Tian* is abundant, your life force and spirit are raised. When the *Qi* is weak and deficient, your entire body's functioning is weakened.

The second purpose of Small Circulation is to use the mind to lead the *Qi* to circulate in the two most important vessels, the Conception and Governing Vessels. According to Chinese medicine, these two vessels are the main vessels which regulate the twelve primary *Qi* channels. If you can use your mind to lead the abundant *Qi* to circulate in these two vessels, then the *Qi* can be distributed throughout the entire physical body through the twelve channels. Physical degeneration can then be slowed. In addition, through this network, the immune system will obtain plenty of *Qi* for its defensive functioning in your body.

To practice Small Circulation, the first step is learning abdominal breathing. In abdominal breathing, the abdominal area moves up and down to pull the diaphragm down and up, helping the lungs to take in air and get rid of carbon dioxide. In addition, through abdominal up and down exercises, *Qi* is recovered from fat. As mentioned in Section 2-2, this kind of exercise is called "back to childhood breathing" (*Fan Tong Hu Xi,* 返童呼吸). The reason for this is that a child uses the abdominal area to breath. This breathing is also commonly known as a "start the fire" (*Qi Huo,* 起火) exercise. Fire means "*Qi.*" Generally, there are two types of "start the fire" exercises— "Normal Abdominal Breathing" (*Zheng Hu Xi,* 正呼吸) which is also called "Buddhist Breathing" and "Reverse Abdominal Breathing" (*Fan Hu Xi,* 反呼吸) which is called "Daoist Breathing." Normally, Normal Abdominal Breathing is more relaxed and Reverse Abdominal Breathing is more aggressive.

After you are familiar with Normal Abdominal Breathing and Reverse Abdominal Breathing, then you must learn "Embryo Breathing" (*Tai Xi,* 胎息) which teaches you how to lead the *Qi* to the real Lower *Dan Tian* and store it there. All of these efforts aim at an abundant store of *Qi* in the Lower *Dan Tian*. Next, I will briefly explain these three practices for Small Circulation. Then, I will summarize the concept of Small Circulation.

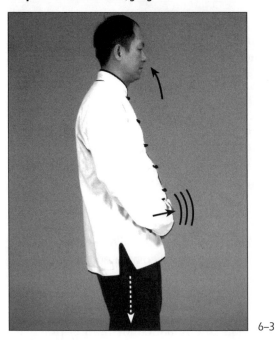
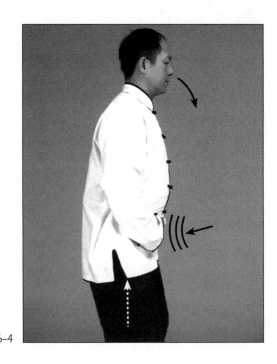

6-3   6-4

Normal Abdominal Breathing and Reverse Breathing

In **Normal Abdominal Breathing, when you inhale, the abdomen is gently pushed out and when you exhale, the abdomen is withdrawn** (Figures 6-3 and 6-4). In order to fill up the *Qi* to an abundant level in the lower abdominal area, **when you inhale you should also gently push your *Huiyin* (Co-1) cavity (or anus) out and when you exhale, you hold it up gently** (Figure 6-5). Remember, you should not tense this area during either inhalation or exhalation unless you are doing some special training such as Hard *Qigong*. Tension in this area can only make the *Qi* circulation stagnant in Small Circulation practice.

In Reverse Abdominal Breathing, when you inhale, the abdomen is gently pulled inward, and when you exhale the abdomen is gently pushed outward (Figures 6-6 and 6-7). Again, the coordination of the *Huiyin* (Co-1) cavity (or anus) is very important. The *Huiyin* cavity is a major gate which regulates the four *Yin* vessels, and therefore controls the *Qi* status of the body. Traditionally, a master will not reveal this secret of *Huiyin* control to any student until he was completely trusted by the master.

When you practice **Reverse Abdominal Breathing, as you inhale you should gently pull your *Huiyin* (Co-1) cavity (or anus) up, and as you exhale you should gently push it out**. Again, you should not tense this area during either inhalation or exhalation unless you are doing some special training such as Hard *Qigong*.

Often, a *Qigong* beginner will mistakenly believe that Reverse Abdominal Breathing is not natural. On the contrary, Reverse Abdominal Breathing is one of our normal breathing habits. Normally, if your emotions are not disturbed or you do not have any intention to energize your muscular power to a higher manifestation of power, you use Normal Breathing. However, when your emotional mind is disturbed, you may change your breathing into Reverse Breathing without realizing it. For example, when you are happy and laugh, you exhale while making the sound of *"Ha,"* and your abdominal area pushes out. When you are sad and cry, you inhale while making the sound of *"Hen,"* and your

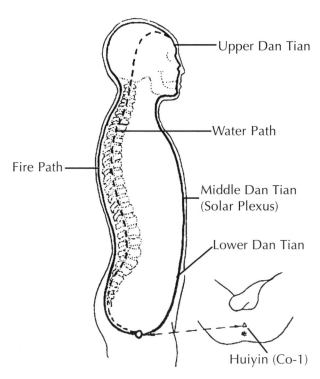

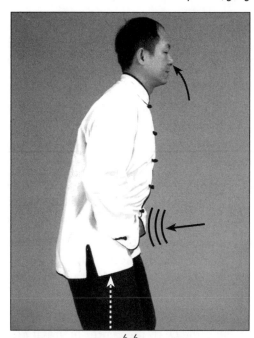

Upper Dan Tian

Water Path

Fire Path

Middle Dan Tian
(Solar Plexus)

Lower Dan Tian

Huiyin (Co-1)

Figure 6–5. The Huiyin Cavity (Co-1)

6-6

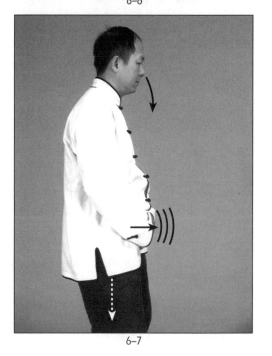

6-7

abdomen is withdrawn. Also, when you are scared, you inhale while holding your abdomen inward.

As mentioned previously, another occasion in which you use Reverse Breathing is when you have an intention to energize your muscular power to a higher, more powerful and spiritual state. For example, if you are pushing a car or lifting a heavy weight, you will use Reverse Breathing. In order to manifest your power to a higher level in martial arts, you must train your Reverse Breathing technique to be more efficient. This is the secret of *Jin* and the way of the Dao.

Often, a *Qigong* or martial arts beginner encounters the problem of tightness in the abdominal area. The reason for this is that in Reverse Breathing, when you inhale the diaphragm is pulling downward while the abdominal area is withdrawing. This can generate tension in the stomach area. To reduce this problem, you must start on a small scale with Reverse Breathing, and only after you can control the muscles in the abdominal area efficiently, gradually relax the area and eliminate the problem. Naturally, this will take time.

Embryo Breathing

As discussed in Section 2-2, according to Daoist research, the Lower *Dan Tian* on the front of the abdominal area is illusory. Therefore, it is called "False *Dan Tian*" (*Jia Dan Tian*, 假丹田). The argument is that, although the front side of the abdominal area can build up the fire or grow elixir (i.e., *Qi*), it cannot store it. Since the front side of the lower abdomen is located on the Conception Vessel, once the *Qi* is built up, it immediately flows into the vessel for circulation. Even though you can build up a stronger and more healthy body, you have not stored abundant *Qi* for longevity or enlightenment cultivation.

In order to store your *Qi* at a more abundant level, you must know the location of the real battery in the body. According to Daoist experience, the "Real *Dan Tian*" (*Zhen Dan Tian*, 真丹田) is at the center of your abdominal area, or the center of gravity (c.g.).

In the same section, we also discussed how we can evaluate the accuracy of the name "Real *Dan Tian*" according to traditional understanding and scientific and logical analysis. To help you understand the importance of Embryo Breathing, you should again review Section 2-2.

After the *Qi* is built up in the lower abdominal area, Embryo Breathing can be used to lead the *Qi* to the center of gravity for storage. In order to reach this goal, the first step is to keep the mind on the real *Dan Tian*. This training is called "keep the mind at the *Dan Tian*" (*Yi Shou Dan Tian*, 意守丹田). According to the theory, the mind can generate an EMF (electromotive force), which can lead the *Qi* or bioelectricity to circulate. Through the mind's thinking, the *Qi* is led. Therefore, if you can keep your mind on the real *Dan Tian*, the *Qi* can be led and stored there.

The question remains, how do we reach this goal in training? The most difficult task is for your mind to feel the center of gravity or the real *Dan Tian*. From my personal experience, I realize that in order to locate this center, when you breath you must first use both the front and the back sides of the abdominal area. The front and the back sides of the muscles must expand and withdraw evenly. After a long period of practice, this training will become a habit, and you will not need too much attention from your mind, i.e., you have reached the level of "regulating without regulating." Then you can move your mind gradually until you have the feel of the center.

Circulate the Qi in the Conception and Governing Vessels

As mentioned earlier, the second main purpose of Small Circulation is to use the mind to lead the *Qi* and to move it around the circuit of the Conception and Governing Vessels. This use of the mind to lead the *Qi* for any purpose is called "using the *Yi* to Lead the *Qi*" (*Yi Yi Yin Qi*, 以意引氣).

It is understood that there are three gates (*San Guan*, 三關) which could cause danger in Small Circulation practice. These three gates are the tailbone (*Weilu*, 尾閭), squeezing spine (*Jiaji*, 夾脊), and jade pillow (*Yuzhen*, 玉枕) (Figure 6-8). Normally, because of the danger involved, the method of opening or widening these gates usually requires the instruction from an experienced *Qigong* master to lead a student step by step until the entire cycle is completed. Because of space limitation in this book, we will leave this subject for the future book: ***Yang's Small and Grand Circulation Meditation***, by YMAA.

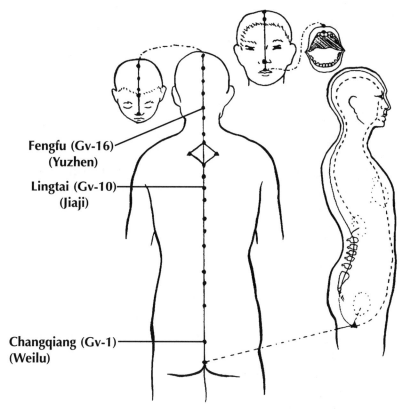

Figure 6–8. The Three Gates in Small Circulation

Grand Circulation

After you have completed the Small Circulation, you should continue your practice through Embryo Breathing to build up the *Qi* in the real *Dan Tian* to a more abundant level. This process can take from twenty to fifty years as you build up your *Qi* to an abundant level for your longevity and enlightenment cultivation practice. Remember, the key to enlightenment is to lead the *Qi* to the brain to activate more brain cells.

In addition, you should also learn how to lead the *Qi* to circulate in the body or exchange it with the *Qi* around you for some special practices. This practice is called Grand Circulation (*Da Zhou Tian,* 大周天). Here, I will briefly introduce three practices which are commonly trained in martial arts *Qigong*.

Four Gates Breathing (*Si Xin Hu Xi,* 四心呼吸)

According to Chinese medicine, there are four gates which regulate the body's *Qi*. Two of these gates are at the center of the palms and are called "labor palace" (*Laogong,* P-8, 勞宮), while the other two are near the center of the soles of the feet and are called "bubbling well" (*Yongquan,* K-1, 湧泉). The *Laogong* cavities belong to the Pericardium Primary *Qi* Channel, which regulates the *Qi* condition in the heart (fire *Qi*). The *Yongquan* cavities belong to the Kidney Primary *Qi* Channel and regulate the *Qi* of the kidneys (water *Qi*). When the *Qi* condition of these two channels is well regulated, the body can be in a state of harmonious balance. Therefore, using meditation to lead the *Qi* to these four gates is a very important practice in Internal Elixir Grand Circulation practice. This kind of training is called Four Gates Breathing.

For the martial artist, learning how to lead the *Qi* to these four gates is also very important. When the *Qi* can be led to the palms, your strikes can be strong, and when the *Qi* can be led to the bottom of the feet, the root can be strong and firm. Four Gates Breathing training is not only beneficial for health but also for martial arts.

Skin Marrow Breathing *(Ti Sui Xi, 體髓息)*

Skin Marrow Breathing is another common practice in Chinese martial arts, especially in internal *Qigong* training. The first purpose of this training is to use the mind, in coordination with Reverse Breathing, to lead the *Qi* to the skin surface to strengthen the Guardian *Qi*. From this training, the immune system can be strengthened, and the sensitivity of the *Qi* through skin can be increased. This is important in internal martial arts. This kind of skin feeling is called Listening *Jin (Ting Jin,* 聽勁*)*.

The second purpose of this training is to lead the *Qi* inward to nourish the bone marrow. From this nourishing practice, the blood cells produced can be more robust (both in quantity and quality). When the blood cells are abundant and healthy, the oxygen, nutrition, and *Qi* can be carried by the blood cells smoothly to every place of the body. Consequently, the life force can be strong. It is known that marrow washing *Qigong* is one of the main keys to longevity. If you are interested in this subject, please refer to the book: **Muscle/Tendon Changing and Marrow/Brain Washing Chi Kung**, by Dr. Yang.

Grand Transportation Gong *(Zhou Tian Mai Yun Gong, 周天邁運功)*

Grand Transportation *Gong* is a practice in which a martial artist learns how to use the mind to lead the *Qi*, following the spine upward to the *Shenzhu* (Gv-12) cavity. It is then divided and spread to the arms for *Jin* manifestation (Figure 6-9). In order to balance the *Qi* leading upward, another flow of *Qi* is also led downward to the bottoms of the feet for rooting.

For *Qigong* practitioners, Grand Transportation includes leading the *Qi* out of the body to exchange with surrounding objects. These objects can be other people, animals, plants or any other natural energy. The naturally surrounding *Qi* is also absorbed into the body for nourishment. Grand Transportation training is a vast subject in Chinese *Qigong* practice.

Spiritual Cultivation

The final goal of still meditation is to seek the most original nature of our spirit. In order to reach this goal, you must first learn to keep your mind in a neutral state, free from emotional bondage. To accomplish this, you must learn how to use your wisdom mind to govern your emotional mind. Slowly and gradually, after a long period of self-regulation and mental cultivation, you will find the balance of *Yin* and *Yang*. From this balance, you can lead your mind to the center of nature, i.e., state of no extremity (*Wuji*, 無極). When you are in this *Wuji* state, the spirit of vitality is raised beyond all emotional disturbance. Only then can spiritual enlightenment be reached.

The first step to spiritual cultivation is learning how to lead the *Qi* from the Lower *Dan Tian* to the brain to nourish the brain cells to a more energized level. Naturally, in order to have abundant *Qi* to nourish your brain, you must first know how to build up and store the *Qi* in the Lower *Dan Tian* using Embryo Breathing. If you do not have plenty of *Qi* stored in the Lower *Dan Tian* to lead upward to nourish your brain, the *Qi* supply to your physical body will be weak.

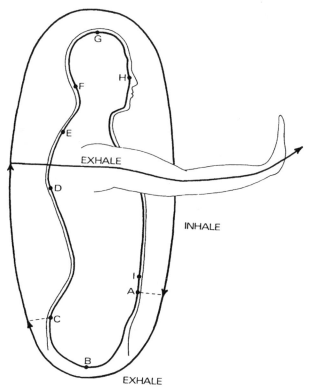

Figure 6-9. Grand Circulation

Consequently, the Guardian *Qi*, which is required to nourish the immune system against negative influences, will also be weak. Naturally, your physical health will be significantly reduced.

The process of leading the *Qi* upward to nourish the brain is called "Return the Essence to Nourish the Brain *Gong*" (*Huan Jing Bu Nao*, 還精補腦功). The more brain cells that are activated and nourished, the higher your spirit can be raised.

To raise your spirit to a higher level, the first step is to keep the spirit at its central residence. This process is called "Keep the Mind at the Spirit" (*Shou Shen*, 守神), and means that you must learn to lead your mind to the third eye (forehead), which is considered to be the residence of the spirit.

The next step is learning how to firm and solidify the spirit. From this process, the spirit can be raised to a stronger level. This process is called "Stabilize the Spirit" (*Ding Shen*, 定神). From the continual nourishment of *Qi* to the brain from the Lower *Dan Tian*, the spirit can grow firm and strong. This process can take many, many years of cultivation and nourishment.

After you reach the goal of stabilizing your spirit, and know how to nourish it to a higher spiritual level, then you should learn how to focus your spirit at your third eye. This process is called "Condense the Spirit" (*Ning Shen*, 凝神). Even while you are focusing, you should not be tense. This process is not as simple as most people think. Normally, when you focus, you will be tense and get a headache. However, if you have practiced meditation for a long time, you will gradually grasp the trick of condensing without tension.

Through condensing practice, the *Qi* will be concentrated at the third eye. It is believed that after a long period of correct meditation with an abundant nourishing of *Qi* to the brain, the spirit can separate from the third eye and gradually become independent. This process is called "Exit

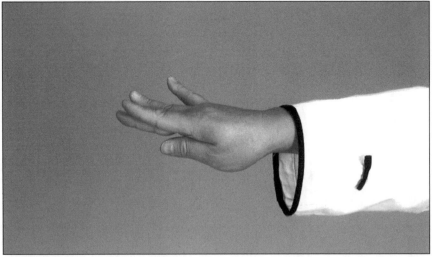

6-10

the Gate" (*Chu Qiao,* 出竅). When this happens, a "baby spirit" is born. You will then continue to nourish this spirit baby until it grows stronger and stronger. It is believed in Buddhist and Daoist society that this spirit baby can eventually grow so strong that it can survive without the existence of the physical body. When this happens, you will escape the routine spiritual path of reincarnation and become a Buddha. Naturally, if your goal is not so high, you may still gain a peaceful spirit and profound comprehension of your life.

6-3. Moving Soft Gong (*Dong Gong,* 動功)

As discussed in previous chapters, in order to have good health and great martial *Jin* you must satisfy two important conditions: a strong and healthy physical body (*Yang*), and abundant *Qi* storage and circulation (*Yin*). If you do not have a strong body but only abundant *Qi*, it is like having a great battery or power supply, yet a poor machine to manifest the stored energy into power. In the same way, if you have a great and strong machine but lack an abundant energy supply, the machine is still useless. Therefore, in order to have powerful *Jin* manifestation, you must have both a healthy and strong physical body and an abundant store of *Qi*.

In this section, first I would like to introduce some stretching and warming up exercises which can loosen up your physical body to the deep joint areas. In addition, through these stretching and warming up exercises, you will be able to stimulate the cells which are in the deep places of the body. Normally, due to lack of stimulation, the *Qi* and blood circulation to these cells is stagnant, which results in the fast degeneration of our physical body. This is the same theory as in some Yoga styles in which stretching is the major part of the practice.

Since White Crane emphasizes the movement of the torso (i.e., spine) and the chest, the stretching and warming up exercises for these areas have become the first step in *Qigong* practice. After stretching and warming up, the Flying Crane *Qigong* set will be introduced.

Before we start the Palm Set of Soft Crane *Qigong*, you should understand a few important points:

1. **The hand forms of White Crane palm should be accurate.** In the White Crane hand form, the thumb and the middle finger are pushed slightly forward while the index finger is straightened and the ring finger and pinkie are lifted softly backward (Figure 6-10). This hand form imitates the wing of a crane. The thumb and index finger are more tensed

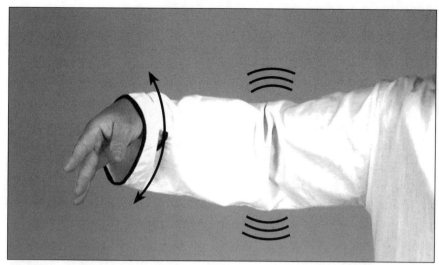

6-11

because this side of the wing encounters the wind while flying. The middle finger is forward but semi-tensed to keep the *Laogong* (*P-8*) cavity opened. The *Laogong* cavity is a major *Qi* gate, and is used to regulate the heart when it becomes too *Yang*. When this cavity is wide open, the heart will not be too *Yang* because of long flying (i.e., long fighting) or too excited emotionally. The middle finger is semi-tensed so it can support the index finger and thumb. However, the ring finger and pinkie are very soft and relaxed. When they are relaxed, the *Qi* can circulate smoothly to the palm in order to support the physical manifestation of flying capability. Without this smooth *Qi* circulation in the palm, the entire hand will be stiff and the flight will not last long.

2. **Smooth and relaxed movement of the chest and the torso is the key to flying.** The Crane is a long distance flyer, and is different from short distance birds such as the sparrow. If you look carefully, you will see that when a sparrow is flying, its wings are fast and stiff. The flapping of the wings is carried out by the muscles in the shoulder area. Therefore, after flying for a while, the muscles are tensed and the flight cannot continue. However, if you look at the flying manner of a long distance bird such as the crane or stork, you will see that the wing flapping is slow and more relaxed, graceful and sweeping. When this kind of bird flies, it uses more of its chest and spine muscles (i.e., torso). In order to go far, the entire body must be relaxed as the great wings glide upon thermal currents. From this you can see that the short distance bird uses its wings to carry its body, while the long distance bird uses its body to carry its body. Therefore, when you practice Soft White Crane *Qigong* and *Jin* manifestation, the chest and the spine must be relaxed yet strong.

A. STRETCHING AND WARMING UP

1. Loosening up the Joints

For stretching, the first step is loosening up the joint areas. The common joints that should be loosened are the wrists, elbows, shoulders, spine, hips, knees and ankles.

When you loosen your wrist joints, shake your elbow sideways while letting the hands swing from side to side (Figure 6-11). This will loosen up the wrist effectively. If you use the muscles near the wrist area to move the hands from side to side, the muscles near the wrist area will be tensed, and the loosening efficiency will be low.

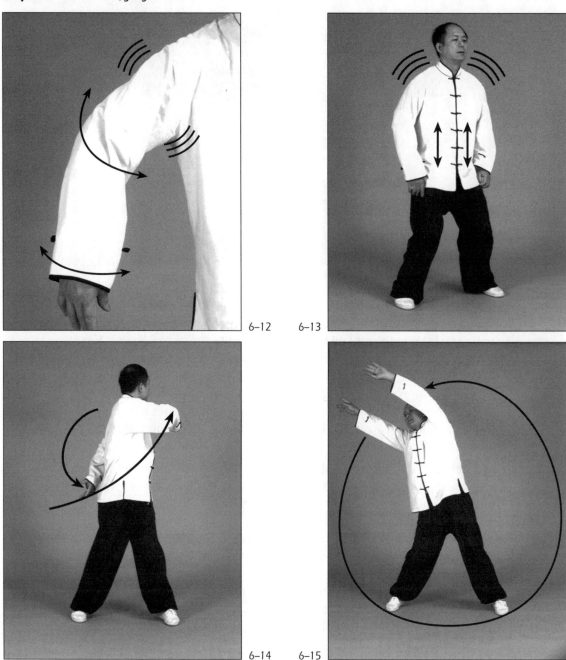

6-12   6-13

6-14   6-15

In the same way, when you loosen up your elbow area, you should move your shoulders and allow your arms to swing around (Figure 6-12). This will loosen up the entire arm area. Next, bounce your body up and down (Figure 6-13). When you do this, you start to loosen your torso. This up and down bouncing motion will also make the joints in the arms reach a deeper loose and relaxed state. This bouncing motion of the body is used to loosen up the joints. It is the most basic *Qigong* exercise. In fact, we can still see these kinds of up and down body bouncing exercises in various dances around the world.

Next, twist your torso from side to side while swinging both of your arms naturally (Figure 6-14). This twisting and swinging exercise will enhance the torso's loosening, especially in the waist area. Then, circle your upper body down, up and around in each direction an equal number of times (Figure 6-15). This will help to stretch and loosen the torso.

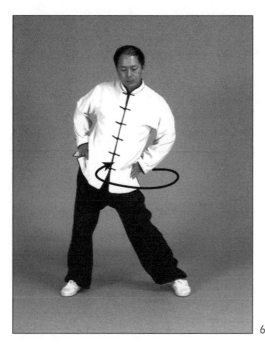

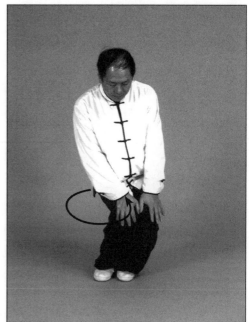

6-16   6-17

Next, circle your waist horizontally, first to one side and then to the other (Figure 6-16). This will loosen the lower back area and the hip joints. Then, squat down slightly and circle both of your knees horizontally in each direction a few times to loosen up the knee joints (Figure 6-17). Finally, circle the ankles of each leg a few times each direction (Figure 6-18). This concludes the loosening and warming up exercises. The number of repetitions for each exercise is up to you. Sometimes, when your body is more tense, you might want to move more. Other times, you may wish to do less.

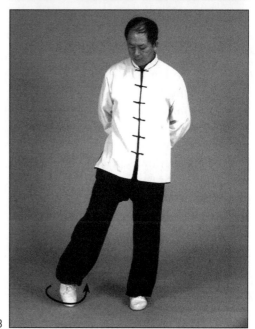

6-18

2. Stretching

After you have loosened up your joints and warmed up, you should start to stretch your physical body. If you stretch your body correctly, you can stimulate the cells into an excited state, and this will improve *Qi* and blood circulation. This is the key to maintaining the health of the physical body. However, when you stretch you should treat your muscles, tendons and ligaments like a rubber band. If you stretch too much too soon, you will break the rubber band. For muscles, tendons and ligaments, that means the tearing off of fibers. However, if you under stretch, it will not be effective. A good stretch should feel comfortable and stimulating.

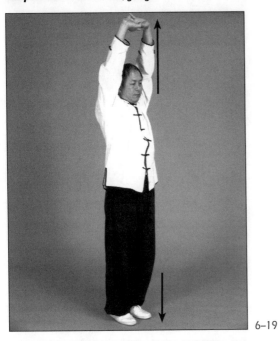 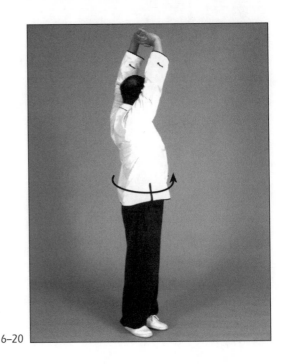

6-19   6-20

Stretching the Torso (Shuang Shou Tuo Tian, 雙手托天)

Theoretically, the first place that should be stretched and loosened is the muscles of the trunk, rather than the limbs. The trunk is at the center of the whole body, and it contains the major muscles which control the trunk and also surround the internal organs. When the trunk muscles are tense, the whole body will be tense and the internal organs will be compressed. This causes stagnation of the *Qi* circulation in the body, and especially in the organs. For this reason, the trunk muscles should be stretched and loosened up before the limbs prior to any *Qigong* practice. Remember, people die from failure of the internal organs, rather than problems in the limbs. **The best *Qigong* practice is to remove *Qi* stagnation and maintain smooth *Qi* circulation in the internal organs.**

For these reasons, many *Qigong* practices start out with movements that stretch the trunk muscles. For example, in the Standing Eight Pieces of Brocade, the first piece stretches the trunk to loosen up the chest, stomach and lower abdomen (which are the triple burners in Chinese medicine). In fact, the following exercise is adapted from the Standing Eight Pieces of Brocade exercises.

First, interlock your fingers and lift your hands up over your head while imagining that you are pushing upward with your hands and pushing downward with your feet (Figure 6-19). Do not tense your muscles, because this will constrict your body and prevent you from stretching. If you do this stretch correctly, you will feel the muscles in your waist area tensing slightly because they are being pulled simultaneously from the top and the bottom. Next, use your mind to relax and stretch out a little bit more. After you have stretched for about ten seconds, twist your upper body to one side to twist the trunk muscles (Figure 6-20). Stay to the side for three to five seconds, turn your body to face forward and then turn to the other side. Stay there for three to five seconds. Repeat the upper body twisting three times, come back to the center, and tilt your upper body to the side and stay there for about three seconds (Figure 6-21), then tilt to the other side. Next, bend forward, touch your hands to the ground and use your pelvis to wave the hips from

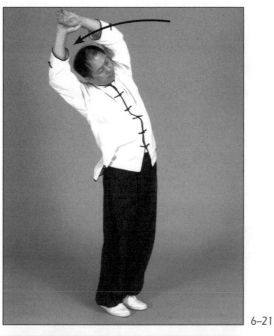

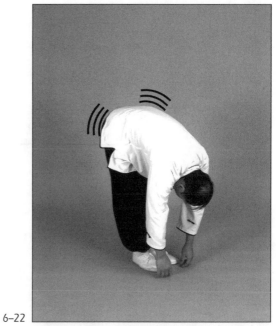

6–21   6–22

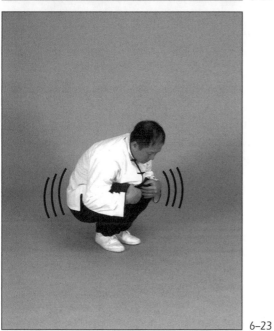

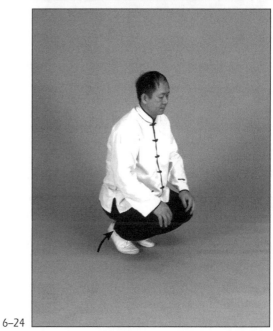

6–23   6–24

side to side to loosen up the lower spine (Figure 6-22). Stay there for three to five seconds. Finally, squat down with your feet flat on the ground to stretch your ankles (Figure 6-23) and then lift your heels up to stretch the toes (Figure 6-24). Repeat the entire process at least three times. After you finish, the inside of your body should feel very comfortable and warm.

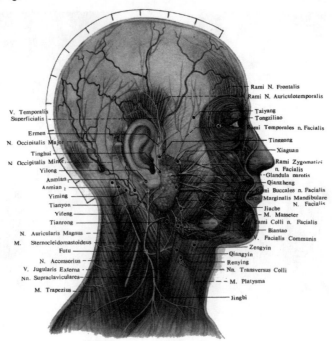

Figure 6–25. The Muscles in the Neck

Stretching and Loosening up the Neck *(Bai He Shen Jing, Na Zha Tan Hai,* 白鶴伸頸，哪吒探海*)*

After you have stretched your torso, next you should stretch your neck. The neck is the junction of the blood and *Qi* exchanging path between the head and the body. Whenever the neck is stiffened or the spine in the neck is injured, this blood and *Qi* exchange will be stagnant. Consequently, your brain will not have proper nourishment. Therefore, in order to maintain your health, you must learn the correct manner of loosening up the neck, including the muscles, tendons, and ligaments.

First, you should stretch the muscles and tendons around the neck and gradually reach to the ligaments, which are hidden deeply between the joints. To stretch the neck muscles and tendons, you should focus on the four biggest muscles/tendons located on the front and the back side of your neck (Figure 6-25). When you stretch your front neck muscles/tendons, you may turn your head backward diagonally while pressing your shoulder backward (Figure 6-26). Start the stretching gently for twenty seconds, then shift the stretching to the rear neck muscles/tendons. When you stretch your rear neck muscles/tendons, simply press your head downward and toward the side (Figure 6-27). Again, stretch for twenty seconds. After you have gone through the four sets of muscles/tendons, repeat from the beginning for another thirty seconds each. You should stretch each muscle/tendon group at least three times. This will provide good stimulation to the muscles/tendons through stretching.

After you have stretched the four neck muscle/tendon groups, extend your head forward with the four muscle/tendon groups evenly stretched (Figure 6-28). To make the stretching more efficient, you may gently push both of your shoulders backward. The goal is to stretch the ligaments instead of the muscles and tendons. Stay in this stretching position for twenty seconds, then turn your head to your left slowly, and then to your right slowly (Figure 6-29). This will help you stretch and loosen up the ligaments in the neck. Repeat the turning two more times on each side.

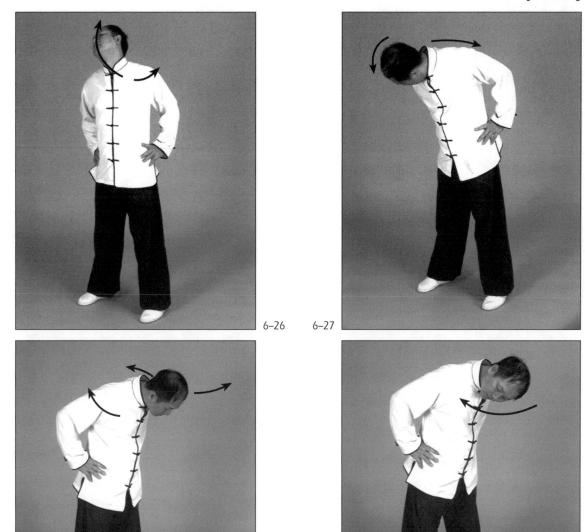

6–26   6–27

6–28   6–29

Finally, gently circle your head to one side on a small scale for about ten times, and then the other side for another ten times (Figure 6-30). You should not circle your neck to its extreme range of motion, since this may damage your cartilage and neck joints. This is a common cause of arthritis in the lower neck area in later life.

3. Loosening Up the Torso and Internal Organs

The torso is supported by the spine and the trunk muscles. Once you have stretched your trunk muscles, you can loosen up the torso. This also moves the muscles inside your body around, which moves and relaxes your internal organs. This, in turn, makes it possible for the *Qi* to circulate smoothly inside your body. Next, I would like to introduce a few torso movements which I believe are the most beneficial *Qigong* exercises in my experience. These movements are practiced in the Southern White Crane style for loosening up the torso and chest.

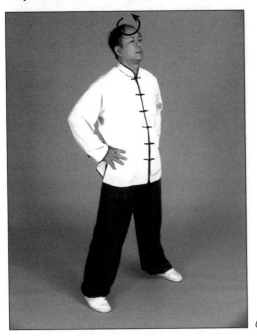 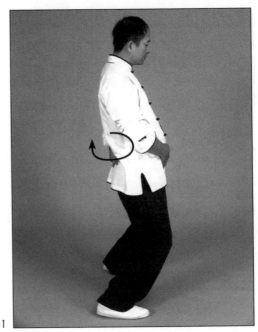

6-30   6-31

Circle the Waist Horizontally (Pin Yuan Niu Yao, 平圓扭腰)

This exercise helps you to regain conscious control of the muscles in your abdomen. The Lower *Dan Tian* is the main residence of your Original *Qi*. The *Qi* in your Lower *Dan Tian* can be led easily only when your abdomen is loose and relaxed. These abdominal exercises are probably the most important of all the internal *Qigong* practices.

To practice this exercise, squat down slightly in the Horse Stance. Without moving your thighs or upper body, use the waist muscles to move the abdomen around in a horizontal circle (Figure 6-31). Circle in one direction about ten times and then in the other direction about ten times. If you hold one hand over your Lower *Dan Tian* and the other on your sacrum, you may be able to focus your attention better on the area you want to control.

In the beginning, you may have difficulty making your body move the way you want. But if you keep practicing, you will quickly learn how to do it. Once you can do the movement comfortably, make the circles larger and larger. Naturally, this will cause the muscles to tense somewhat and inhibit the *Qi* flow, but the more you practice the sooner you will again be able to relax. After you have practiced for a while and can control your waist muscles easily, start making the circles smaller and also start using your *Yi* to lead the *Qi* from the Lower *Dan Tian* to move in these circles. The final goal is to have only a slight physical movement, but a strong movement of *Qi*.

There are four major benefits to this abdominal exercise. First, when your Lower *Dan Tian* area is loose, the *Qi* can flow in and out easily. This is especially important for martial arts *Qigong* practitioners who use the Lower *Dan Tian* as their main source of *Qi*. Second, when the abdominal area is loose, the *Qi* circulation in the large and small intestines will be smooth and they will be able to absorb nutrients and eliminate waste. If your body does not eliminate effectively, the absorption of nutrients will be hindered and you may become sick. Third, when the abdominal area is loose, the *Qi* in the kidneys will circulate smoothly and the Original Essence stored in the kidneys can be converted more efficiently into *Qi*. In addition, when the kidney area is loosened, the kidney *Qi* can be led downward and upward to nourish the entire body. Fourth, these exercises eliminate *Qi* stagnation in the lower back, healing and preventing lower back pain. Furthermore, this exercise can also help you rebuild the strength of the muscles in the waist area.

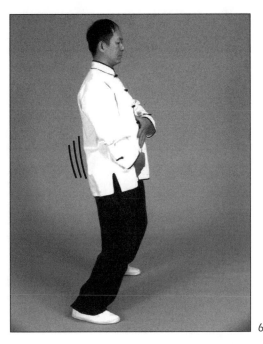

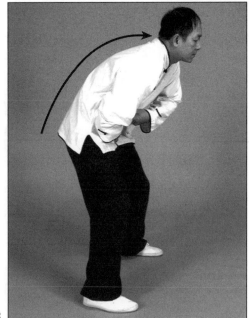

6-32   6-33

Waving the Spine and Massaging the Internal Organs
(*Ji Zhui Bo Dong, Nei Zang An Mo,*
脊椎波動，內臟按摩)

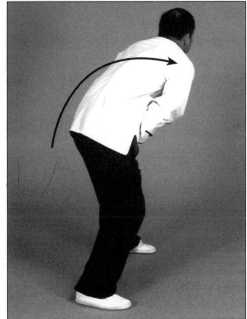

6-34

Beneath your diaphragm is your stomach, on its right is your liver and on its left is your spleen. Once you can comfortably do the movement in your lower abdomen, change the movement from horizontal to vertical and extend it up to your diaphragm. The easiest way to loosen the area around the diaphragm is to use a wave-like motion between the perineum and the diaphragm (Figures 6-32 and 6-33). You may find it helpful when you practice this to place one hand on your Lower *Dan Tian* and your other hand above it with the thumb on the solar plexus. Use a forward and backward wave-like motion, flowing up to the diaphragm and down to the perineum and back. Practice ten times.

Next, continue the movement while turning your body slowly to one side and then to the other (Figure 6-34). This will slightly tense the muscles on one side and loosen them on the other, which will massage the internal organs. Repeat ten times.

This exercise loosens the muscles around the stomach, liver, gall bladder and spleen, and therefore improves the *Qi* circulation in these areas. It also trains you to use your mind to lead *Qi* from your Lower *Dan Tian* upward to the solar plexus area.

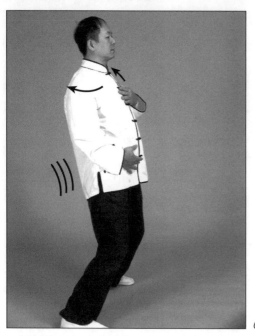
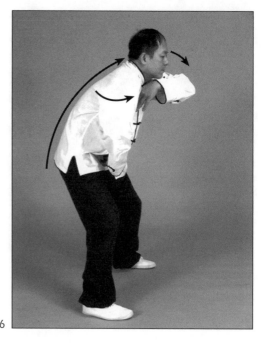

6-35   6-36

Thrust the Chest and Arc the Chest *(Tan Xiong Gong Bei, 袒胸拱背)*

After loosening up the center portion of your body, extend the movement up to your chest. The wave-like movement starts in the abdomen, moves through the stomach and then up to the chest. You may find it easier to feel the movement if you hold one hand on your abdomen and the other lightly on your chest. You should also coordinate with the shoulders' movement. Inhale when you move your shoulders backward (Figure 6-35) and exhale when you move them forward (Figure 6-36). The inhalation and exhalation should be as deep as possible and the entire chest should be very loose. When you move your spine, you should be able to feel the vertebrae move section by section. Repeat the motion ten times.

This exercise loosens up the chest and helps to regulate and improve the *Qi* circulation in the lungs. It also teaches Martial Arts *Qigong* practitioners to lead *Qi* to the shoulders in coordination with the body's movements. In White Crane martial applications, *Jin* (power) is generated by the legs or waist, directed by the pelvis and manifested by the hands. In order to do this, your body from the waist to the hands must be soft and connected like a whip. Only then will there be no stagnation to hold back the power.

White Crane Waves Its Wing *(Bai He Dou Chi, 白鶴抖翅)*

Once you have completed the loosening up of the chest area, extend the motion to your arms and fingers. First, practice the motion with both arms ten times and then do each arm individually ten times. When you extend the movement to the arms, you first generate the motion from the legs or the waist and direct this power upward. It passes through the chest and shoulders and finally reaches the arms (Figures 6-37 and 6-38). When you practice with one arm, you also twist your body slightly to direct the movement (Figures 6-39 and 6-40).

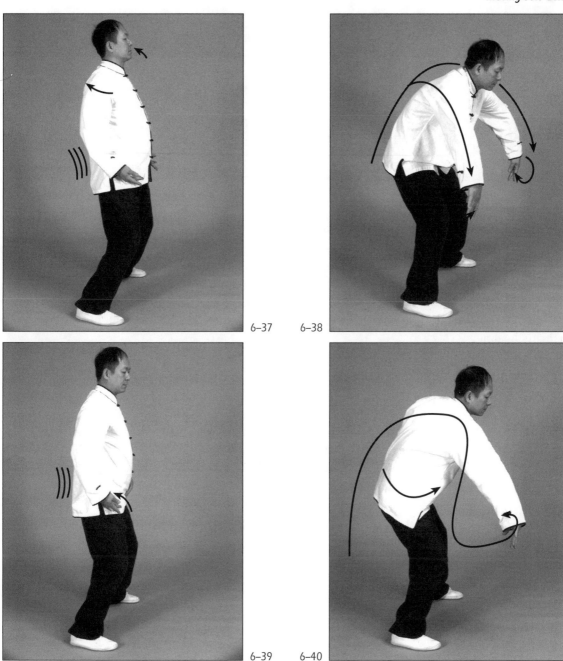

6–37   6–38

6–39   6–40

These exercises will loosen up every joint in your body from the waist to the fingers. These exercises are in fact the fundamental practice of *Jin* manifestation in the Soft Styles of Chinese martial arts.

B. FUNDAMENTAL PRACTICES

Before introducing Flying Crane *Qigong*, you should first be familiar with some basic and fundamental training. From this practice, you will be able to build up a firm foundation for White Crane Soft *Qigong*.

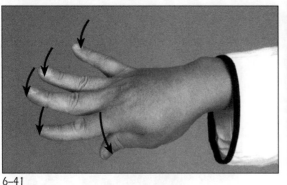

6-41

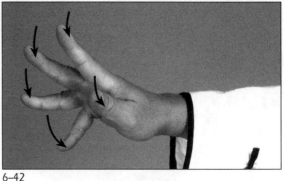

6-42

1. Finger and Wrist Gong (*Zhi Wan Gong*) 指腕功

Finger and wrist *Gong* specializes in training a White Crane practitioner how to loosen up the joints in the fingers and wrists. The same exercises can also be used to strengthen the tendons/muscles and ligaments of the finger and wrist joints. Next, we will introduce five basic movements which can serve these purposes. The soft joint exercises have commonly been used to expedite the healing process for the finger and wrist joint injury. They can also be used for arthritis healing.

a. Waving the Fingers (*Zhi Bo Gong*) 指波功

Waving the fingers practice specializes in training the base joints of the five fingers. The first purpose is to loosen up these joints so the *Qi* can circulate to the finger tips. The second purpose is to build up the endurance and the strength of the tendons/muscles and ligaments in these joints. When you practice for the first goal, your joints must be as relaxed as possible. However, if you are aiming for the second goal, then the exercises should not be as loose and relaxed. Only you can decide if you would like to loosen or build up the endurance and strength of these base joints.

To practice, first bend your thumb forward without bending the second thumb joint. Immediately follow with bending the rest of the fingers. Again, when you bend these fingers, you are only bending the base joints while keeping the other two joints straight (Figure 6-41). Repeat the exercises 30 to 50 times.

Next, reverse the waving moving by starting from the pinkie and finally reaching the thumb for 30 to 50 repetitions (Figure 6-42). You may practice these exercises with both hands at the same time.

If you practice these exercises for loosening up, your hands should be as relaxed as possible. However, if you intend to build up the strength of these joints, you must slightly tense up the trained areas. If you are using these exercises for healing, you should be as relaxed as possible instead of tensing up.

b. Closing the Fingers or Octopus Gong (*Zhang Yu Gong*) 章魚功

Closing the Fingers practice aims for a moving connection from the wrist to the finger tips. Again, you may practice this exercise in either a hard or soft manner. The soft way is to loosen up and relax the joints while the hard way is to build up the strength of the joints, especially those joints located in the palms.

When you practice, first gently push both of your wrists inward toward the center of your chest (Figure 6-43). Next, expand both of your arms to the sides while moving your wrists out-

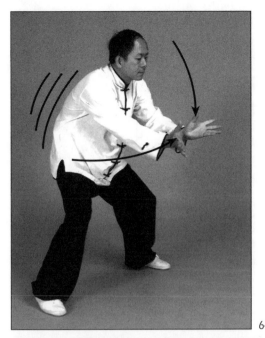

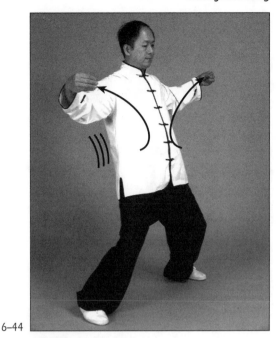

6-43   6-44

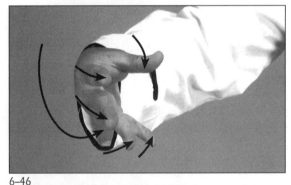

6-45

6-46

ward (Figure 6-44). When you are doing this, curl your palms inward and let the fingers follow the curling motion until they touch each other. In fact, the entire movement of the hand is just like an octopus' swimming motion (Figures 6-45 to 6-47).

After you have practiced for some time and have connected your shoulder, elbow, wrist and finger joints like a soft whip, you should start moving from the waist and the chest areas. The idea is to build up a smooth

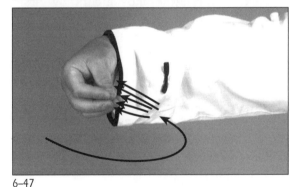

6-47

and relaxed connection through the joints from the waist area to the finger tips.

c. Side Spreading (*Wai Hua Gong*) 外化功

The purpose of side spreading practice is to train the entire arm's clockwise and counterclockwise circling motions. When the arms are circling, you also rotate your wrists. From this training, many defensive hand techniques can be developed. In fact, these exercises can be considered one of the most important and basic moving practice sets for the arms and wrists.

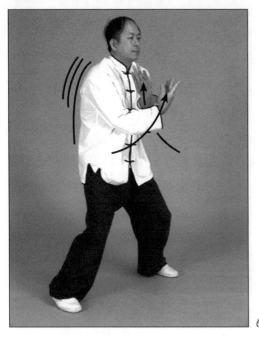

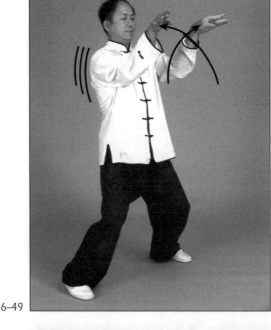

6–48   6–49

When you practice, first inhale, arc your back and withdraw your chest while scooping both of your arms upward with fingers pointing upward and palms facing you (Figure 6-48). Next, exhale and expand both of your arms to the sides while repelling with both of your hands (Figure 6-49). As you do this, straighten up your torso and thrust your chest out. Repeat these repelling movements 30 to 50 times.

Next, reverse the movements by first crossing both of your arms right in front of your upper chest with fingers pointing upward and palms facing you, and inhale deeply (Figure 6-50). Next, exhale and circle both arms down and then to the sides while bending your wrists and pointing the fingers downward (Figure 6-51). Again, repeat 30 to 50 times.

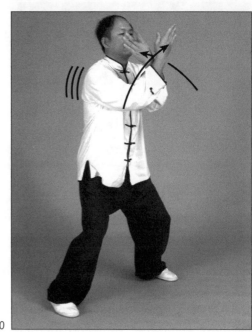

6–50

d. Downward Dropping

(Chen Chi Gong) 沈翅功

The purpose of this training is learning to use the sinking motion from the wrist and forearm area to seal, to restrict, or even to control the actions of the opponent's upper limbs. For example, in the Small Wrap Hand (*Xiao Chan Shou,* 小纏手) *Qin Na,* once you use your left hand to wrap the opponent's grabbing fingers, your right wrist's sinking action is very critical to making the control effective (Figure 6-52).

When you practice, first inhale and arc your back and withdraw your chest while scooping both of your arms upward with the fingers pointing upward (Figure 6-53). Next, exhale and move both of your arms forward and then downward (Figures 6-54 and 6-55). As you do this, straight-

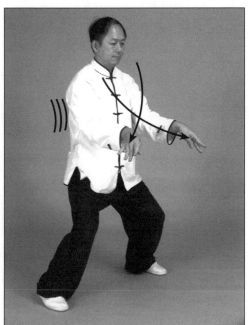

6–51

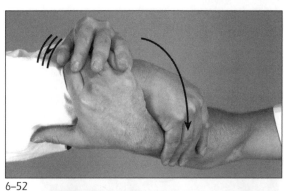

6–52

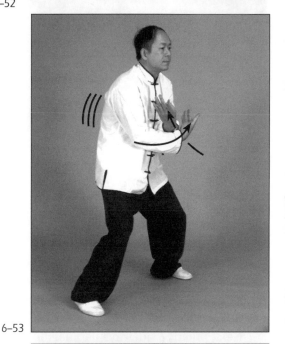

6–53

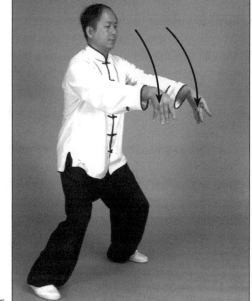

6–54

6–55

en up your torso and thrust your chest out. Repeat this downward dropping movement 30 to 50 times.

After you have practiced for a long time, slowly and gradually replace the muscular movements with relaxed and soft actions and a concentrated mind.

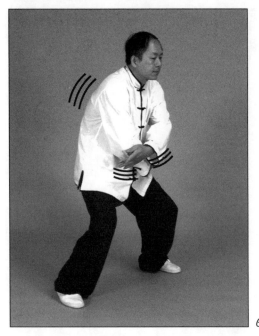
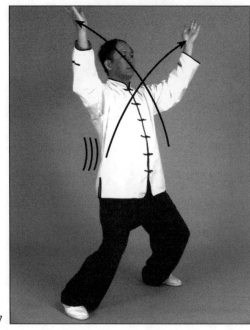

6-56   6-57

2. **Arm Flapping Gong** (*Pu Chi Gong*) 撲翅功

Arm Flapping *Gong* is to train a White Crane practitioner how to coordinate body movements with the flapping action of the arms. The flapping movement is generated by the waist and the action is manifested from the fingers.

First, practice the upward flapping. In this training, inhale, arc your back and withdraw your chest while placing both of your arms right in front of your chest area (Figure 6-56). Next, exhale and flap both of your arms upward and to the sides (Figure 6-57). As you do this, straighten up your torso and thrust your chest out. Repeat this flapping 30 to 50 times.

Next, practice sideways flapping. In this training, again inhale, arc your back and withdraw your chest while placing both of your arms right in front of your chest area (Figure 6-58). Next, exhale and flap both of your arms sideways (Figure 6-59). As you do this, straighten up your torso and thrust your chest out. Repeat this flapping 30 to 50 times.

Finally, practice the downward and sideways flapping. In this training, again inhale, arc your back and withdraw your chest while placing both of your arms right in front of your chest area (Figure 6-60). Next, exhale and flap both of your arms downward and sideways (Figure 6-61). As you do this, straighten up your torso and thrust your chest out. Repeat this grabbing 30 to 50 times.

When you practice this flapping exercise, you should use the tendons of the joints more than the muscles. This means you should be as relaxed as possible. The entire motion is just like a whip; the power is generated from the waist and ends up at the fingers.

3. **Coiling Gong** (*Chan Zhuan Gong*) 纏轉功

Coiling *Gong* is to train the coiling motion of your hands and wrists. In any soft martial style, coiling is a crucial and fundamental movement for techniques. When you train this *Gong,* you are imagining that your arm is coiling like a snake around a tree branch, soft, sticking and adhering.

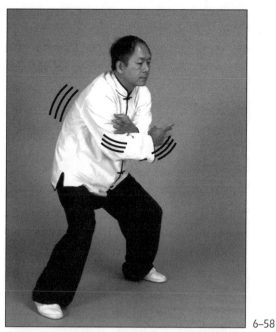
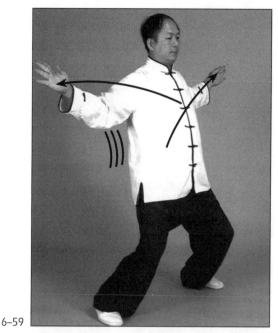

6-58   6-59

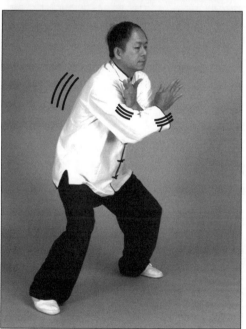
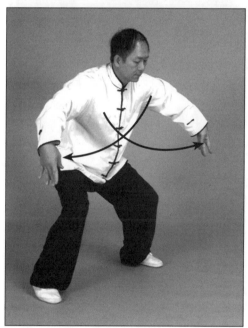

6-60   6-61

When you practice, place your left hand on your Lower *Dan Tian* area. This will help you feel the motion of the waist, which is used to direct the coiling action. First, inhale and generate the coiling action from the waist area, arc your back and withdraw your chest (Figure 6-62). Next, exhale, straighten up your torso and thrust your chest out while coiling your right hand outward (Figure 6-63). Repeat this coiling exercise 30 to 50 times, then change the coiling direction for 30 to 50 times.

Next, repeat the same coiling practice for the left arm. In order to make the coiling effective, you must be soft and relaxed. Only then can your arm stick and adhere to the branch. If you remain stiff, your arm will lose contact with the branch and the coiling purpose will be lost.

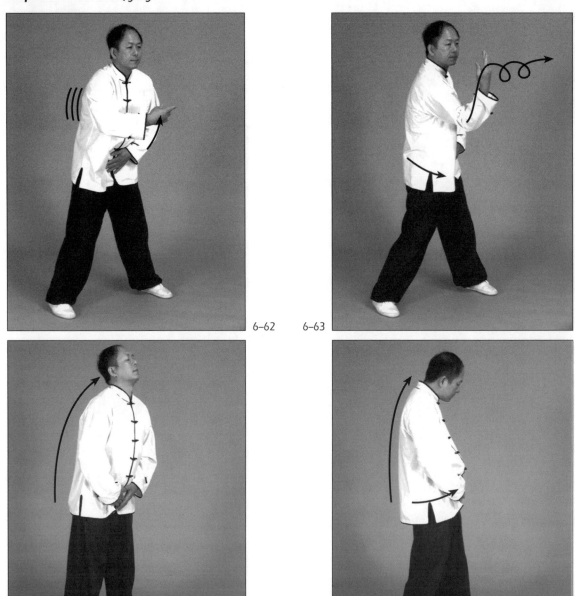

6–62   6–63

6–64   6–65

4. Crane Neck Gong *(He Jing Gong)* 鶴頸功

Crane Neck *Gong* is to train a White Crane beginner how to loosen up the neck joints. This is a crucial part of the *Jin* training. In Soft *Jin* manifestation, if the neck is stiff, the power can be trapped in the head and generate a headache. When you manifest your *Jin* as a soft whip, every section of joints, including your neck, should be loose and relaxed.

In this training, you generate a small and gentle waving motion from the waist area and let this wave pass through the spine and neck to reach the crown of the head (Figure 6-64). The wave motion should be small and all of the joints relaxed. Wave your neck forward 20 times and then gradually turn your head to the side to repeat the same waving motion (Figure 6-65).

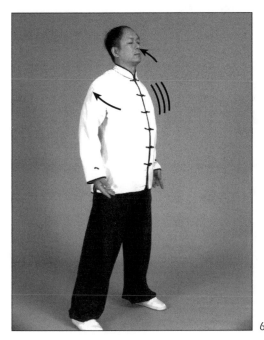 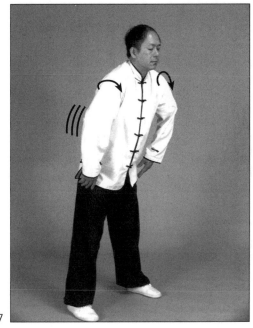

6-66   6-67

5. Soothe the Lung Gong (*Shu Fei Gong*) 舒肺功

This exercise is commonly used to soothe the spine and chest area right after *Qigong* training or White Crane martial sequence training. This exercise is especially important in Hard *Qigong* and *Jin* training. From this exercise, all of the joints in the spine and chest area will be loosened up, which allows the blood and *Qi* circulation to expedite the recovery process.

When you practice this *Gong,* first inhale, thrust your chest out, shoulders gently pushing backward, and generate a waving motion from the waist area (Figure 6-66). Next, exhale and pass the motion upward through the spine to the chest and circle your shoulders out (Figure 6-67).

This motion is like when you sigh and make the sound of "*Hen.*" When you are sighing, your body will generate a similar motion. This motion allows you to loosen up your torso and chest and therefore the stagnant *Qi* and emotion can be released easily. White Crane imitates this body motion to relax the torso and chest.

C. Flying Crane Gong (*Fei He Gong*) 飛鶴功

Flying Crane *Gong* includes twelve pieces. When you practice this set, you should treat the entire body like a soft whip, one unit that moves in a wave. In order to reach this goal, the joints must be loose and the movements soft and relaxed. All the movements originate either from the waist or from the legs and flow continuously, comfortably and gently from joint to joint to the finger tips. It is also very important that your hands be formed in the Crane wings described earlier. This *Qigong* set is the foundation for Soft White Crane *Jin*. Without this training, neither the Soft nor Soft-Hard *Jin* manifested will be sharp and penetrating.

When you train this set, imagine that you are a crane perched on the tip of a very tall stalk of bamboo. This is a common sight in China. When the wind blows, the Cranes retain their stability and root by opening their wings to maintain balance. Once you have this image, you will be able to maintain good balance and your root can grow deeper and deeper.

At the beginning of each piece, imagine that the wind blows weakly. Therefore, the movements of the wings (i.e., arms) are very small. Gradually, imagine that the wind blows stronger and stronger. In order to maintain your balance, the scale of the wings' movement becomes larger. When the scale reaches its maximum, stay there for a minute or so and then gradually reduce the scale of movement until the wind ceases, and the sweep of your wings also ceases.

In this practice, you may use either Normal Abdominal Breathing or Reverse Breathing. You may choose either phase of flight for inhalation and the opposite phase for exhalation. For example, when you swing your arms forward and backward, you might inhale or exhale when you swing forward, so long as you do the opposite as the arms swing back. Breathing is only a strategy for leading the *Qi*. You may adapt the breathing any way you like.

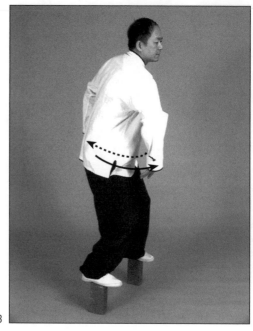

6-68

First, you should practice the entire set on the ground. After you have practiced for a long time, and you feel comfortable and natural in your movements, lay a pair of bricks on the floor and stand on their spines as you repeat the same training. As you do this, the root in your mind should be under the brick instead of only under your feet. Later, you may then stand on the crown of the bricks (Figure 6-68). If you master this training, continue to stand on two bricks and then three bricks. Naturally, this is extremely difficult.

1. Forward and Backward Flying (*Qian Hou Xiang*) 前後翔

Forward and Backward Flying trains the waving movement of the spine. The waving motion can begin either in the legs or waist, and continues past the shoulders and elbows to finally reach the finger tips.

Double Wing Flying (*Shuang Chi Fei*) 雙翅飛

When you do Double Wing Flying, place both of your hands beside your body naturally, palms facing backward. Start the movement either from the legs or from the waist. If you stand on bricks, you should start the movement from the waist at first, since it is easier. After practicing for a long time, you should slowly bring the movement lower than the waist, until finally reaching the bottom of the feet.

Begin on a tiny moving scale. The movement follows the spine upward, to the shoulders, elbows and fingers (Figure 6-69). Slowly and gradually make the scale of the flying bigger and bigger, until both of your hands reach the same height as your shoulder (Figures 6-70 and 6-71). You should feel the movement of every joint.

Fly at the maximum scale of movement for a minute or so, then slowly reduce the scale little by little. Imagine the wind growing weaker and weaker. Finally, the wind ceases and you end your movement. Stand still, breathing comfortably and naturally for a minute.

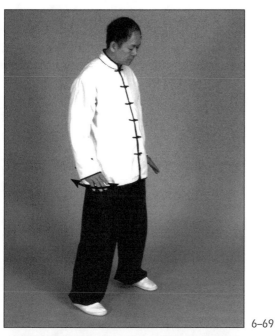

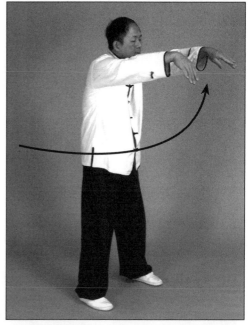

6-69   6-70

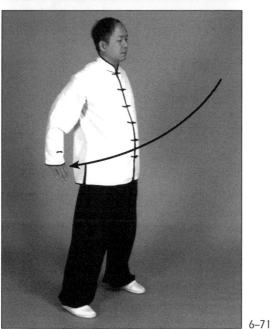

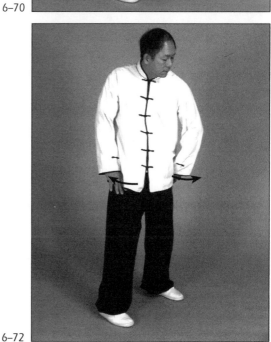

6-71   6-72

Single Wing Flying (Dan Chi Fei) 單翅飛

After a minute of rest from Double Wing Flying, continue with Single Wing Flying. In this training, imagine the wind is blowing from the side, and you must twist your body when you fly in order to balance.

Again, start with a weak wind. That means a small scale. Sway one arm forward while the other one moves backward, and then reverse the directions (Figure 6-72). When you move both arms back to the sides of your body, inhale, arc your back and hold in your chest. When they swing away from your body, exhale, straighten out your torso and thrust out your chest. Again, slowly increase the scale of the swinging until both arms are

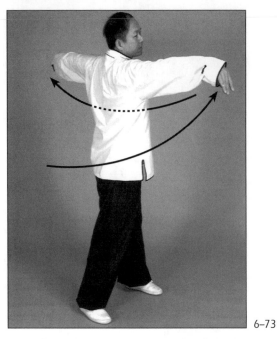
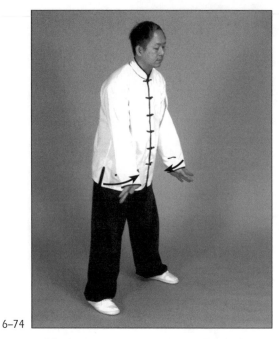

6-73   6-74

the same height as the shoulders (Figure 6-73). Swing there for a minute or so and then gradually decrease the scale until the movement ceases and the arms return back to the sides of the waist. Stand still and breathe comfortably and naturally for a minute.

2. Left and Right Flying (*Zuo You Xiang*) 左右翔

Left and Right Flying is to swing the wings sideways. The entire training specializes in the practice of chest and spine coordination. Again, the movement can either start from the waist or from the legs.

Double Wing Flying (*Shuang Chi Fei*) 雙翅飛

In Double Wing Flying, begin with both arms dropped naturally at the front of your abdomen, palms facing each other. First, inhale, arc your back and hold in your chest slightly. From this torso movement, swing the arms inward on a small scale at first (Figure 7-74). Next, exhale, straighten out your back while thrusting your chest and swing your arms outward to the sides (Figure 6-75). Slowly and gradually increase the scale of your arms' swinging until both arms meet above your head (Figure 6-76). Keep swinging on this maximum scale for a minute or so, and then slowly and gradually decrease the scale until both arms return to the beginning position. Stand still and breath comfortably and naturally for a minute.

Single Wing Flying (*Dan Chi Fei*) 單翅飛

After a minute of rest from Double Wing Flying, continue with Single Wing Flying. In this training, imagine the wind is blowing from the side.

Again, start with a weak wind. Sway one arm inward and the other outward, and then reverse the direction. As you swing to one side inhale, and as you swing to the other side exhale (Figure 6-77). In Single Wing Flying, the torso and the chest movements are very difficult. However, you should continue to train until the body is able to move first, and

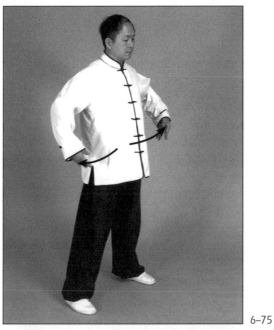

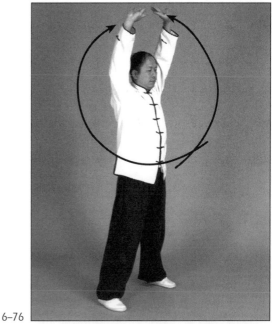

6–75   6–76

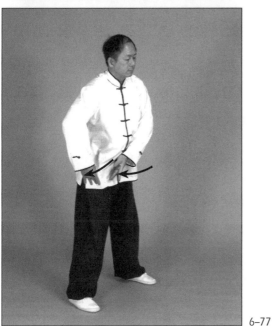

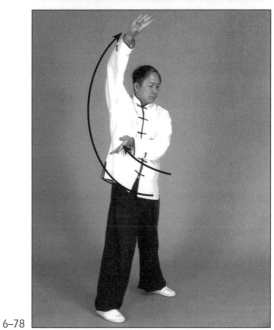

6–77   6–78

the arms simply follow the body's movements. Again, slowly increase the scale of the swinging until the arms reach the top of the head (Figure 6-78). Keep swinging on this maximum scale for a minute or so and then gradually decrease the scale until the movement ceases and the arms return back to the sides of the waist. Stand still and breath comfortably and naturally for a minute.

3. Straight Backward Flying (*Zhi Hou Xiang*) 直後翔

Straight Backward Flying aims to strengthen the ligament and tendon structure of the upper chest. In order to reach this goal, the chest is opened and then closed. Naturally, to do the action correctly, coordination of the spine movement is always important.

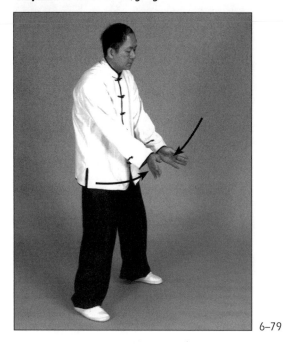

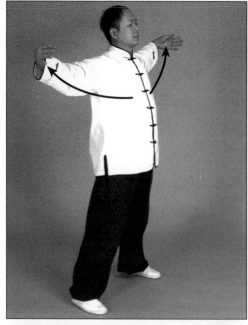

6–79   6–80

Double Wing Flying

(Shuang Chi Fei) 雙翅飛

Start with hands in front of the abdominal area, palms facing each other. As before, generate the motion from the sacrum's backward motion by moving the pelvis backward to open the *Mingmen* (Gv-4, 命門) cavity. This action generates a wave motion upward to the *Shenzhu* (Gv-12, 身柱) cavity on the upper back area, and then passes to the shoulders and finally opens up the arms and hands. Begin with a slight movement. Imagine that the wind blows weakly, but is gradually growing stronger (Figure 6-79). Gradually, the wings' opening and closing becomes bigger, and both arms are raised upward gradually to the height of the chest area

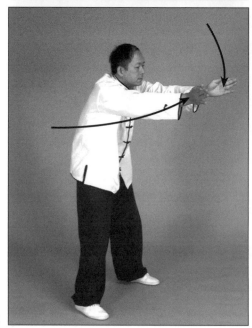

6–81

(Figures 6-80 and 6-81). Fly like this for a minute or so and then gradually lower your arms as the scale of opening and closing becomes smaller until both arms cease moving right in front of the abdomen. Stand still and breath comfortably and naturally for a minute.

Single Wing Flying *(Dan Chi Fei)* 單翅飛

As before, after your rest, simply fly one arm first and follow with the other. Again, begin with a slight movement. Imagine that the wind is blowing weakly (Figure 6-82). Gradually, the wings' opening and closing becomes bigger, and the arms raise up gradually to the

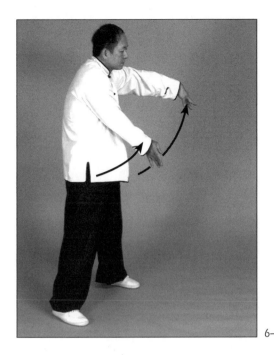

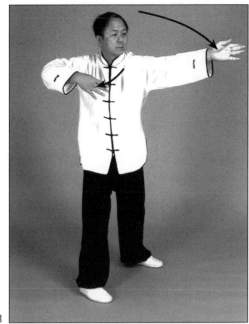

6-82   6-83

height of the chest area (Figure 6-83). Fly
for a minute or so and then gradually lower
your arms as the scale of opening and closing becomes smaller until both arms cease
moving right in front of the abdomen.
Stand still and breathe comfortably and
naturally for a minute.

4. Internal Circular Flying-Vertical Palm
(*Nei Yuan Xiang-Shu Zhang*)

內圓翔‧豎掌

This flying is again for strengthening the
structure of the ligaments and tendons in the
upper chest. In order to reach this goal, the
chest is again opened and then closed.
Naturally, to do this action correctly, coordination with the spine's movement is always
important.

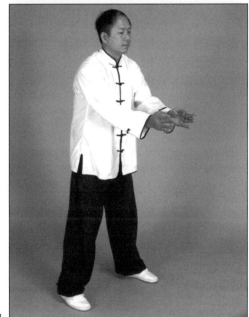

6-84

Double Wing Flying (Shuang Chi Fei) 雙翅飛

The motion of this flying is very similar to that of the last piece. When you start, place
both of your arms in front of your chest with the palms facing each other (Figure 6-84).
Again, inhale and generate the motion from the waist area controlled by the pelvis. This
motion is then led upward and reaches to the fingers. When this motion reaches the
shoulder area, exhale and use the motion to generate a circling motion in the arms

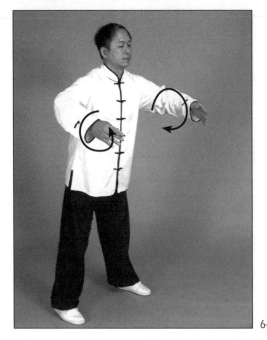

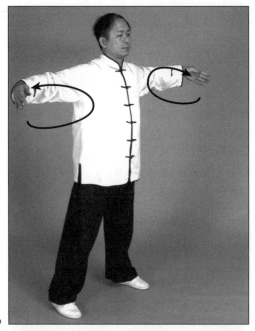

6–85   6–86

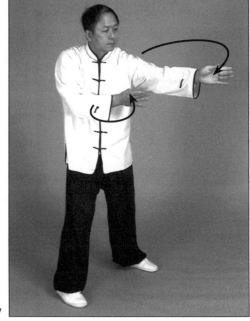

(Figure 6-85). Begin on a small scale and gradually increase the size of the circle (Figure 6-86). Practice for a minute with this big circle, and then gradually and slowly reduce the scale of the circle until both arms completely stop. Drop both of your arms and rest for a minute.

6–87

Single Wing Flying *(Dan Chi Fei)* 單翅飛

After a rest, raise both of your arms again.

However, this time you fly with alternating arms. Again, start on a small scale and gradually increase until the circle is big (Figure 6-87). Naturally, the body's movement is slightly different from that of the Double Wing Flying. In Single Wing Flying, you must turn your body from side to side to generate a sort of circular swinging motion. When you reach the biggest scale, stay there for one minute and then gradually reduce the scale until both arms stop in front of your chest. Drop both of your arms beside the waist and rest for a minute.

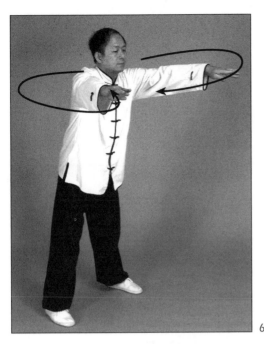

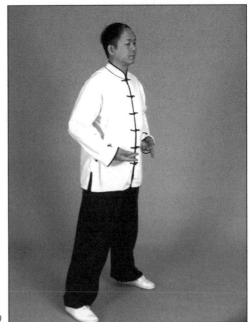

6–88   6–89

5. Internal Circular Flying-Horizontal Palm (*Nei Yuan Xiang-Pin Zhang*)

内圓翔· 平掌

The body and the arm movements of this piece are exactly the same as in the last piece. The only difference is that the palms are facing downward instead of facing each other. Again, start on a small scale with double arms, and then change to a single arm (Figure 6-88).

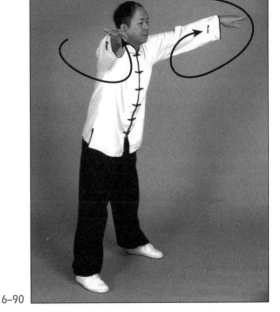

6–90

After you have completed the last two pieces, you should combine them into one motion. When you combine it with Double Wing Flying, it is called "Eagle Attacks Its Prey" (老鷹撲食). When you do this, place both of your hands right in front of the waist area with the palms facing upward (Figure 6-89). Begin the motion from the waist area again by controlling the pelvis, inhale, thrust your upper chest out and open both of your arms, palms facing each other. When the wave motion reaches the upper chest, exhale, circling both of your arms to the sides and then forward until the palms are facing downward (Figure 6-90). Finally, inhale and withdraw the arms back to the chest area to repeat the exercise.

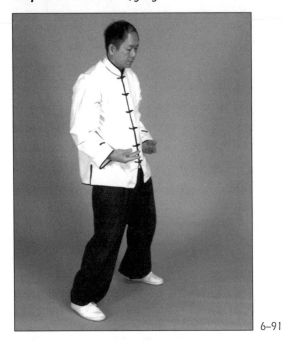

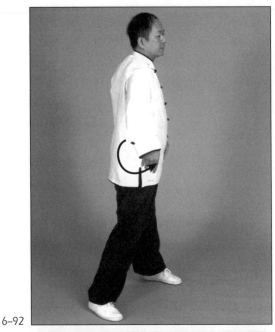

6–91   6–92

When you combine it with Single Wing Flying, it is called "Lion Rotates the Ball" (獅子滾球). Again, place both of your hands right in front of your abdomen area (Figure 6-91). Next, inhale, twist your body and generate a circular whipping motion from the waist area (Figure 6-92). When the motion reaches the right shoulder, exhale and circle your right arm out and return it to the chest area (Figure 6-93). Repeat the same process for the left arm. You should repeat these right arm and left arm circular motions 30 times each. After completing the practice, rest for a minute or so.

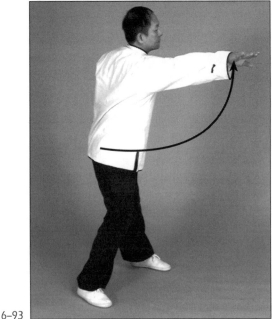

6. External Circular Flying-Vertical Palm

(*Wai Yuan Xiang-Shu Zhang*) 外圓翔・豎掌   6–93

This piece is very similar to the fourth piece. It again aims for strengthening the structure of the ligaments and tendons in the upper chest. The difference is that the direction of the circle is reversed.

Double Wing Flying (*Shuang Chi Fei*) 雙翅飛

When you start, place both of your arms in front of your chest with the palms facing each other (Figure 6-94). Inhale, arc in your spine and withdraw your chest (Figure 6-95). Next, exhale, thrust your chest out while extending your arms forward and then sideways (Figure 6-96). When the arms reach to the sides, inhale, arc your spine and withdraw your chest and continue the circling until hands return to the center line in front of your chest. Begin circling on a small scale and gradually increase to a large circle. Practice for a

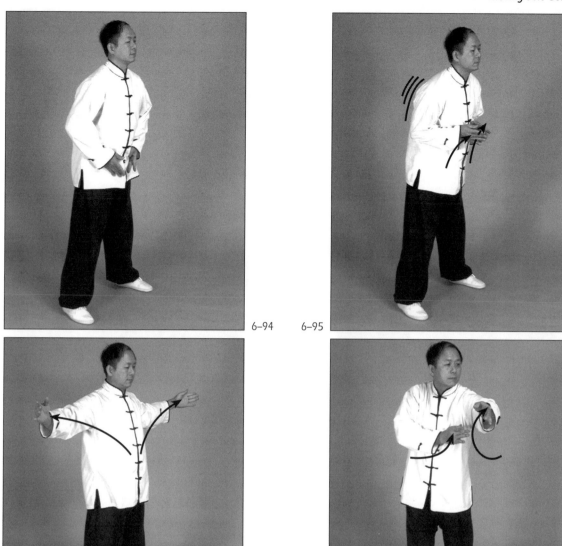

6–94   6–95

6–96   6–97

minute with this big circle and then gradually and slowly reduce the scale of the circle until both arms have completely stopped. Drop both of your arms and rest for a minute.

Single Wing Flying (Dan Chi Fei) 單翅飛

After a rest, raise both of your arms again, however, this time you fly with alternating arms. Again, begin on a small scale that gradually grows larger (Figure 6-97). Naturally, the body's movement is slightly different from that of the Double Wing Flying. In Single Wing Flying, you must turn your body from side to side to generate a sort of circular swinging motion. When you reach the biggest scale, stay there for one minute and then gradually reduce the scale until both arms stop in front of your chest. Drop both of your arms beside the waist and rest for a minute.

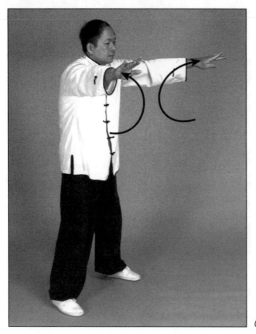

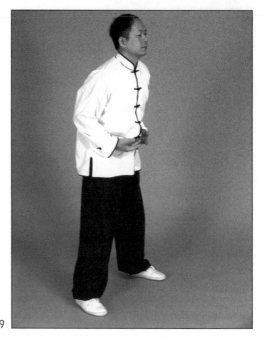

6-98   6-99

7. External Circular Flying-Horizontal Palm (*Wai Yuan Xiang-Pin Zhang*) 外圓翔‧平掌

The body and the arm movements of this piece are exactly the same as in the last piece. The only difference is that the palms are facing downward instead of facing each other. Again, start on a small scale with double arms, and then switch to single arm (Figure 6-98).

After you have completed the last two pieces, you should combine them into one motion. For Double Flying, it is called "Large Bear Swimming in the Water" (大熊游水). When you do this, place both of your hands right in front of the abdominal area with the palms facing upward (Figure 6-99). Begin the motion from the waist area with the control of the pelvis, inhale, arc your back and withdraw your chest (Figure 6-100). Next, exhale, generate the motion from the waist with the control of the pelvis and extend both of your arms forward until both palms are facing downward (Figure 6-101). Continue your arms' circular motion, inhale, arc your back and withdraw your abdominal area again to repeat the second movement. Repeat 30 times each.

When you combine this with Single Wing Flying, it is called "Left and Right to Open the Mountain" (左右開山). Again, place both of your hands right in front of your abdominal area. Next, inhale, turn your body to your left while starting to circle your right arm (Figure 6-102). Exhale, slowly and gradually rotate your body to your right while turning your right arm until the palms are facing downward and your body is facing to your right (Figure 6-103). Repeat the same process for the left arm. You should repeat these right and left arm circular motions 30 times each. After completing the practice, rest for a minute or so.

8. Backward Circular Flying (*Hou Yuan Xiang*) 後圓翔

Backward Circular Flying is to train a practitioner to extend the motion from the waist or leg through the spine and the chest to the arms. Although previous pieces also serve the same purpose, the muscles which control the circling are different.

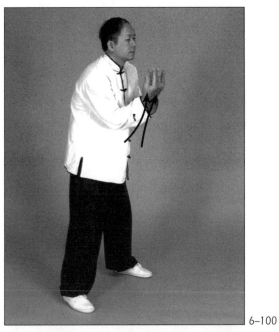
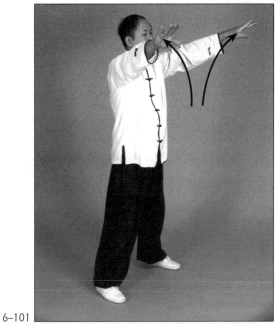

6-100   6-101

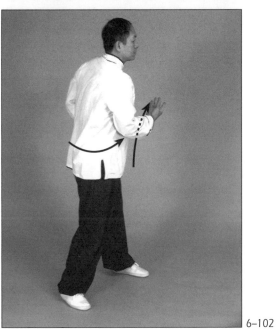
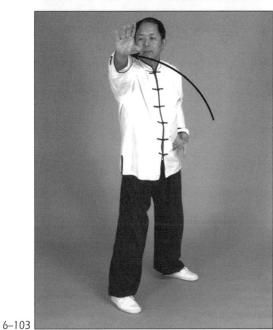

6-102   6-103

Double Wing Flying (Shuang Chi Fei) 雙翅飛

When you do this piece, first place both of your hands with the palms facing each other right in front of your abdominal area (Figure 6-104), inhale deeply while generating the waving motion from the sacrum and extend it upward to the spine, to the shoulders and

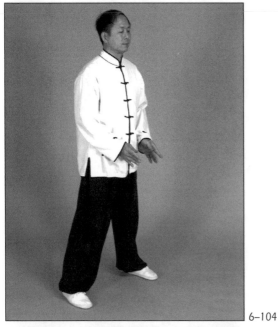
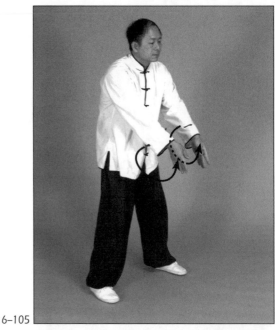

6–104   6–105

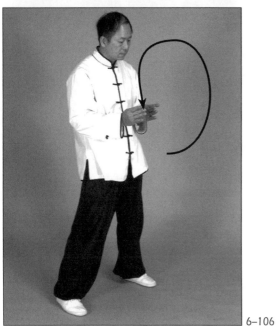
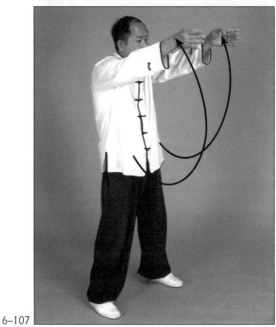

6–106   6–107

then to the arms. Move your hands down and then forward (Figure 6-105). Next, exhale and thrust your chest out while circling your hands back to the abdominal area (Figure 6-106). Start circling on a small scale and slowly and gradually increase the circle of both hands (Figure 6-107). Stay circling on the large scale for a minute or so, then gradually reduce the circle and finally stop at the front of the abdomen. Rest for a minute or so.

Single Wing Flying (Dan Chi Fei) 單翅飛

After Double Wing Flying, repeat the same motion except this time add the body's twisting action, which leads only a single hand to circle (Figure 6-108). Start again with a smaller circle and gradually increase the scale of the circle (Figure 6-109). Keep circling on a large scale for a minute or so and then gradually reduce the circle until the hands stop right in front of the abdominal area. Again, rest for a minute or so.

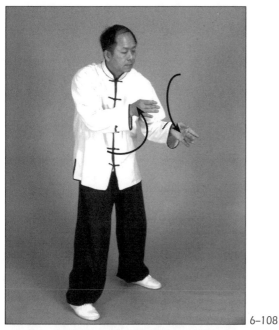
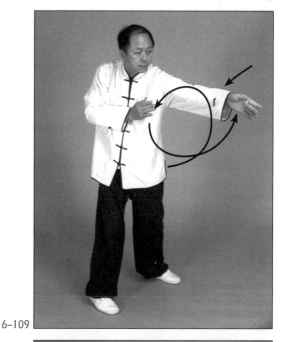

6-108   6-109

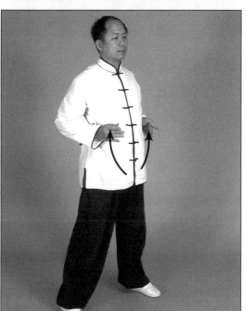
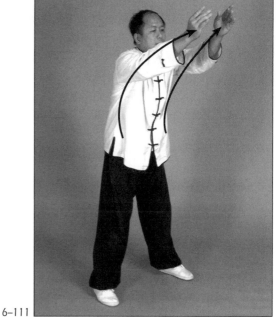

6-110   6-111

9. **Forward Circular Flying** (*Qian Yuan Xiang*) 前圓翔

This piece is exactly the reverse of the last piece.

Double Wing Flying (*Shuang Chi Fei*) 雙翅飛

Again, place both of your hands right in front of your abdominal area. First, inhale, generate the motion from the sacrum and thrust your chest out, raising up your hands (Figure 6-110). Next, exhale, following the motion of the spine, and extend and circle your arms forward. Finally, inhale and circle back to repeat the motion. You should start with a small circle and gradually increase the scale (Figure 6-111). Continue this large circle for a minute or so, then gradually reduce the circle until both hands are stopped right in front of the abdomen area. Rest for minute or so.

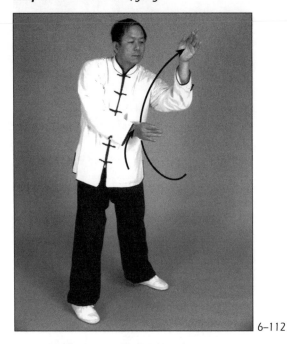 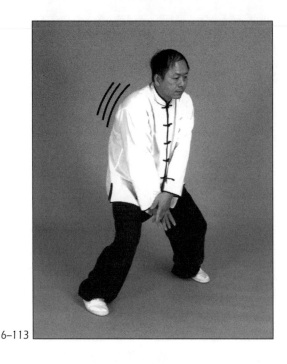

6-112   6-113

Single Wing Flying (Dan Chi Fei) 單翅飛

The motion of this Single Wing Flying is similar to the Single Wing Flying of the last piece. The difference is that the direction for circling is reversed. Again, you should start with a small circle and gradually increase to a big circle (Figure 6-112). Keep circling on the large circle for a minute or so and then gradually reduce the circle until stopped. Rest for a minute or so.

10. Upward Flapping (Shang Pu) 上撲

Upward Flapping imitates the upward flapping motion of a crane. The purpose of this flapping is to train a practitioner to connect the spine and chest movements to the hands.

Double Wing Flapping (Shuang Pu) 雙撲

When you practice this piece, first squat down and place both of your hands in front of your abdominal area with the palms facing downward (Figure 6-113). Next, inhale and generate a wave motion from the sacrum. The movement passes through the spine, through the shoulders and then to the arms. Following the body's motion, flap both of your arms up and to the sides while exhaling (Figure 6-114). Again, begin on a small scale and gradually increase to a bigger scale. Stay there for one minute or so. After you finish it, drop both of your arms beside your waist and rest for a minute or so.

Single Wing Flapping (Dan Pu) 單撲

Single Wing Flapping is similar to the Double wing flapping. However, the body should twist slightly to the side whenever the single arm is flapping upward (Figure 6-115). Practicing Single Wing Flapping is much harder than Double Wing Flapping. After you have practiced for a minute or so, gently drop your arms to the side of your body and rest for a minute or so.

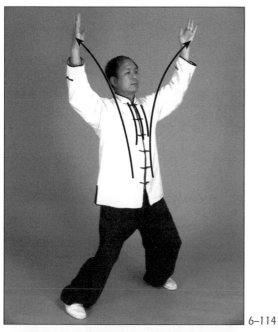
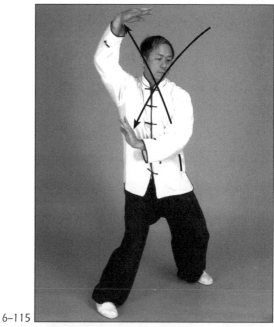

6-114   6-115

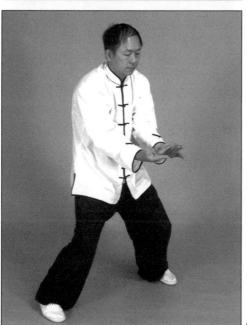
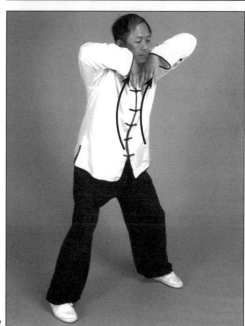

6-116   6-117

11. Downward Flapping (*Xia Pu*) 下撲

Downward Flapping swings both of your hands downward right in front your waist area. Again, you are aiming for the connection and coordination of the body and the upper limbs.

Double Wing Flapping (*Shuang Pu*) 雙撲

When you practice this piece, again squat down with both hands naturally dropping right in front of your abdominal area (Figure 6-116). Generate the body motion from the sacrum, inhale and thrust out your chest while raising both of your arms upward (Figure 6-117). Next, exhale, arc your torso and withdraw your chest while swinging both of your

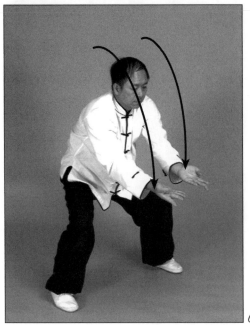
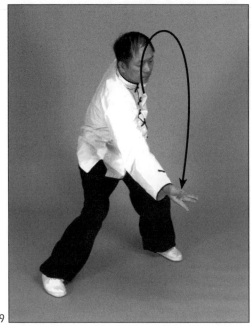

6-118   6-119

hands downward (Figure 6-118). As usual, begin on a small scale and then gradually increase. When you reach a large scale, practice for a minute or so and then gradually reduce. Finally, drop both of your arms beside your body and rest for a minute or so.

Single Wing Flapping (Dan Pu) 單撲

The action of Single Wing Flapping is the same as that of Double Wing Flapping, except this time you add a sideways body twisting motion to generate the Single Wing Flapping power. Again, start on a small scale and gradually increase to a big scale and stay there for a minute or so (Figure 6-119). Finally, reduce the scale and end with both arms dropped naturally beside your body. Rest for a minute or so.

12. Baby Crane Waves Its Wings (You He Dou Chi) 幼鶴抖翅

This last piece is a recovery movement which can help you loosen your spine and chest, which may be tight from the training. In order to make your body as relaxed as possible, the scale of movement is comfortable and natural.

Double Wing Waving (Shuang Dou Chi) 雙抖翅

When you practice this piece, first place both of your hands in front of your chest area with the palms facing downward. Inhale deeply and generate a soft and relaxed motion from the sacrum, thrusting your chest out while raising your body and both elbows slightly (Figure 6-120). Your hands and wrists should be following the movement of the elbows and stay relaxed. Next, exhale, squat down, arc your back and withdraw your chest while lowering both of your elbows and allowing both hands to follow the elbows' movement downward (Figure 6-121). Repeat 30 times, drop both of your arms naturally and rest for a minute.

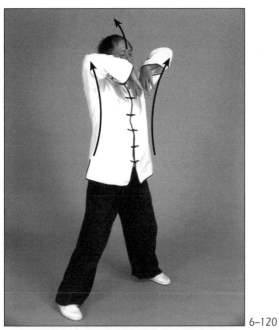
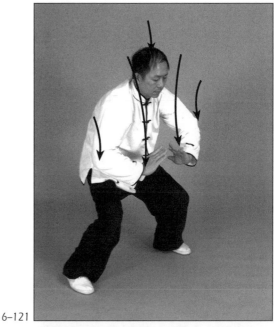

6-120   6-121

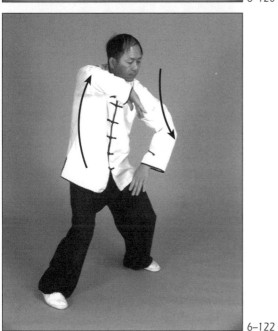
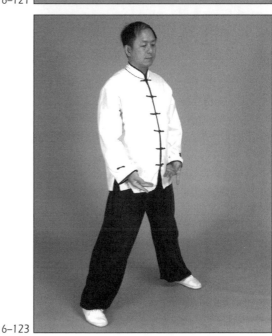

6-122   6-123

Single Wing Waving (Dan Dou Chi) 單抖翅

After you have finished the Double Wing Waving, practice the same movement with a single hand. That means that one hand is waving upward while the other is waving downward (Figure 6-122). Again, you should use the body to lead and the arms just follow the waving motion. Practice for a minute or so and then rest for a minute.

After you have completed this set, stand up comfortably (Figure 6-123). Next, generate movement from the sacrum upward through the spine, over the shoulders and finally circle both of your hands naturally and smoothly (Figure 6-124). This final recovery form is able to relax your torso significantly.

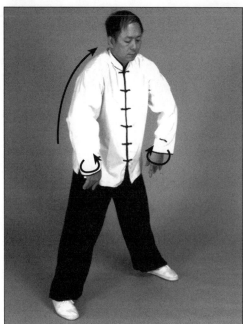

6-124

Part III

White Crane Jin

白鶴勁

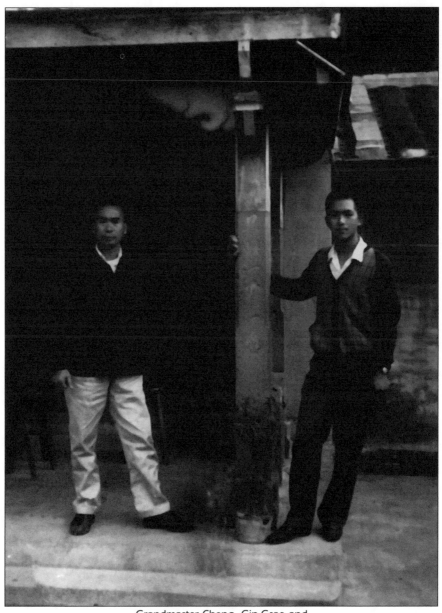

Grandmaster Cheng, Gin-Gsao and
Dr. Yang, Jwing-Ming, 1964

Chapter 7

Theory of Jin

勁理

7-1. Introduction

In Chapter 1, it was mentioned that martial power, or *Jin*, can generally be divided into three categories: **Hard *Jin*** (*Ying Jin*, 硬勁), **Soft-Hard *Jin*** (*Ruan-Ying Jin*, 軟硬勁) and Soft *Jin* (*Rou Jin*, 柔勁). Among these, Hard *Jin* uses the most muscular power, followed by Soft-Hard *Jin* and finally Soft *Jin*. But no matter which *Jin*, in order to manifest maximum power you must have both the strength of the physical body (*Yang*) and a sufficient supply of smoothly circulating *Qi* (*Yin*). The external physical strength manifested in specific external movements is called "**External *Jin***" (*Wai Jin*, 外勁); it is a *Yang* manifestation of *Jin*. The internal *Qi*'s build up and circulation is called "**Internal *Jin***" (*Nei Jin*, 內勁); it is the *Yin* manifestation of *Jin*. When this internal and external coordinate and support each other harmoniously and efficiently, it is called "**the unification of internal and external**" (*Nei Wai He Yi*, 內外合一).

You should also understand that *Jin* can be again divided into *Yang Jin* 陽勁) (commonly called "**Attacking *Jin***" (*Gong Jin*, 攻勁) which is aggressive and used for an attack, and *Yin Jin* (陰勁) (commonly called "**Defensive *Jin***" (*Shou Jin*, 守勁) which is defensive. There is another category of *Jin* which is neither for attacking nor defending; it is called "**Non-attacking and Non-defending *Jin***" (*Fei Gong Fei Shou Jin*, 非攻非守勁). No matter which category of *Jin*, when the *Qi* is manifested into a physical form, it is called "**Emitting *Jin***" (*Fa Jin*, 發勁).

In the next section, we will first define what *Jin* is and how different *Jins* can be classified, and will follow with a theoretical analysis and discussion of how *Jin* can be manifested. Then, in section 7-3, the concepts of "external *Jin*" and "internal *Jin*" will be explained. From understanding this chapter, you will have a better idea of why Martial Arts *Qigong* is so important to Chinese martial arts training and how Martial Arts *Qigong* is related to *Jin* manifestation.

7-2. Theory

In this section, first let us define what *Jin* is and how different Jins are classified. From this, you will be able to grasp a clear concept of the *Jin*. Then, in order to help you understand how *Jin* can be manifested from an idea (i.e., mind), a scientific and logical model will be discussed.

General Definition of Jin

Theoretically, in order to activate the muscles to generate force or power, the mind must lead the *Qi* to the area where the muscles should be energized. For example, when you push a car, you must first generate an idea, and from this mind, an electromotive force (EMF) is generated. From this EMF the *Qi* (or bioelectricity) is led to the muscles for energization. Through the nervous system (a highly electrically conductive system) the muscles are stimulated and contract, thereby generating action.

To make the concept of *Jin* more clear, let us examine how the Chinese define *Jin*. The Chinese dictionary gives two main meanings for "*Jin*." The first is "strong, unyielding, muscular;" this is usually applied to powerful, inanimate objects. For example, "*Jin Gong*" (勁弓) means a strong bow and "*Jin Feng*" (勁風) means a strong wind. It can also be applied to more abstract feelings of strength, as in "*Jin Di*" (勁敵) which means a strong enemy.

Jin has often been confused with *Li* (力) which is commonly used to express power or externally manifested muscular force. Using the previous illustration, we can see *Li* is explicit and is shown externally, while *Jin* is more implicit and internal—you must **feel** it to sense its strength. You can't tell the strength of a bow by looking at it, rather you must pull it to see if it has the potential to generate a lot of power. Once it emits an arrow, the strength of its *Jin* is shown by the power (*Li*) of the arrow. (For inanimate objects, *Li* refers to inherent strength or power.) Another quality often associated with *Jin* is the feeling of a strong, pulsed flow. An example is "*Jin Feng*" (勁風) (a strong wind)—never steady, it moves this way and that, over and around obstacles and when it surges, trees bend and houses are knocked down.

The second dictionary definition of *Jin* is "*Qi-Li*" (氣力) or "*Li-Qi*" (力氣), which refers to muscles which are supported by *Qi*. Using only your muscles is considered *Li*. However, **when you use your concentrated Yi (mind) to lead the muscles to do something, Qi will flow to where you are concentrating and enliven the muscles.** This is considered *Jin*. The Chinese martial arts emphasize using *Yi* and concentration, so whenever *Jin* is mentioned in this book, it means "*Qi-Li*."

There are many types of *Jin*, but the one thing they all have in common is that they all deal with the flow of *Qi*. The most obvious type of *Jin* is "**manifest Jin**" (*Xian Jin*, 顯勁), where you can see something happening, as when you push someone. Sensing another person's motion or energy is also considered a type of *Jin*. In fact, in the highest levels of "**sensing Jin**" (*Jue Jin*, 覺勁), you actually sense the *Qi* flow of your opponent and thereby know his intentions. These sensing Jins are enhanced by increasing the *Qi* flow to your skin. In general, the higher the level of *Jin*, the more *Qi* and the less *Li* is used.

In the martial arts, it is said that *Jin* is not *Li*. This means that although you must use your muscles (*Li*) every time you move, *Jin* is more than just muscular strength. There are several different kinds of manifest *Jin*. When you rely primarily on muscular strength, but also use *Qi* and your concentrated mind, it is considered "Hard *Jin*" (Figure 7-1). This kind of *Jin* is usually easily visible as tensed muscles. When muscle usage is reduced and both *Qi* and muscles play equal roles in the *Jin*, it is called "Soft-Hard *Jin*." When muscle usage is reduced to a minimum and *Qi* plays the major role, it is called "Soft *Jin*." Soft-Hard *Jin* and especially Soft *Jin*, are usually expressed in a pulse. Soft *Jin* is often compared to a whip, which can express a great deal of force in a very short time, concentrated in a very small area. When you snap a whip, it stays loose as it transmits a wave or pulse of energy along its length to the tip. Similarly, when you use Soft *Jin* your muscles stay relatively relaxed as you transmit a pulse of energy through your body. This is done with the tendons and the ends of the muscles, supported by *Qi*.

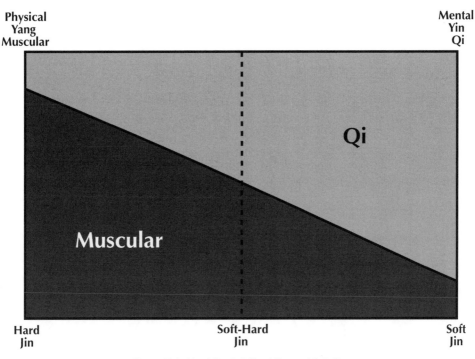

Figure 7–1. Hard Jin, Soft-Hard Jin, and Soft Jin

When a Soft *Jin* is manifested, the emission of *Jin* is a relatively short, smooth and relaxed pulse of energy, without any angular changes in direction. The pulse can be long or short, near the body or at a distance. It can be a sudden contraction and expansion as you bounce the opponent away, or an even sharper "spasm" as you strike or break something. In all cases, *Jin* uses *Li,* because *Li* is necessary any time you move, but the muscles must be supported by *Qi*.

Figure 7-2 may help you understand the difference between *Jin* and *Li*. In this figure, the vertical coordinate represents the depth to which power can penetrate and the horizontal coordinate represents the elapsed time. The areas under the curves represent the power generated for each curve. We assume that the areas under the curves are the same, i.e., the power generated for each curve is equal. In curve 1, the power is generated, reaches its maximum, stays at the maximum for the time t^1 and then drops to zero. Without strong *Qi* support, this is a typical example of *Li* — muscular strength predominates and penetration is limited. With *Qi*, it is considered "Hard *Jin*."

In curve 2, both muscles and *Qi* are involved and the power is at its maximum for the shorter time t^2. Since the power generated is the same as with curve 1, the peak has to reach higher, which means there is greater penetration. In order to do this, the muscles must be relaxed to allow the *Qi* from either the local area or the Lower *Dan Tian* to flow smoothly to support them. This is the general idea of "Soft-Hard *Jin*." In Soft-Hard *Jin*, commonly the body is soft and relaxed so the *Qi* can be led to the area where the *Jin* will be manifested. Once the *Qi* arrives, a slight but sharp muscular tension is intentionally generated and the power is manifested.

In curve 3, the time t^3 in which the power is generated is even shorter. The muscles must be extremely relaxed to generate and express this sharply penetrating power. In order to reach a deep penetrating power, **speed is a crucial key for successful Soft *Jin* manifestation**. Naturally, *Qi* plays the predominant role in this "soft" *Jin*. Curve 3 is typical of *Taiji Jin*. From the point of view of muscle usage, curve 1 is like a wooden staff, curve 2 is like a rattan staff and curve 3 is

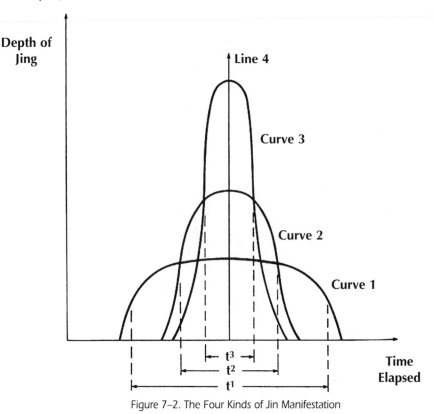

Figure 7–2. The Four Kinds of Jin Manifestation

like a whip. The wooden staff is stiff like tensed muscles, the rattan is more flexible and the whip is soft, its power sharp and focused.

Even curve 3, which is a very high level of power, is still not the highest power in the martial arts. The highest level of the *Qi* manifestation into *Jin* can be represented by line 4. In this level, the muscular strength is reduced to minimum and the *Qi* plays the major role of the power manifestation. When a martial artist has reached this level, he can transport his *Qi* into his enemy's body through the acupuncture cavities to shock organs and cause damage or death instantly. The time used is extremely short and the penetration is deeper than is possible with *Jin* or *Li*. This is known as the skill of "Pressing Cavity" (*Dian Xue,* 點穴) or "Pressing Primary *Qi* Channel" (*Dian Mai,* 點脈).

From the above explanation, you can see that **Li can be considered closer to Hard *Jin*** in which muscular strength plays the major role in power manifestation. **It is said that *Li* or Hard *Jin* is derived from the bones and muscles. The *Qi* is supported from the local area. Soft-Hard *Jin* and Soft *Jin* originate from the tendons and are supported strongly by *Qi* which is generated in the Lower *Dan Tian*.** Since the tendons are emphasized in the Soft-Hard *Jin* and Soft *Jin*, the muscle fibers can be relaxed, allowing the *Qi* to flow through them and support them. If your force is derived from the bones, there is a strong tendency for you to resist and meet your opponent's force directly. When your force is derived from the tendons it is easier to be flexible and elusive, to disappear in front of the opponent's attack and to appear at his weak spot.

Now let us summarize the differences between *Li*, or Hard *Jin*, and Soft *Jin*:

1. **Hard *Jin*, or *Li*, has shape, while Soft *Jin* has no shape or form**. This means that Hard *Jin* or *Li* can be seen easily, but that Soft *Jin* must be felt. The storing of energy and the preparation for moves, as well as the actual emission of energy, can be more subtle with

Soft *Jin* because it is done with the body and Lower *Dan Tian* rather than the arms. With Hard *Jin* or *Li* the muscles of the arms and shoulders tend to be the major source of energy and this is more easily seen.

2. **Hard *Jin*, or *Li*, is square, while Soft *Jin* is round.** In Chinese, square means clumsy, stiff, stubborn and straightforward; while round implies smooth, flexible, alive and tricky. This means that when Hard *Jin* or *Li* is used, it is sluggish and stiff, whereas when Soft *Jin* is used, it is smooth, agile and alive.

3. **Hard *Jin*, or *Li*, is stagnant, while Soft *Jin* is fluid.** It is also said that **Hard *Jin*, or *Li*, is slow, but Soft is swift.** Because Hard *Jin* or *Li* emphasizes muscular contraction, the muscles are stiffer and respond more slowly. Since Soft *Jin* is more relaxed it is easier to change direction. The actual emission of energy is more restrained and controlled, so you can be more subtle and can deal more easily with changes in the situation.

4. **With Hard *Jin*, or *Li*, power is diffuse, but the power of Soft *Jin* is concentrated.** When using just the muscles, it is hard to concentrate the energy. When you train Soft *Jin* you emphasize relaxation and moving from the center of your being. This allows you to concentrate all of your energy into a very small space and time.

5. **Hard *Jin*, or *Li*, floats, but Soft *Jin* is sunk.** This has two interpretations. First, when you use muscular strength, you emphasize the arms and shoulders and your movements tend to be angular and jerky. This makes it easier to lose your connection with the ground. With Soft *Jin*, especially in *Taijiquan,* the arms and body are relaxed and energy is derived from the waist, legs and Lower *Dan Tian.* When your attention is on your legs, it is easier to keep firmly in contact with the ground. Since your center and source of motion are more removed from the opponent than is the case with Hard *Jin* or *Li*, it is easier to avoid throwing yourself at the opponent, which would break your root. A second interpretation of this saying is that with Hard *Jin* or *Li* the power is more from the surface, while with Soft *Jin* the power is more internal. That is, the tendons, from which Soft *Jin* is derived, are relatively more internal than the muscles. After long training, the *Qi* which supports Soft *Jin* comes from deep within the body.

6. Hard *Jin*, or *Li*, is dull, but Soft *Jin* is sharp. This implies that Hard *Jin* or *Li's* power stays on the surface while Soft *Jin* penetrates deeply. Since the approach and the methods of training Soft *Jin* are more refined and internal than is the case with Hard *Jin* or *Li*, it is possible to be more precise in the application of force and to have the force penetrate more deeply into the opponent.

The above discussion has offered you an understanding of how to define *Jin*. Next, let us analyze exactly how *Jin* can be manifested from a scientific point of view.

Mind, Qi, and Jin

First, we should discuss in more detail the relationship of the mind, *Qi* and physical actions of our body. Part of the theory discussed is a hypothesis derived from my personal understanding and study of both western scientific discovery and eastern *Qigong* experience. This section is only to offer you a reference or different point of view for your thinking.

1. Mind:[1-11]

We already know that an action is first initiated from an idea or thought and from this thought, the EMF (i.e., electromotive force) is generated which leads the *Qi* (i.e., bioelectricity)

$$\text{Yi} \longrightarrow \text{Qi} \longrightarrow \text{Jin or Action}$$
$$\text{(mind)} \quad \text{(bioelectricity)} \quad \text{(power manifestation)}$$

Figure 7–3. Jin Manifestation From the Mind

to circulate to the muscles for energization (Figure 7-3). Though this concept is very simple, the scientific understanding and explanation is more difficult.

First, let us examine the brain. Currently, many scientists believe that we probably understand only 10% of the capacity of our brain. That means we are still in the infancy of understanding this center of our being. It also implies that we still cannot use today's science to fully understand our brain functions.

I have heard it said that normally, we use only 32-35% of our brain cells. This means that we do not use our brain at its full capacity. We still do not know what will happen and how much the brain can demonstrate if we were capable of using more than 35% of its abilities. Theoretically, in order to activate more brain cells for functioning, we must provide more *Qi* (bioelectricity), nutrition and oxygen to the brain. Brain cells consume more of these necessities than other cells. We know that every brain cell consumes at least 12 to 18 times more oxygen than regular cells. From this ratio, we can assume that every brain cell will probably consume 12 to 18 times more nutrition and bioelectricity. Therefore, in order to activate more brain cells for functioning, we must provide the required extra *Qi*, nutrition and oxygen.

From several thousand years of *Qigong* practice in China, Buddhist and Daoist *Qigong* meditators have understood that in order to raise the brain (or spirit) to a higher spiritual level, the first task is learning how to build up an abundant storage of *Qi* in the Lower *Dan Tian* (human battery). The second task is learning how to lead the *Qi* through the Thrusting Vessel (*Chong Mai*, 衝脈) (i.e., spinal cord) to the brain efficiently through meditation.

Third, according to the EEG (Electroencephalogram) machine, four groups of different brain waves (oscillating electrical currents) are classified, with different activities involved during the testing. Normally, brain waves are classified according to frequency bands in cycles per second (Hz). These four categories are (Figure 7-4)[12]:

1. Beta activity (above 13 Hz): occurs in bursts in the anterior part of the brain and is associated with mental activity

2. Alpha activity (8-13 Hz): Relaxation, is abolished by attention

3. Theta activity (4 to less than 8 Hz): Drowsy and asleep

4. Delta activity (below 4 Hz): Deep Sleep and coma

From these recordings, we can see that when we are awake or getting involved in heavy thinking (Beta), the activity is busy and the signals are weak (i.e., amplitude is low). We can roughly

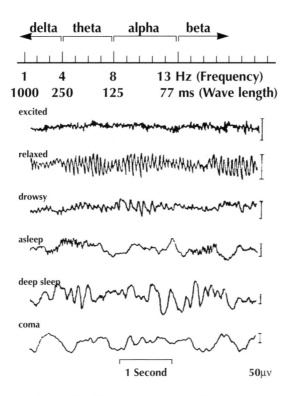

Figure 7–4. Typical Brain Wave Patterns From a State of Excitement to One of Deep Coma

see that on average there are 13 or more thoughts per second passing through our brain. Once we are relaxed (Alpha), although the signals are still weak, the number of oscillations is significantly reduced. Furthermore, the amplitude is increased. This means that when you are relaxed, your mind is more clear, calm and peaceful. This implies that concentration is increased. When you are in a drowsy or sleeping state, the number of oscillations is also reduced, but the thoughts are more irregular (Theta). Once you are in a deep, sound sleep (Delta), the number of oscillations is reduced to only a few and the oscillation amplitude is also significantly increased. According to science, we know that the power of oscillation is as follows:[13]

$$P \propto \text{Frequency}^2 \times \text{Amplitude}^2$$

This implies that, when you are in a deep, sleeping state, although your conscious mind is not heavily involved in thought (i.e., frequency reduced), the brain cells are obtaining a heavy supply of nutrition, oxygen and *Qi* nourishment. In this calm state, there is less distortion or disturbance in the brain. Under these extremely calm and relaxed conditions, if you are able to control your consciousness without falling asleep, you can build up a better sensitivity for energy correspondence with the outside world. This is one of the desired states in meditation practice; there are also other states which correspond to different meditation goals.

In such meditation, you are trying to reach the stage at which the brainwaves are between Theta and Delta. This means that it seems you are sleeping, yet your conscious mind is still governing the being. According to Chinese meditation, this is the state of **semi-sleeping** or a **self-hypnotic** state. In this state, the brain's sensitivity or energy correspondence with other brain waves or natural vibrations reaches a peak. It is in this stage that a meditator seeks for the connection between his spiritual being and the spirit of nature.

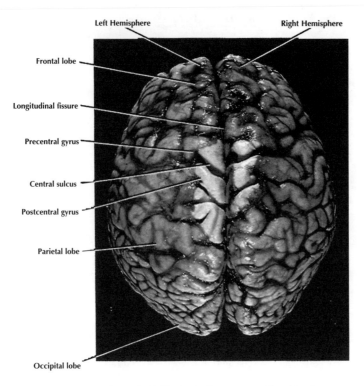

Left Hemisphere   Right Hemisphere

Frontal lobe

Longitudinal fissure

Precentral gyrus

Central sulcus

Postcentral gyrus

Parietal lobe

Occipital lobe

Figure 7–5. The Brain Encompasses Two Hemisphere

If we look at the brain's structure, we can see that it is encompasses two hemispheres (Figure 7-5). According to our understanding, different portions of the brain control specific thought processes. Between the two hemispheres is a place which is called the "**spiritual valley**" (*Shen Gu,* 神谷) by Chinese Daoists. The reason for this name is because Chinese *Qigong* meditators believe that this valley is the residence of the spirit. The spirit residing here is called "**valley spirit**" (*Gu Shen,* 谷神).

The pituitary and pineal glands, located near this area are called "mud pills" (*Ni Wan,* 泥丸) because they are shaped like pills made from mud (Figure 7-6). The spiritual valley is therefore called "**mud pill palace**" (*Ni Wan Gong,* 泥丸宫). According to Chinese *Qigong* meditation experience, these mud pills produce energy which can bring your spiritual energy to a higher level. Naturally, these meditation practitioners did not understand that this energy is raised because of the production of **human growth hormone** (HGH) from the pituitary gland and perhaps even **melatonin** from the pineal gland. What they practiced was to lead the *Qi* or bioelectricity from the Lower *Dan Tian* (i.e., human battery) through the spinal cord (i.e., Thrusting Vessel) to the mud pills (i.e., pituitary and pineal glands) to activate the production of the elixir (i.e., life force or hormone). From this practice, more brain cells can be activated and become functional. Eventually, the energy level and the functioning of the brain will become stronger. When this training reaches a high level, an aura or halo can sometimes be seen in the dark over the crown of the head. According to physics, this halo might be explained as the light generated from the interaction between the charges on the head and the surrounding air molecules which are ionized (Figure 7-7).

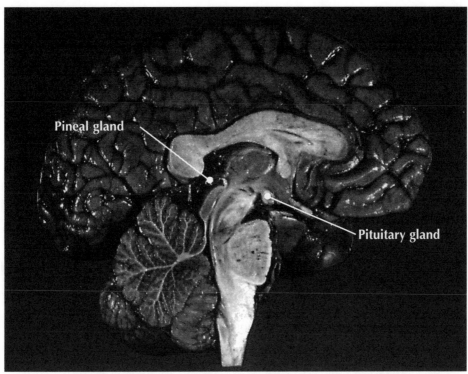

Figure 7–6. The Pituitary and Pineal Glands (Mud Pills) in the Spiritual Valley

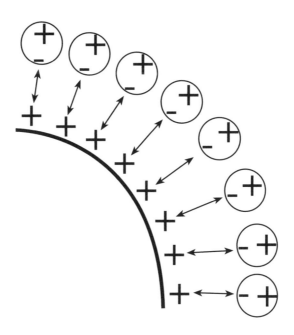

Figure 7–7. Ionization of Air Molecules by Static Charges

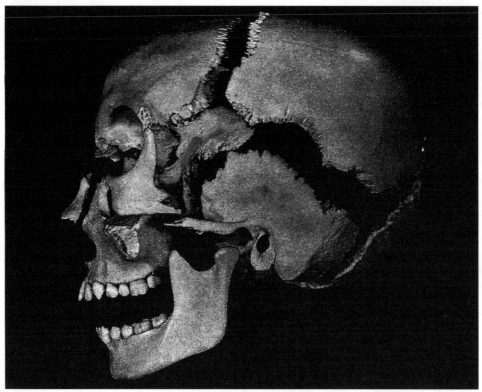

Figure 7–8. The Structure of a Human Skull

In meditation practice, the mind leads the *Qi* to the third eye or upper *Dan Tian* constantly. The main purpose of this training is to open the third eye, allowing your spirit to exit and enter your being easily. This allows you to communicate with the natural spirit and energy easily. If you look at the structure of the brain and the skull, you will see that there are several places where the skull can be separated into pieces (Figure 7-8). If you pay attention to the structure of the brain and the skull, you can see that the energy trapped in the spirit valley can easily penetrate through these connecting places and communicate with the outside world. From past experience, the crack on the top of the head is a wide open gate for the spiritual energy to line up with the earth's energy. There are two other places where the energy residing in this valley can communicate with the outside. These are at the front and back ends of the valley.

Even though there is a skull crack in the rear, because our thoughts usually "aim" forward to correspond with the sensing of our eyes and ears, the energy transmitted to and from the rear is not strong. In both the West and the East, energy from the front side of the brain is stronger and able to feel or sense outside energy. For this reason, this place is commonly called the "**third eye**" (West) or "**Upper *Dan Tian***" (*Shang Dan Tian,* 上丹田). Unfortunately, the structure of the skull at the forehead is very compact and strong. The spiritual energy is trapped on the front side of the valley. Because of this, Buddhists and Daoists in the past have tried to open this third eye using the mind's concentration and spiritual up lifting. They have discovered that through still meditation, they can build up an amount of *Qi* that can penetrate the bone barrier. Theoretically, *Qi* is bioelectricity. If there is a great amount of energy accumulating on the front side of the valley, a great electrical potential difference can be generated between the spiritual valley and outside of the third eye. We know that bones are piezoelectric material and that the electrical conductivity of the bone acts like a semi-conductor.[14, 15, & 16] When the potential difference is built to a level, the bone can become electrically conductive and therefore the energy can communicate with the outside world.

It is believed in Daoist and Buddhist society that if your spirit can leave your body and become stronger and independent, once your physical body is dead, this spirit can be independent and avoid the path of reincarnation. Then, one can embark on the path to becoming a Buddha or divine being.

Recent reports in the media have suggested that scientists have discovered the energy between the two hemispheres of the brain communicate with each other. When more of the brain cells are activated and promoted to a more energized state, the energy trapped in the valley will be stronger and therefore, the brain wave correspondence with other brains or with nature will be stronger. This implies that the space between the two hemispheres of our brain (i.e., spiritual valley) acts as an energy resonance chamber. Normally, once a person enters a deep meditative or hypnotic state, he or she can sense or understand things which cannot be answered when he or she is awake.

From this, you can see that the more you can concentrate in a relaxed meditative state, the clearer and more wise you will be, simply because you can concentrate your mind and find your being better. Every time you practice your meditation and intend to open your third eye, you are also leading the *Qi* through the pituitary gland. This will slow down the aging process by maintaining growth hormone production. From the public announcements in 1990 from medical institutes such as the Medical College of Wisconsin and National Institute on Aging, we now understand that through injection of synthetic human growth hormone, we can possibly live up to 120 years old.[17,18,& 19] It is also said in Chinese Daoist society that "(if one dies) before 120, it is young"[20].

Personally, I believe that if modern bioenergetic and spiritual science continues to develop, in the next few decades the idea of living 120 years or more will not be surprising for most people. In the last twenty years, we have already seen a giant leap in our scientific development in understanding the functioning and the basic structure of the human mind and body. For example, the invention of the SQUID (Superconducting Quantum Interference Devices) developed in the late 1980's (the most sensitive magnetic field detector) can detect magnetic fields which are 100 million times weaker than the magnetic field strength of the Earth. With this machine, we have entered a new era of understanding our brain functions. In fact, from past experience with *Qigong* enlightenment meditation in Chinese monasteries, there is reason to believe that the key to health, longevity and happiness depends on the condition of the spirit which resides in the brain. With this new technology, we have started to open the mysterious gate to understanding our brain's function.

From the above discussion, we can conclude:

1. In order to energize your spiritual resonance chamber (spiritual valley) to a more sensitive state which allows you to communicate with other beings or with nature, you must first learn how to build up abundant *Qi* in the Lower *Dan Tian*. This can be done with the correct meditation methods.

2. To extend your life span, you must learn how to lead the *Qi* through the spinal cord upward to the pituitary gland to improve hormone production. When you do this, the energy state in the spiritual valley will be raised to a more sensitive state.

3. When the energy in the spiritual valley reaches a high level, through concentration of the third eye, you will be able to exit your spirit. You will also be able to exit your spirit through the *Baihui* (Gv-20) cavity (crown).

4. When the energy of the brain is stronger, the spirit can be raised. When the spirit is raised, the entire being will have its center. This will allow your mind to govern your *Qi*

more efficiently. The EMF (electromotive force) generated by the mind will then be strong. When EMF is strong, the *Qi* led can be strong. Naturally, the physical manifestation of the *Qi* can also be strong.

2. Qi:

According to our latest understanding, we believe that *Qi* is bioelectricity circulating in our body and existing in all living things.[14] *Qi* affects our thinking, health, spirit, longevity and is our life force. Because *Qi* is bioelectricity, our body is actually a living electrical circuit. In order to keep *Qi* smoothly flowing in this circuit and have a long life, we must consider several things.

A. **Smooth the *Qi* flow in this circuit.** That means the circuit should have a low electrical resistance. We know that fat accumulated in our body is one of the main causes of electrical resistance. Although we need some fat to store energy, we must learn how to eliminate unnecessary fat which may cause resistance to the necessary *Qi* circulation. According to Chinese medical science, we know that we have twelve primary *Qi* channels, which are called *Jing* (經).[21] One end of these twelve channels connects to our toes and fingers and the other end connects to our twelve internal organs. From *Jing* there are thousands of smaller secondary *Qi* channels, like capillaries, called *Luo* (絡) which lead the *Qi* to the skin surface and the bone marrow. The *Luo* also manage communications between the internal organs. If there is too much fat accumulated on these paths, the *Qi* circulation will be stagnant and sickness can result. These primary and secondary *Qi* channels are considered to be rivers and streams in Chinese medicine in which the *Qi* flows like water. One of the best ways for reducing resistance within these circuits is through relaxed movements.

B. **High regulating capability of the capacitors.** According to Chinese medicine, in order to maintain smooth *Qi* circulation, there are eight *Qi* vessels existing in our body. These vessels act as reservoirs which can regulate the *Qi* circulating in the twelve channels (rivers). These vessels also act as capacitors, which are commonly used as "regulators" in electrical circuits. If these vessels have failed or are incapable of regulating the *Qi* in the circuit, then the *Qi* circulating in the rivers may encounter sufficiency problems. Naturally, the internal organs which require a proper *Qi* supply can be affected and become sick. Therefore, maintaining the function of the *Qi* vessels is one of the main goals of *Qigong* practice.

C. **Abundant storage of *Qi* in the battery.** Even if you have healthy conditions in all vessels and circuits, if you do not have a good battery which can build up and store the *Qi*, then there is no origin for the *Qi* supply. Naturally, the level of your life force will also be downgraded. From Part I, we already know that the Lower *Dan Tian* is our battery. Therefore, learning how to build up the *Qi* in the Lower *Dan Tian* and store an abundant level has always been a subject of *Qigong* practice.

D. **Maintain the strong managing force for the circuit.** Finally, even if you have an abundant level of *Qi* in the Lower *Dan Tian,* healthy conditions of the eight vessels and smooth circulation of the *Qi* in the twelve channels, but do not have efficient management to direct the energy, this energy will not be used efficiently and can even be used in the wrong way. The managing center of our being is our brain. From thinking, the Electromotive Force (EMF) is generated which can therefore direct the circulation of the *Qi* and make it circulate as wanted, smoothly and efficiently. In order to make this managing center wise and powerful, the brain must be nourished. Through proper nourishment, the functions of the brain can be raised to a more active and efficient level.

Naturally, the spirit (*Shen,* 神) which resides in the brain can also be raised. This spirit is the center of our spiritual being and can lead us to the *Yin* world (or *Yin* space) which is still beyond our understanding.

3. Jin:

Our physical body is a machine which manifests our mind and *Qi* into action. Normally, we do not use our muscles to their maximum capability or efficiency unless there is a special reason, such as pushing a car or lifting a heavy weight.[22] Theoretically, in order to make our physical body demonstrate its greatest potential, we must first provide *Qi* or bioelectricity, which is the energy source of power manifestation. As explained earlier, in order to have stronger *Qi*, you need a meditative mind which can generate a stronger electromotive force (EMF). Through this concentration, your spirit can be raised to a higher focusing stage from which you can govern your entire being more efficiently. When this happens, you will be able to manifest your physical power to its maximum.

Different actions require activation of different groups of muscles. In order to manifest the *Jin* required for each individual martial arts style, different groups of muscles are emphasized. For example, you may have practiced jogging for a long time and can jog ten miles a day. However, if you try weight lifting, you will realize that your jogging potential does not necessarily provide you with any advantage in weight lifting over and above your balance, endurance, and heart and lung capacity. The reason for this is simply because you are using different muscle groups for different activities.

Therefore, in order to make the *Jin* manifested more powerful and effective, the first task is not just to build up the *Qi* abundantly or to lead the *Qi* circulating in your body smoothly and strongly. The first task is also to build a stronger **physical** body and greater muscular strength which are required for your *Jin* manifestation. If you have a strong energy supply but a weak machine, how do you expect your energy to be demonstrated efficiently and effectively? The energy will tear the machine to pieces. Thus, the first step in *Jin* training is learning how to move accurately according to the style and making the physical body stronger. The physical body is as deep as the bones and as superficial as the skin. Without this physical conditioning first, the intention of *Jin* manifestation will be in vain.

As discussed earlier, different types of *Jin* require different parts of the body. For example, Hard *Jin* uses more muscles, while Soft-Hard *Jin* and Soft *Jin* use more tendons. Therefore, learning the right method of conditioning your physical body is the first task of *Jin* training. In the next section, we will discuss more of this external *Jin* training.

7-3. External Jin and Internal Jin

In order to understand *Jin*, you must first know what both external *Jin* and internal *Jin* actually are. As mentioned earlier, external *Jin* is an external action which can be seen externally. It includes the structure of the physical frame (i.e., bones and joints) and the muscles which make the movements. External *Jin* also includes the practice of the movements which show the special characteristics of the individual style. From external *Jin* manifestation, we can normally see the specialties of a style and the kind of *Jin* it manifests.

Internal *Jin* is the practice of how to store the *Qi* in the body and how to use the concentrated mind to energize the physical body to a more highly efficient level. For Hard *Jin*, the first step in internal *Jin* training is to use the concentrated mind to energize the muscles using local *Qi*. For

Soft-Hard *Jin* and Soft *Jin*, the first step for internal *Jin* practice includes cultivating *Qi* at the Lower *Dan Tian,* leading it to circulate in the two main vessels (i.e., Small Circulation) and finally learning to lead the *Qi* to the limbs as support for the external *Jin*.

In this section, we will discuss the training theory and methods of both external *Jin* and internal *Jin*. However, though theory and methods can offer you a concept of how and what to train, they cannot offer you the correct feeling of the practice. Furthermore, according to past martial arts training experience, there are many dangers that can emerge, especially at the profound levels of Soft *Jin*. Normally, high skills and deep levels of *Jin* training should be taught or directed only by a qualified master.

A. EXTERNAL JIN (*Wai Jin,* 外勁)

1. Hard Jin (*Ying Jin,* 硬勁)

In external Hard *Jin*, first the strength and endurance of the skin, muscles and tendons are built up. In order to reach this goal, the methods and theory introduced in the Muscle/Tendon Changing (*Yi Jin Jing,* 易筋經) are adopted.

By using concentration, the local muscles and tendons are tensed and then relaxed. This method is commonly seen in Hard *Qigong*. In this training, the breath is typically held for a few seconds after the muscles reach their extreme of tension or energy manifestation. The purpose is to lead the *Qi* to the muscles, skin and even beyond. Due to the tension, the blood and *Qi* circulation is stagnant and/or slowed down, which provides nutrition, oxygen and *Qi* to the cells for multiplication. More muscle cells are thereby produced to handle the work demanded. A typical result of this is larger muscles and tendons.

There are two major kinds of muscles, white muscles and red muscles, which carry out orders from our mind. In general, red muscles relate to the endurance of your body and fine motor coordination, while white muscles handle speed and strength. The "color" of the muscle is determined by its capillary density, the red having a much higher capillary density than the white at any given volume. The red muscles are sometimes referred to as "slow-twitch" muscles, because they operate at relatively low nerve frequencies at small peak tensions. They are also highly fatigue resistant. Your heart is an example of this type of muscle. White muscles are sometimes called "fast-twitch" muscles. These muscles are responsible for any large movement of your body. They operate at higher nerve frequencies, with higher peak tensions.[22 & 23] Although both types of muscles are found interwoven throughout the body, speed and power are generally the domain of the white muscles. These muscles can develop a "memory" depending on how they are trained. If strength is over trained, normally speed suffers and vice-versa. Therefore, in order to train for speed without having a negative impact on strength, the tendons near the joints are the key. If we compare strength and quality of the muscles and tendons, you will see that tendons are much stronger than muscles. For example, the strength and endurance of the tendons in our fingers allows us to hang our body or even raise it up. We are even able to hold the entire weight of our body on the toes of single foot comfortably, mainly because of the strength of the tendons. The tendons are much stronger than the muscles in our body. When you wish to train for speed, the most important factor is to keep the muscles as relaxed as possible, allowing the ligaments and tendons to do the work.

In Hard *Jin*, more muscles than tendons are conditioned. Therefore, muscular body increases can be seen. It is also because of this that the styles which emphasize more Hard *Jin* are considered "external styles." Normally, in order to build up Hard *Jin* to a higher level, Hard *Qigong* practices are required.

Often the movements of *Qigong* are specially designed for the purpose of Hard *Jin*'s manifestation. They also demonstrate the special characteristics and martial purposes of the style.

2. Soft-Hard Jin (*Ruan Ying Jin,* 軟硬勁)

If we consider the special characteristics of Soft-Hard *Jin*, we can see that in the manifestation of Soft-Hard *Jin*, at first the action is soft and the physical body is very relaxed. However, right before reaching the target, the physical body is suddenly tensed.

From this, we can see that at the beginning of the *Jin*'s emission, usage of the muscles is reduced significantly while tendons are given more attention. The main reason for this is to provide good conditions for smooth *Qi* circulation. However, when the target is almost reached, a sudden tension of the muscles is used to prevent the over-stretching of the ligaments. Over-stretching of the ligaments in such a short pulse is the main cause of many joint injuries in *Jin* manifestation practice.

If you think clearly, you can see that in Soft-Hard *Jin* manifestation, first the speed muscles are used and when the action reaches the target, the power muscles immediately take over. From this alternative usage of the both kind of muscles, power can be stronger and more penetrating.

In order to lead the *Qi* to circulate, correct breathing habits must also be cultivated. Moreover, through correct breathing techniques, the *Qi* is led through the joints to enter the bone marrow when the body is soft and led outward through the sides of the bones to support the muscles' action when the body becomes tensed. In order to reach this goal, the breathing is soft and deep. Often, in order to harden the muscles at the end of the action, holding the breath is also commonly employed in the training.

To provide optimal physical conditions for the manifestation of external *Jin*, the *Qigong* patterns are used to relax the muscles and coordinate the breathing at first and then to tense up the muscles at the end of the action. Also, body conditioning for Hard *Jin* and Soft *Jin* is often trained independently. Once a practitioner has grasped the essence of the training, he or she will be able to mix them skillfully and naturally. It is said: "When it is needed to be hard, it can be hard. When it is required to be soft, it can be soft. Soft and hard can support each other skillfully. Then it is called understanding the *Jin*."[24]

3. Soft Jin (*Rou Jin,* 柔勁)

Physically, Soft *Jin* emphasizes the tendons, ligaments and marrow. The health of the bone marrow is considered very important since it is the bone marrow which can store and release the *Qi* in the limbs. In *Taijiquan,* it is said: "condense the *Qi* to the bone marrow" (凝氣於髓). This means to store the *Qi* to the bone marrow before the *Jin* is emitted.

Since in Soft *Jin* stiff muscular power is not emphasized, the speed muscles and tendons are heavily trained. In addition, in order to prevent injury of the ligaments caused by the fast, jerking emission of *Jin*, the strength and endurance of the ligaments must be conditioned. In order to reach this goal, Moving Soft *Qigong* was designed to exercise the tendons and ligaments. In Part II of this book, you should have obtained a clear idea of how Moving Hard *Qigong* is adopted into the Hard *Jin* and how the Moving Soft *Qigong* is used as the foundation of Soft *Jin*.

Since speed is the main factor in this power's manifestation, the entire body must act as softly as a whip. Normally, Soft *Jin* is more penetrating than the other two kinds of *Jin*. Naturally, its theory and training methods are also the hardest. In a fight, normally **to be soft is difficult and to be hard is easy.** In order to be soft, both the mental and physical selves must be relaxed. However, this is no easy task when the situation happens.

Danger of External Jin Manifestation:

When you train *Jin*, you must also consider the possibility of danger caused by the methods of training or from improper practice. Theoretically, to be too hard all the time is not good for *Qi* circulation and to be too soft without knowing the hard can also cause swift degeneration of the physical body. The best training for health is to train both hard (*Yang*) and soft (*Yin*).

Next, we will summarize **some of** the possible dangers which can be caused from *Jin* training. This is not an exhaustive list and YMAA would be very interested in obtaining feedback from the reader in order to update it in future volumes.

1. Hard Jin (*Ying Jin*, 硬勁)

The first concern in Hard *Jin* training is the over development of the muscles. Due to the constant tensing of the muscles in Hard *Jin* training, muscles will be built up to a highly developed level. This can cause the body's *Qi* to manifest too strongly and can make the internal organs too *Yang*. Normally, after a martial artist trains Hard *Jin* for several years, the physical body will be over developed and the *Qi* state will be very *Yang*. If he or she stops the training or gets old, the physical body can degenerate very fast. The consequences of this can be high blood pressure, nervousness or uncontrolled impulses, or even stroke. This kind of phenomena is well known as "energy dispersion" (*San Gong*, 散功) in Chinese martial society. Normally, in order to prevent this problem, a practitioner will turn into softer training and also begin practice on the internal side. That is why it is said: "External style is from external to internal and from hard to soft."

Normally, in the *Jin* emitting training, damage to the ligaments is also a serious concern. However, the advantage of Hard *Jin* is that because the muscles are tensed, the ligaments are well protected. However, one of the most serious problems encountered in Hard *Jin* training is actually injury to the spine. The reason is that when you are emitting Hard *Jin*, the muscles of the torso are very tense. In order to emit power strongly, the torso's twisting power is necessary. That means the joints in the vertebrae will be twisted under heavy pressure (Figure 7-9). This could result in joint damage in the spine, especially in the lower back area. This is commonly seen in those who have practiced Hard *Jin* for some time. Therefore, how to move the spine in order to relax the joints and to repair this damage has become a critical part of Hard *Jin* training.

2. Soft-Hard Jin (*Ruan Ying Jin*, 軟硬勁)

Compared with the other categories of *Jin* manifestation, Soft-Hard *Jin* is probably the least dangerous. This is because, when Soft-Hard *Jin* is manifested, it is soft at first and right before the power reaches the opponent's body, the physical body is suddenly tensed up. In this case, the body is not tense all the time and therefore the muscles will not be over-developed. Problems caused from "energy dispersion" will be naturally eliminated.

Moreover, since the physical body is tensed right before the contact, the ligaments in the joint areas are also well protected. Though the penetrating power generated is not as great as that generated by Soft *Jin*, it is significantly greater than that of Hard *Jin*.

3. Soft Jin (*Rou Jin*, 柔勁)

In Soft *Jin* manifestation, the entire body is soft all the time. Therefore, the problem of "energy dispersion" does not exist. However, the risk of damaging the ligaments in Soft *Jin* manifestation is the greatest among the three categories. This is because the muscles and tendons remain

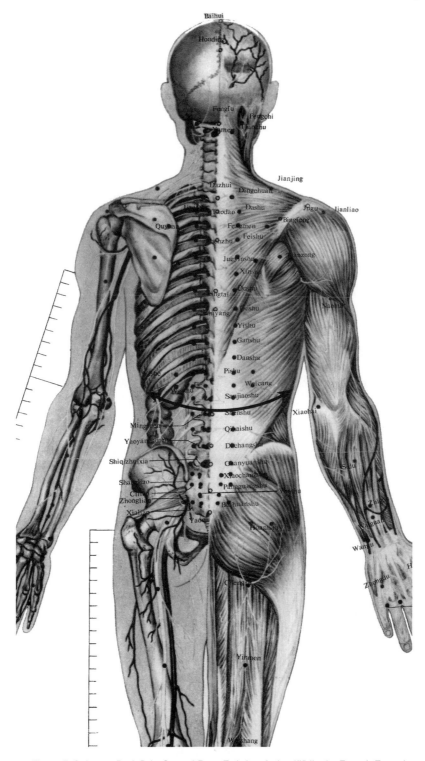

Figure 7–9. Lower Back Pain Caused From Twisting Action While the Torso is Tensed

soft and relaxed, even when power is manifested. If the method is not correct, the ligaments in the joint areas can be torn. In the worst case, the ligaments can be detached from the bones.

In order to prevent damage to the ligament areas, the entire body must act like a whip. You whip the power out through the arms. You must also know the correct timing and method to pull it back right before you tear the ligaments. When you pull back, at the moment of pulling back, the muscles and tendons are tensed for a short time, protecting the ligaments at this critical moment. However, to a beginner or non-proficient martial artist, it is very difficult to catch the correct timing. Also, many *Jin* manifestations cannot be manifested in this whip-like manner simply because the angles manifested are not proper for whipping. Therefore, these *Jin* are normally applied with Soft-Hard *Jin* or hard *Jin*. From this, you can see that in order to learn the correct manner for manifesting Soft *Jin*, an experienced master is necessary.

In addition, in order to manifest Soft *Jin* to its maximum, internal *Qi* cultivation and circulation remain the most critical part of the training. Unfortunately, this cannot be understood or done easily by beginners or non-proficient martial artists. In order to understand the internal side of Soft *Jin* manifestation, the training of Small Circulation and Grand Circulation must be done. Otherwise, the Soft *Jin* manifested will remain merely external.

B. INTERNAL JIN (*Nei Jin,* 內勁)

Internal *Jin* is the energy or *Qi* which is the essential origin of the power or *Jin*. Without great amounts of energy and its circulation, the *Jin* manifested will remain external. This means that the *Qigong* training to build up the *Qi* storage and to use the concentrated mind to lead the *Qi* to complete the Small Circulation and Grand Circulation are key issues.

1. Hard Jin (*Ying Jin,* 硬勁)

For Hard *Jin* manifestation, the first step of internal *Jin* training is learning how to concentrate the mind and use the local *Qi* to energize the muscles and tendons. There is no difference from when you concentrate your mind to push a car or lift a heavy object. However, through practice and concentration, the contribution of the local *Qi* to the *Jin* manifestation can be significantly increased. Normally, in order to make the power manifest strongly, Reverse Abdominal Breathing is employed. Moreover, often a belt is used to tighten the abdominal area. In this case, when the power is manifested and the abdomen is pushing outward, through the resistance of the belt, the power can be manifested more efficiently.

Later, when a practitioner has completed training the Small Circulation and Grand Circulation, he can then apply the *Qi* from the Lower *Dan Tian* to the physical body for energization. Naturally, in order to lead the *Qi* smoothly and strongly, the body should be relaxed. This means, more and more, that Hard *Jin* manifestation will be shifted into the Soft-Hard *Jin* or Soft *Jin*. That is why martial artists in the external styles begin with hard and external and gradually change into soft and internal.

2. Soft-Hard Jin (*Ruan-Ying Jin,* 軟硬勁)

For Soft-Hard *Jin*, the cultivation of the *Qi* in the Lower *Dan Tian,* Small Circulation and Grand Circulation are important. Although by using the local *Qi*, the Soft-Hard *Jin* can be manifested efficiently, by using the Lower *Dan Tian Qi* the power manifested will be much more proficient and complete.

A belt on the abdominal area is also often used at the beginning stage of Soft-Hard *Jin* training. However, when Lower *Dan Tian Qi* is used, in order to free the restrictions on *Qi* circulation, the belt will be removed.

3. Soft Jin (*Rou Jin*, 柔勁)

The main energy support for the Soft *Jin* comes from the Lower *Dan Tian*. Local *Qi* is not used since the tension of the muscles and tendons is not required. In order to have Soft *Jin* reach its most efficient state, internal *Jin* is required. It is also from this internal cultivation of the *Qi* that spiritual enlightenment can be reached. A belt is seldom used in Soft *Jin* manifestation. To practice the internal cultivation and circulation of *Qi*, you may refer to the book: **Yang's Small and Grand Circulation Meditation**, to be published shortly.

Unification of the External Jin and Internal Jin

Unification of the external *Jin* and the internal *Jin* means to apply the internal *Jin* to the external *Jin* manifestation. When you are doing this, the mind, breathing and the coordination of the *Huiyin* cavity movement are essential keys to the unification. With correct practice, power can be manifested to its maximum level. Traditionally, in order to reach a great level for the *Jin* manifestation, more than ten years of correct practice both external and internal is required.

In addition, you must also learn how to coordinate the sounds. Different sounds are commonly used for *Jin* manifestation. As explained in Section 4-4, from uttering sounds, the spirit can be raised and the *Qi* can be led efficiently. There are many sounds used in Chinese martial arts. However, the two sounds, "*Hen*" and "*Ha*," are the most common and important in *Jin* manifestation. "*Hen*" is considered as *Yin*, which can lead the *Qi* inward for storage and outward to emit *Jin* with some power reserved. "*Ha*" is an extremely *Yang* sound which can raise your spirit to a high level; it is therefore commonly used to manifest attacking power. If you are interested in knowing more about the applications of these two sounds, please refer to **Tai Chi Theory & Martial Power** (formerly *Advanced Yang Style Tai Chi Chuan, Vol. 1.*), by YMAA.

The final and ultimate goal of *Jin* manifestation is to apply the *Jin* into the opponent's body. In order to do this, you must train yourself until you have a **sense of enemy**. This means that whenever you emit your *Jin*, you are imagining that you are actually fighting with someone. Through this imagination, the spirit can be raised and the *Qi* can be led efficiently. Therefore, the internal and external are unified.

References

1. *High Technology Business,* p. 3, July-August, 1989.

2. *The Blood-Brain Barrier in Health and Disease,* Bradbury, M. W., et al., eds., 1986.

3. *Brain Imaging,* Bradshaw, J. R., 1988.

4. *Inside the Brain,* Calvin, W. H. and Ojemann, G. A., 1980.

5. *Functions of Brain,* Coen, C. W., ed., 1985.

6. **The Wonder of Being Human,** Eccles, John. and Robinson, D. N., 1985.

7. *Human Brain and Human Learning,* Hart, Leslie, 1983.

8. *The Human Brain,* Nolte, John, 1981.

9. *Brain and Mind,* Oakley, David, ed., 1985.

10. *Neurobiology,* 2nd ed., Shepherd, G. M., 1988.

11. *High Brain Functions*, Wise, S. P., 1987.

12. *The New Encyclopedia Brittanica*, Vol. 4, Encyclopedia Brittanica Inc., 1993.

13. *Fundamentals of Physics*, David Holliday and Robert Resnick, p. 308, John Wiley & Sons, Inc. New York, NY, 1970.

14. *The Body Electric*, Robert O. Becker, M.D. and Gary Selden, William Morrow and Company, Inc., New York, 1985.

15. *Live Invisible Current,* Albert L. Huebner, East West Journal, June 1986.

16. *Healing with Nature's Energy,* Richard Leviton, East West Journal, 1986.

17. **"Effects of Human Growth Hormone in Men Over 60 Years Old,"** *New England Journal of Medicine,* Daniel Rudman, July, 1990.

18. **"The Foundation of Youth,"** *Harvard Health Letter,* Vol 17, Number 8, June, 1992.

19. **"The Hormone That Marks Your Body 20 Years Younger,"** Bill Lawren, *Longevity,* Oct. 1990.

20. 一百二十謂之夭。

21. *Acupuncture*, A Comprehensive Text, Shanghai College of Traditional Medicine, Eastland Press, Chicago, 1981.

22. *Mechanics of Muscle*, 2nd Edition, Daniel J. Schneck, New York University Press, p. 19, 1992.

23. *Skeletal Muscle – Structure and Function*, Richard L. Lieber, Williams & Wilkins, p. 15, 1992.

24. 當軟則軟，該硬則硬，軟硬相濟，是爲懂勁。

Chapter 8

White Crane Jin Patterns

白鶴勁

8-1. Introduction

As mentioned previously, there are four different major Southern White Crane styles and one Northern White Crane style currently existing in Chinese martial arts. All of these styles have their own different ways of manifesting power, and each emphasizes different types of power manifestation. Consequently, the *Jin* patterns in each style can also be somewhat different. In this chapter, only those *Jin* which are trained by the Ancestral Southern White Crane (Trembling Crane or Shaking Crane) will be discussed. Although the *Jin* patterns introduced here are used for Southern White Crane, in fact, you may adopt more than half of them into any other martial style. The basic theory and the principles of manifesting *Jin* remain the same.

In White Crane *Jin* training, many *Jins* can be executed in either a hard way or a soft way. Generally, for these *Jins,* you start out hard and gradually become soft. However, many others can **only** be performed in either a hard way or a soft way. Others are executed softly at the beginning of the *Jin* emission and turn hard at the end.

Before we introduce the different *Jin* patterns in White Crane, again I would like to remind you that *Jin* includes external *Jin* (*Wai Jin - Yang*) and internal *Jin* (*Nei Jin - Yin*). The internal *Jin* is the *Qigong* training which we have discussed in Part II of this book, and the external *Jin* is the moving patterns which will be introduced in this chapter. To make your *Jin* manifestation clear, sharp and penetrating, you must train both types. You should understand that without the internal, *Jin* is only the external movement without a strong energy foundation. Without the correct body action or movements, the *Jin* manifestation will be stagnant and its efficiency will be reduced.

Finally, you should recognize that White Crane practice routines are constructed from a sequence of *Jin* patterns. From each *Jin* pattern, many applications are derived. Normally, how to apply the *Jin* patterns into martial applications is kept secret by the master. How deep a White Crane practitioner understands these applications depends on individual ability in White Crane styles. It also depends on personal martial arts experiences. Although the number of *Jins* is limited, the applications can be countless and profound.

In the next section, I will introduce the White Crane *Jin* patterns by dividing them into three categories: neutral *Jins*, offensive *Jins* and defensive *Jins*.

8-2. White Crane Jin Patterns

Before the introduction of different *Jin* patterns, you should know an important thing. External *Jin* patterns are only the body's movement. From this movement, power is generated and then directed to different parts of the body for either neutralization or attack. Therefore, with the same body movements, power can be manifested in different hand or leg forms depending on the target or the purpose of the action. For example, although they use the same body movement, the hand forms for attacking the eyes are different from those for attacking the throat or the chest. The leg forms attacking the groin and the shin are also different. Therefore, how to apply the body movement into actual fighting situations is a living art which must be pondered and figured out by yourself, since there can be countless applications from the same body movements.

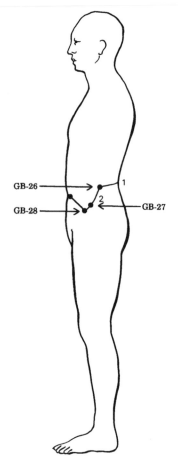

Figure 8–1. The Girdle Vessel (Dai Mai)

I.   Neutral Jin (non-offensive and non-defensive)

Neutral *Jin* is a *Jin* of neither defense (*Yin*) nor offense (*Yang*). It is the practice of self sensitivity, which can provide a deep foundation for manifesting both defensive and offensive *Jin*.

1.   Steady Jin (*Wen Jin*, 穩勁)

Steady *Jin* is generated from balancing, centering and rooting. Therefore, it can be called a combination of balancing *Jin*, centering *Jin* and rooting *Jin*. Steady *Jin* is heavily practiced in all Chinese martial arts styles. The reason is that if you are not steady and rooted, any *Jin* manifestation will be weak and useless.

In order to have good balance, you must learn how to expand your *Qi* circulating in the Belt Vessel (or Girdle Vessel) around your waist area (Figure 8-1). The more you can expand the *Qi* horizontally from the waist area, the more you can balance yourself.

Only after you have balanced yourself, can you find your center. The center includes your mental center and your physical center. From mutual coordination through the mind, you can center yourself comfortably.

After you have found the center, you can be rooted. When you train your rooting, your mind should be under your feet. Start with a couple of inches and then grow deeper and deeper. All of this training is explained in Part II in the Still Hard *Qigong* section. You should refer to this section for details.

After you are rooted, you look for steadiness of your body. That means you can keep your balance, center and root when an external force invades your body or when you are emitting power for an attack. From this, you can see that Steady *Jin* is the foundation both for Neutralization *Jin* (i.e., Defensive *Jin*) and for Attacking *Jin* (i.e., Offensive *Jin*).

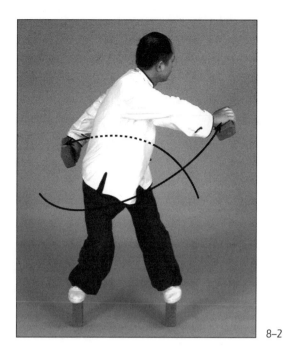

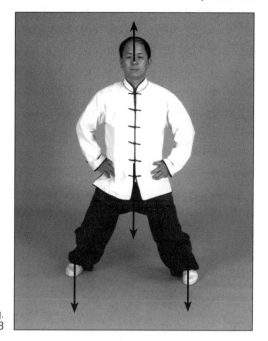

8–2   Fig.
        8–3

Steady *Jin* training can be divided into Hard Style and Soft Style training. In Hard Style training, you train according to the description of the Still Hard *Qigong* explained in Part II. After you have trained for a long time, you carry weights in your hands and swing them around while standing on bricks (Figure 8-2). You may practice with a partner.

In Soft Style Steady *Jin* training, first you must learn how to move your body softly, especially your spine. That means your torso must be relaxed to the vertebrae. In addition, you must learn how to use your waist to direct the power either for neutralization or for an attack. In order to reach this goal, the waist area must be extremely relaxed. When the waist is relaxed and soft, your opponent's power landing on your upper body can be dissolved at the waist area. Consequently, your root is protected. Other than practicing the softness of the torso through the Soft *Qigong* introduced in Part II, you must also practice with a partner. Pushing hands practice with a partner in the internal Chinese martial styles is very effective for this training.

2. **Pressing Upward Jin** (*Ding Jin,* 頂勁)

Pressing Upward *Jin* is used to raise the spirit of vitality. When you practice this *Jin*, first inhale deeply through the abdomen and then lead the *Qi* downward to the bottom of the feet, while also leading the *Qi* upward to the top of your head. It is said in the *Taiji* classics: **If there is a top, there is a bottom; if there is a front, there is a back; if there is a left, there is a right. If the mind wants to go upward, this implies considering downward.**[1] Force and counter force are mutually balanced against each other. In order to raise your spirit, you must first have a firm root. Therefore, Pressing Upward *Jin* is the reverse side or the result of Rooting *Jin* (Figure 8-3).

Commonly in Hard Style training, you imagine that you are using both of your hands to push upward at the sky. This is called **"Both Hands are Holding the Heaven Posture"** (雙手托天勢) (Figure 8-4). In this practice, you imagine the heavens are falling down and you use your power to push them upward. Naturally, this kind of practice is physically demanding. However, from this practice, the spine is straightened upright and the upward and downward *Qi* are balanced.

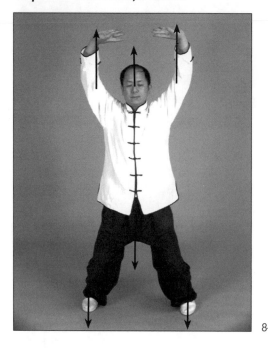 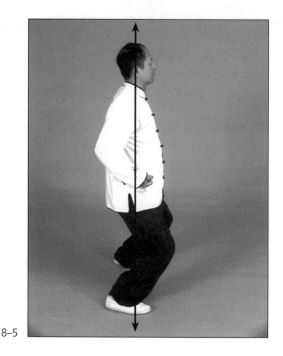

8-4   8-5

In Soft Style training, this kind of training is called: "**Insubstantial (Energy) Leads the Head Upward *Jin*"** (虛領頂勁) (Figure 8-5). That means you imagine that there is an invisible force to lead the energy upward. For this practice, your spine must be straight and relaxed. This implies that your torso should remain relaxed and soft.

3. **Trembling Jin or Shaking Jin** (*Zhan Jin,* 顫勁) (*Dou Jin,* 抖勁)

Trembling or Shaking *Jin* is the most fundamental and also the most important and unique *Jin* in White Crane style. From this *Jin*, many other *Jins* can be manifested. This *Jin* imitates the shaking power of a dog when it gets out of the water or a crane's trembling power after the rain.

In order to have good, powerful shaking, the root must be firm. The power can be generated from the bottoms of the feet, then pass through the joints in the ankles, knees, hips and spine, then manifested on the surface of the body (Figure 8-6). The shaking power can also be generated from the waist's twisting which is controlled by the pelvis and then brought through the spine, and manifested on the skin's surface (Figure 8-7).

In order to have significant and powerful *Jin*, the muscles must be relaxed. All the action comes from the twisting power of the tendons in the joint areas. From this, you can see that Trembling *Jin* or Shaking *Jin* is the soft side of training in Southern White Crane.

4. **Winding Jin** (*Pan Jin,* 盤勁)

Winding *Jin* combines the balance and rooting of the body. Remember, when you are balanced, you will find the center, and when you have the center, you can be rooted. Finally, only when you are rooted can the spirit be raised. From this, you can see that the first step for training Winding *Jin* is the balance of the physical and mental bodies. As we know, there are eight vessels in our body. Expect for the Belt Vessel, all vessels are lined up with the torso. The Belt Vessel is the only one in which the energy is expanding outward parallel with the ground when you are standing (Figure 8-8). Theoretically, in order to have good balance, you would like to expand the *Qi* as wide as possible. The key to training *Qi* expansion from the Belt Vessel has already been discussed in Part II.

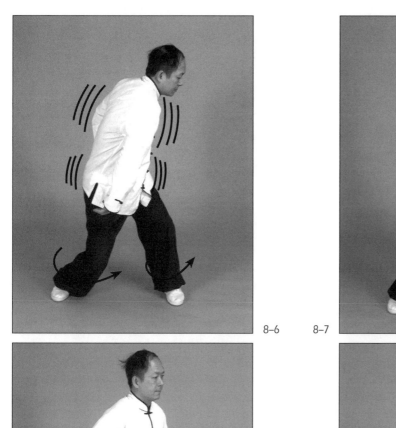

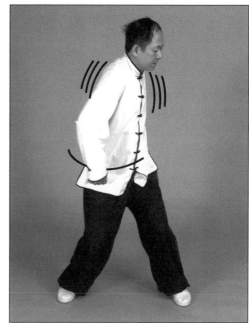

8–6   8–7

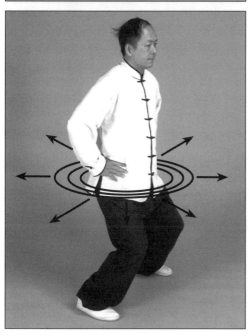

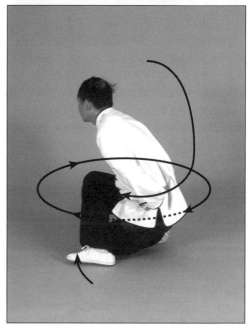

8–8   8–9

Winding *Jin* can be trained both in the arms and the legs. When it is trained for legs, as mentioned earlier, it is used to train root and the stability of the stances. Naturally, from this training, the strength and endurance of the joints such as the ankles, knees and hips will be built to a stronger level. When you train Winding *Jin* for the leg, first you stand in the Horse Stance with both hands beside the waist (Figure 8-8). Next, rotate your body either to the right or to the left while squatting down (Figure 8-9). When you train this, you should have a feeling like a snake winding down to the ground and even underneath, firm and steady. After you stay there for a few seconds, turn your body back to Horse Stance and squat down to the other side. If you are a beginner, you should train only a few times. Only if your joints become stronger should you increase the number of squat times.

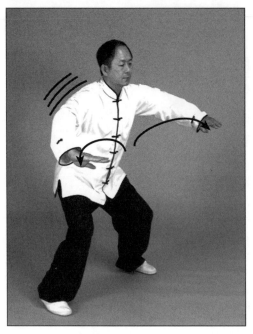
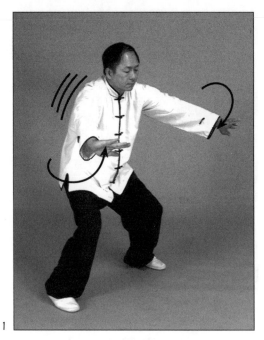

8-10   8-11

When you train your arms, you are actually training how to use your waist to direct the circular motions of the arms and hands. This kind of circular motion originates from the winding power of the rooted legs, is controlled by the waist and is finally manifested to the arms. This entire body's winding power is just like a spring, twisted and wound. When this winding strength is manifested, it becomes a strong circular attacking or defensive *Jin*. From this, you can see that Winding *Jin* is the foundation of many White Crane *Jins* in which horizontal circular motions are the source of the *Jins*' manifestation.

When you practice this Winding *Jin*, first generate the winding power from the twisting of the legs, directed by the waist to reach the arms and hands. You may first practice both arms winding. This is simpler, since both arms offer you a more balanced and symmetrical feeling (Figure 8-10). You should practice circling to one side first and then to the other side (Figure 8-11). You must practice **until you have the feeling that from the legs (root), through the waist and to the arms, the body acts like a soft whip**. That means from your legs, to the waist and to the hand, the body acts as one unit, continuous and smooth. After you have mastered the movements of both arms' winding practice, you should practice the single arm form (Figures 8-12 and 8-13). Again, you should practice both directions.

5. **Listening Jin** (*Ting Jin,* 聽勁)

Listening means "skin's listening" or "skin's feeling" instead of listening with the ears. Listening *Jin* is popularly trained in Chinese soft martial styles. In the soft martial styles, sticking (or Adhering) *Jin* and Coiling *Jin* are heavily emphasized. In order to adhere and coil efficiently and effectively, the sensitivity of the skin is the most important factor for successful sticking and coiling.

Normally, this kind of Listening *Jin* can be trained through skin-marrow internal elixir *Qigong* training. From skin breathing *Qigong* training, the sensitivity of the skin can be improved. You should refer to Part II for skin-marrow *Qigong* practice.

Another way of training Listening *Jin* is through the so called "Bridging Hands" (*Qiao Shou,* 橋手) practice with a partner. Bridging hands training starts with harder contact for beginners.

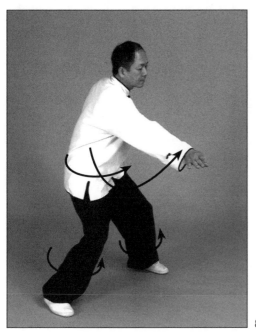 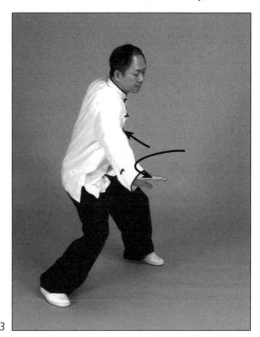

8–12   8–13

Only after a person has mastered the basic bridging techniques will he gradually become softer and softer. When Qiao Shou becomes extremely soft, it is no different from the practice of *Taiji* "Pushing Hands."

6. **Understanding Jin** (*Dong Jin,* 懂勁)

Understanding *Jin* is the capability of understanding what your skin "hears." If, through the feeling of the physical contact, you still cannot understand your opponent's intention for every movement, you are not listening well. Only if you understand your opponent's intention can you then respond accordingly.

Normally, Understanding *Jin* must be built up from the experience of sticking hands (Bridging Hands) practice. Start with slow communication, and gradually become familiar with the language. Often, different opponents have different ways of communication; therefore, in order to increase your experience, you must practice with many different partners. Remember, the more experience you have, the better your understanding will be.

II. **OFFENSIVE JIN** (*Yang Jin*) 攻勁 (陽勁)

Offensive *Jin* is mainly used for attack. When *Jin* is initiated, it can be manifested from the fingers, the blade of the hands, the palms, wrist, fists, forearms, elbows, shoulders, back, chest, hips, thighs, knees, the blade of the feet, the soles, heels, or toes depending on the techniques.

Offensive *Jin* can be classified as pure *Yang Jin* or *Yang-Yin Jin*. In the attack of a pure *Yang Jin*, the power generated is completely emitted and is aimed at the opponent's body, while in *Yang-Yin Jin*, part of the power is reserved either to prevent disadvantageous situations or for the initiation of a second strike.

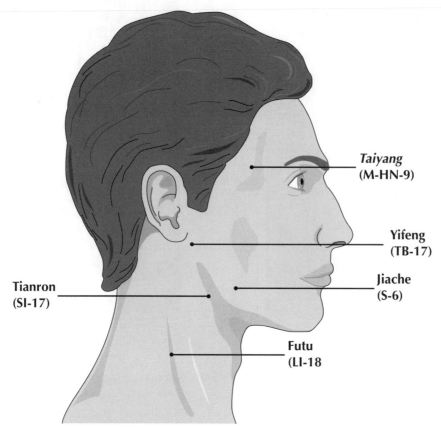

Figure 8–14. The Taiyang (M-HN-9), Yifeng (TB-17), Jiche (S-6), Tianron (SI-17), and Futu (LI-18) Cavities

A. JIN MANIFESTED ON ARMS OR BODY 手勁與身勁

1. Pecking Jin (*Zhuo Jin*, 啄勁)

Pecking *Jin* is a Soft-Hard *Jin* and is one of the major *Jins* which must be learned in Southern White Crane, especially in the Eating Crane style. Pecking *Jin* is using the finger tips, which are formed as the beak of a bird, to attack the opponent's vital areas such as eyes, temples (*Taiyang*, M-HN-9, 太陽), sides of the neck (*Futu*, LI-18, 伏兔 or *Tianron*, SI-17, 天容), under the ears (*Yifeng*, TB-17, 翳風), sides of chin (*Jiache*, S-6, 頰車), etc. (Figure 8-14). As with other *Jin* manifestation, many different hand forms are commonly used depending on the vital areas being attacked and the angles of attacking.

General hand forms which are used for Pecking *Jin* are:

a. Formation of thumb and index finger as a beak (Figure 8-15)

b. Formation of thumb, index and middle fingers as a beak (Figure 8-16)

c. Formation of five fingers as a beak (Figure 8-17)

d. Formation of four fingers

    i. Crane Wing (*He Chi*, 鶴翅) (Figure 8-18)

    ii. Hammer Hand (*Chui Shou*, 捶手) (Figure 8-19)

    iii. Gong Word Hand (*Gong Zi Shou*, 弓字手) (Figure 8-20)

    iv. Phoenix Eye Hand (*Feng Yan Shou*, 鳳眼手) (Figure 8-21)

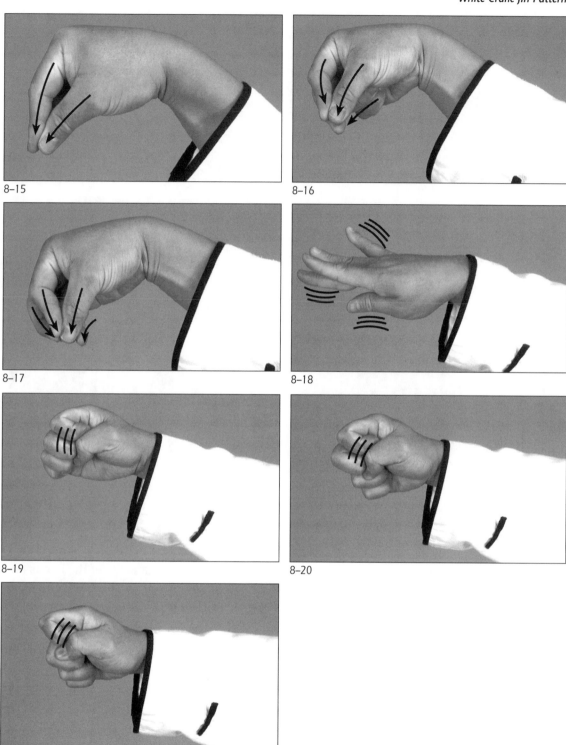

8–15

8–16

8–17

8–18

8–19

8–20

8–21

Since the main goal of the pecking is to generate sharp penetrating power, a jerking motion generated from the body is necessary. Generally, when you are in a situation which allows you to apply Pecking *Jin*, the distance between you and your opponent is short range. In such a short range, the timing is urgent and therefore power is often generated from the waist and the shoulders instead of from the legs.

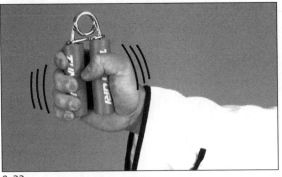

8–22

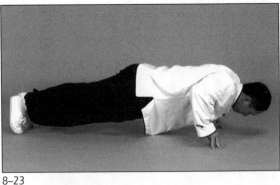

8–23

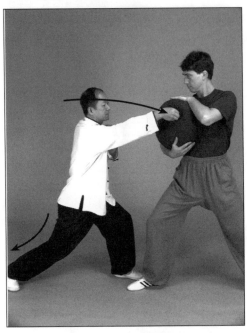

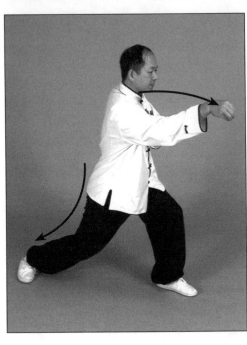

8–24   8–25

In order to apply pecking efficiently, the fingers' strength and endurance must first be trained. In addition, the inner physical structure of the tendons and ligaments in the hands must be strong. Normally, this can be done by grabbing training and finger push ups. For grabbing training, you can use a spring, which is available in most sport shops (Figure 8-22). In finger push ups, simply push up by using your fingers. In order to build up the endurance of the tendons and ligaments in the hands, stay half way up in the push up position for a minute, and gradually increase the time to three minutes (Figure 8-23).

Once you have the strength and endurance required, place a cushion or a pile of tissue on the target and generate jerking power to peck the target (Figure 8-24). The power can be generated either from waist or the shoulders (Figure 8-25). The reason for sitting on a chair is that, as mentioned earlier, Pecking *Jin* is normally applied when you and your opponent are in short range. The timing is urgent and the power generated from the waist or shoulder is necessary. That means Pecking *Jin* is a short *Jin* instead of a long *Jin*.

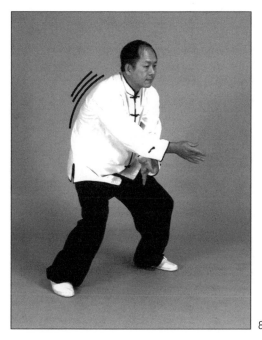

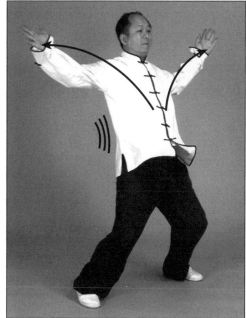

8–26   8–27

2. Developing (Expanding) Jin

(*Zhan Jin,* 展勁)

Developing or Expanding *Jin* can either be a Hard *Jin* or a Soft Hard *Jin*. This *Jin* is to train the expanding power of the bow formed from the chest muscles. As mentioned earlier, in order to generate great power, the muscles in the torso and the chest are treated as the two biggest bows in our body. If you know how to store the power in these two bows and manifest it efficiently, the power generated will be strong. This *Jin* specializes in the training of the chest bow. Naturally, the coordination of the spine is critical to make this *Jin* manifest correctly and efficiently.

8–28

In this training, first place both of your arms right in front of your chest (Figure 8-26). Inhale deeply and then exhale. When you exhale, jerk your arms outward to the sides suddenly and powerfully (Figures 8-27 and 8-28). To prevent injury, you should start with minor jerking strength until someday your chest muscles and tendons are strong enough to apply more power in the jerking.

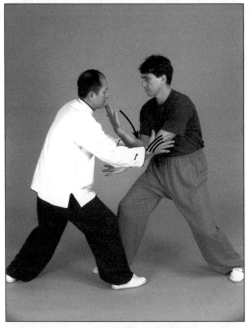
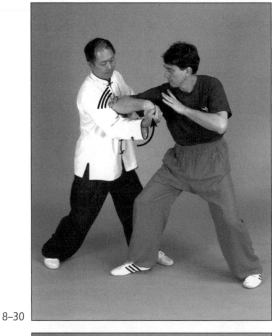

8–29   8–30

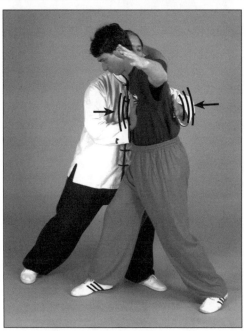
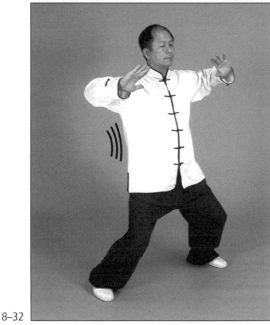

8–31   8–32

3. Squeezing Jin (*Ji Jin,* 擠勁)

Squeezing *Jin* can be either Hard or Soft-Hard. The action of Squeezing *Jin* is reversed from Expanding *Jin*. The purpose of squeezing is to lock or to seal the opponent's arm movement by squeezing his elbows inward (Figure 8-29). This Squeezing *Jin* can also be applied on other occasions such, as *Qin Na* on the wrist (Figure 8-30) or squeezing the solar plexus to seal the breath (Figure 8-31).

This *Jin* originates from the muscle contraction from the front chest area, and the force is extended to the arms and hands. When you train, first open your arms while thrusting your chest out (Figure 8-32). Inhale deeply and then exhale while squeezing both of your forearms toward each other (Figure 8-33). In order to increase the squeezing strength, you may squeeze a ball between your palms.

– 274 –

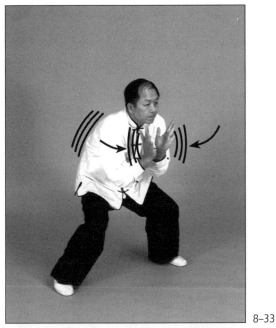

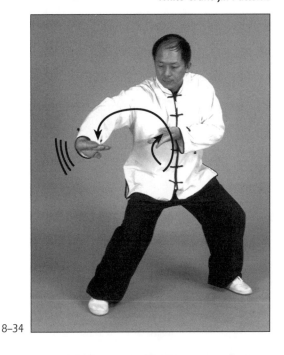

8-33   8-34

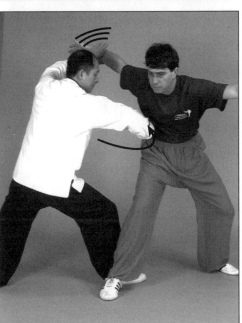

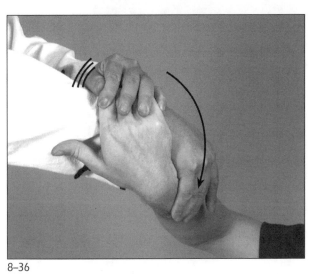

8-36

8-35

4. **Filing Jin** (*Cuo Jin*, 挫(搓)勁)

Filing *Jin* can be manifested as either Hard or Soft-Hard. There are many ways to manifest Filing *Jin*. The first way is to file horizontally with a circular motion (Figure 8-34). The target of filing normally is the tendons on the sides of the waist or the lower ribs (Figure 8-35). The second way of filing is downward, which can be used to control the wrist (Figure 8-36) or the elbow in *Qin Na*. Finally, the filing action can be used against the front or the sides of the neck (Figure 8-37).

It does not matter which way the Filing *Jin* is applied, the motion is generated from the waist (or legs) with the torso's twisting, and is then extended to the arms for the filing (Figure 8-38). The way of manifesting the *Jin* horizontally is different from filing downward vertically. You must practice until you feel the manifestation of the *Jin* is smooth and comfortable.

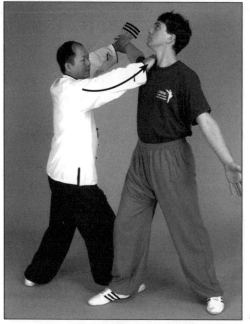

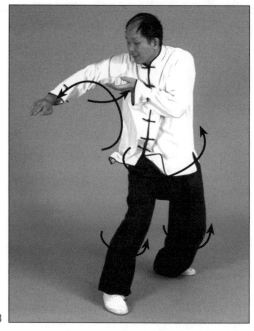

8–37   8–38

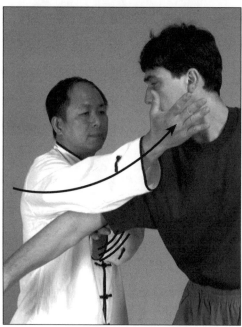

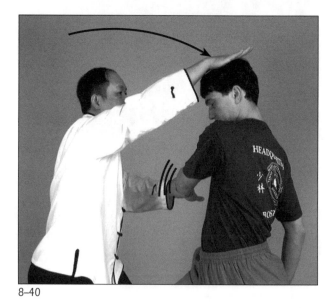

8–40

8–39

5. Flapping Jin (*Pai Jin,* 拍勁)

Flapping *Jin* is a Soft *Jin* in which the palms on either side are used to slap the opponent in the face, crown of the head, or groin. When the face, especially the front side of the face or ear, is slapped by a conditioned hand, dizziness can be generated (Figure 8-39). When the crown of the head (*Baihui,* Gv-20, 百會) is slapped, especially at midnight, serious damage can be caused (Figure 8-40). This is because the *Qi* is strongly flowing is this area. Any shock or disturbance can damage the brain easily. Finally, when the groin is slapped, a serious pain or even death can be caused (Figure 8-41). The reason for this is that the liver primary *Qi* channel passes through the bottom of the groin (Figure 8-42). When the groin is attacked, the shock can cause the liver to tense and be damaged.

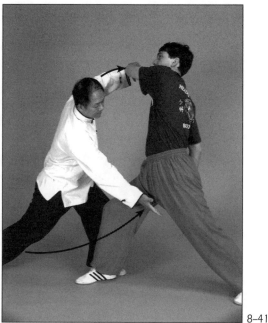

8–41

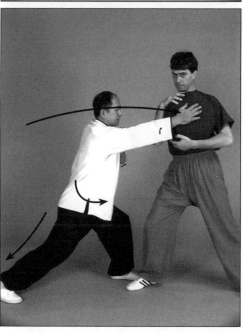

8–43

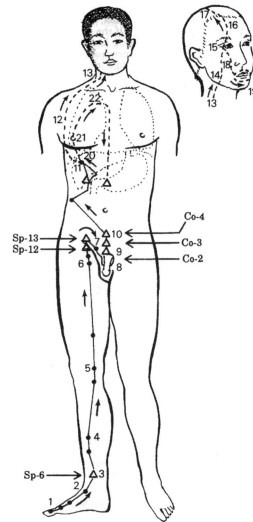

Figure 8–42. The Liver Primary Qi Channel

When you train Flapping *Jin*, again the whipping action is generated from the legs or waist and finally reaches to the hands. You can first place a pad or cushion on the imaginary target and learn how to slap it (Figure 8-43). Gradually, make the pad thinner and thinner as your hands grow stronger. When you train, you should be careful to not cause injury deep inside your hands. If there is any injury, it may cause arthritis later in your life.

6. Throwing Jin (*Pao Jin,* 抛勁)

Throwing *Jin* can either be Hard, Soft-Hard, or Soft depending on the purpose of manifestation. When it is used for hard techniques, it is used to pull out the opponent's root and throw him or her away (Figure 8-44). When it is used as Soft-Hard or Soft, it is used to jerk the *Jin* forward for attacking (Figure 8-45). This *Jin* is also used to hurl darts, a hidden weapon, at the opponent (Figure 8-46).

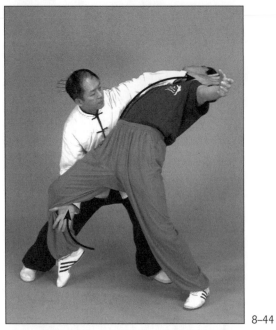

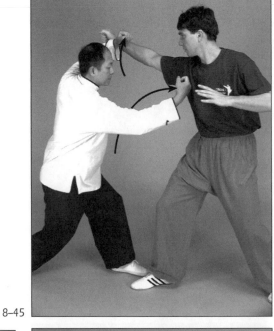

8–44   8–45

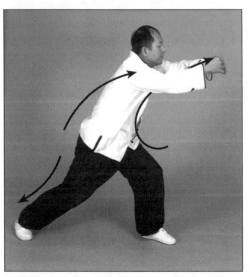

8–46

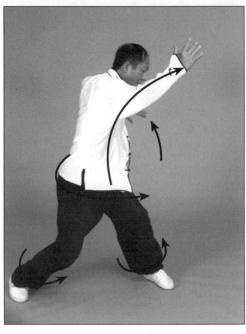

8–47

When you apply this *Jin*, the power is generated from the root. A firm root is the key to the power. You may train this *Jin* by throwing sideways (Figure 8-47) or forward (Figure 8-48).

8–48

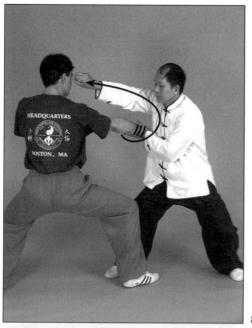
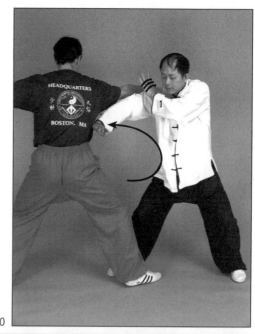

8-49   8-50

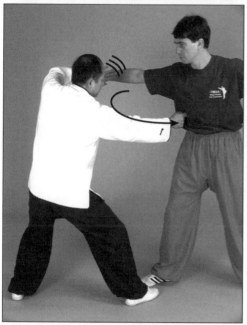
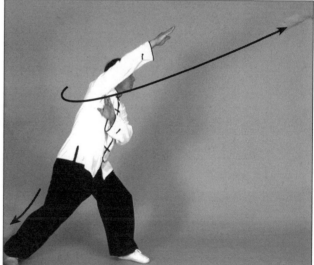

8-52

8-51

7. Swinging Jin (*Shuai Jin*, 甩勁)

Swinging *Jin* can be a Soft *Jin* or a Soft-Hard *Jin*. Normally, the direction of the swinging is sideways. The actual movement uses the same moving foundation as sideways Winding *Jin*. The power is generated from the legs or waist by twisting. This is like a spring is wound and coiled. Next, from the action of the reverse twisting, the power is swung outward for an attack. Swinging *Jin* can be used to peck the opponent's vital areas as shown earlier, for example, the temple (Figure 8-49). It can also be used to side cut the opponent's waist area with the edge of the palm (Figure 8-50) or the side of the ribs with the phoenix eye (Figure 8-51). This *Jin* was commonly used to throw darts in ancient times (Figure 8-52).

In order to prevent joint injuries in the shoulders and elbows, at the beginning of the training, the shaking motion generated from the legs or waist is manifested only to the elbows. Later, the swinging motion is then extended to the finger tips.

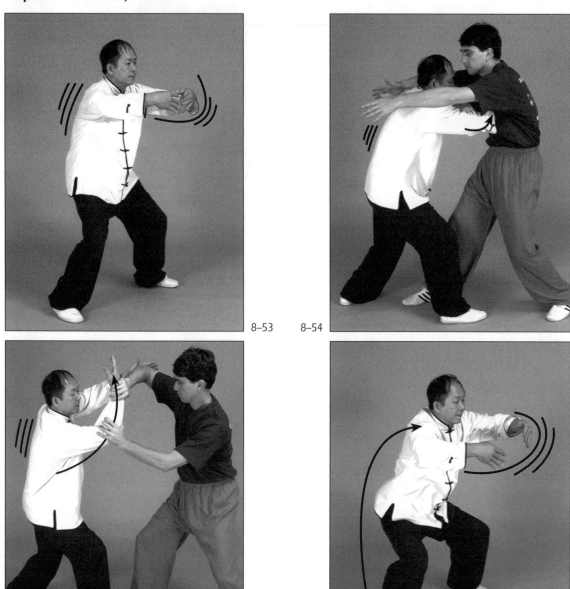

8–53   8–54

8–55   8–56

8. Arcing Jin or Wardoff Jin *(Gong Jin,* 拱勁 *) (Peng Jin,* 掤勁 *)*

Arcing *Jin* can be a Hard or Soft-Hard *Jin*. Arcing *Jin* acts like an inflated beach ball that can bounce power away. In order to reach this goal, the chest is arced inward and the upper back is arced backward, while the arms are arced outward (Figure 8-53). Arcing *Jin* can be used against the opponent's embracing (Figure 8-54) or to roll the opponent's pushing away (Figure 8-55). Arcing *Jin* is commonly used in the Soft Styles, and is the essential key to neutralization.

When Arcing *Jin* is used as a hard technique, the power derives from the upper chest and the arms. When it is used for Soft-Hard *Jin*, the action originates from the legs or the waist while the spine is arced backward and the arms are bounced forward (Figure 8-56).

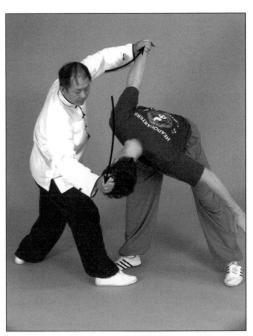

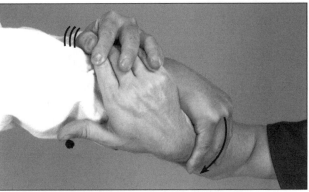

8–58

8–57

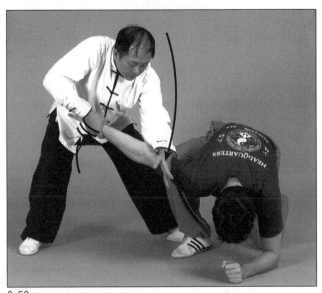

8–59

9. Sinking or Dropping Jin (*Chen Jin,* 沈勁) (*Zhui Jin,* 墜勁)

Externally, Sinking *Jin* is commonly used as a Hard *Jin* and internally, it is used as a Soft *Jin*. When it is used for Hard *Jin*, usually you grab a part of your opponent's body and force it to move downward. For example, if you have grabbed your opponent's hair or clothes, you pull it down to make him fall (Figure 8-57). Hard Sinking *Jin* can also be used for *Qin Na* to push the opponent's wrist (Figure 8-58) or elbow downward (Figure 8-59).

Normally Soft Sinking *Jin* is to prevent your opponent from lifting your body upward and throwing you down, as in wrestling. To prevent this, first make your body extremely soft, so your opponent does not have a firm structure to connect his grabbing area to your root. Next, use your mind to lead the center of gravity downward to the ground. This Soft Sinking *Jin* is extremely important in Chinese wrestling practice.

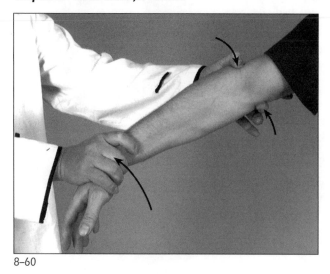

8–60

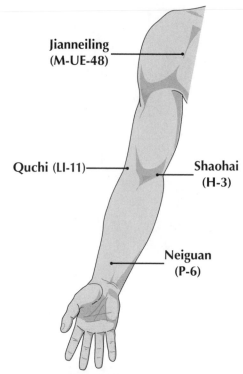

Figure 8–61. The Jianneiling (M-UE-48), Quchi (LI-22), Shaohai (H-3), and Neiquan (P-6) Cavities

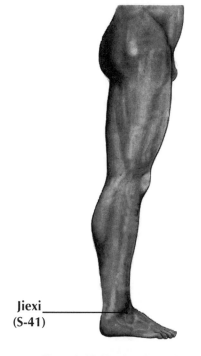

Jiexi (S-41)

Figure 8–62. The Jiexi Cavity (S-41)

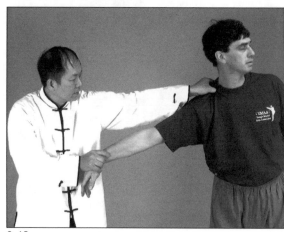

8–63

10. Plucking or Grabbing Jin (*Kou Jin,* 扣勁) (*Cai Jin,* 採勁)

Plucking *Jin* can be Hard or Soft-Hard. When it is hard it is used to immobilize the opponent's movements. Commonly, small joints such as the wrists, elbows, shoulders and ankles are used (Figure 8-60). When one of these joints is grabbed and controlled, you have placed your opponent into a disadvantageous position for your further attack. When the joints are locked, normally grabs are made to the cavities, which can cause numbness in your opponent. The common cavities used are: *Neiguan* (P-6) (內關), *Quchi* (LI-11) (曲池), *Shaohai* (H-3) (少海), *Jianneiling* (M-UE-48) (肩內陵), and *Jiexi* (S-41) (解溪)(Figures 8-61 and 8-62). In addition, some tendons, such as those in the shoulders and the sides of the waist, are also used to control the opponent by this Hard *Jin* (Figure 8-63).

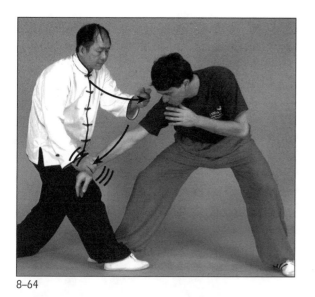
8–64

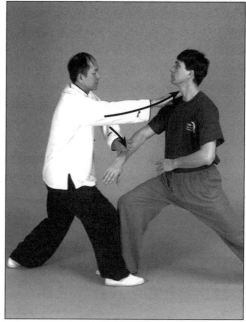
8–65

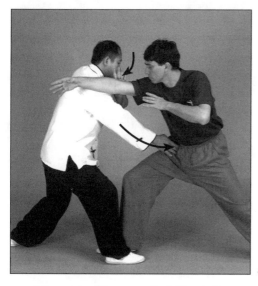
8–66

When plucking as a Soft-Hard *Jin*, once the joint is grabbed, immediately pull your opponent strongly downward, sideways, or upward to set up an attacking opportunity for yourself. In this case, the grabbing is soft and the pulling is hard. For example, once you have grabbed your opponent's wrist, immediately pull down to expose his face for your further attack (Figure 8-64).

This *Jin* is commonly trained in any Chinese martial style which uses grabbing, such as Eagle, White Crane, Tiger, Snake, and Praying Mantis. The first step in training this *Jin* is to train the fingers' grabbing power as discussed previously.

11. Sting Jin (*Ci Jin*, 刺勁)

Sting *Jin* can be manifested as a Soft-Hard or Hard *Jin*. The purpose is to use the fingers' piercing and penetrating forward thrusting power to attack opponent's vital areas such as the eyes, throat (Figure 8-65) or *Shuxi* (N-CA-6) (鼠蹊)(Figure 8-66).

In order to make the stinging effective, the fingers should be conditioned. However, if you do not know the proper method to condition your fingers, you should not do so. There are six primary *Qi* channels on your fingers. Without the correct training methods and herbs for the training, the sensitivity of the eyes can be damaged. The reason for this is that all of the twelve pri-

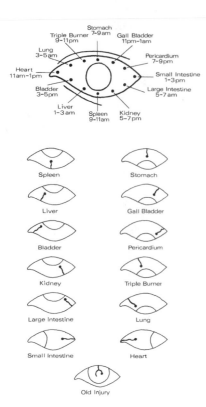

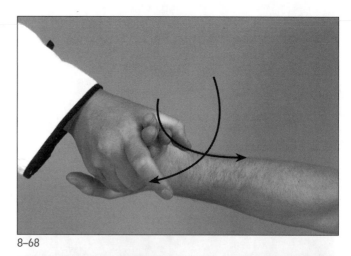

8-68

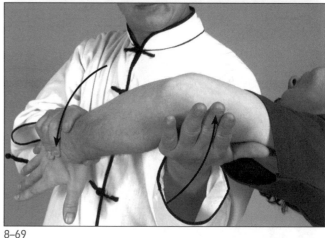

8-69

Figure 8-67. Eye Diagnosis of the Injuries in the Primary Qi Channels

mary *Qi* channels are connected to the eyes (Figure 8-67). Since we do not need such special training for our defense today, we will not discuss the training methods here.

12. Thrusting Jin (*Chong Jin*, 衝勁)

Thrusting *Jin* is a very fast moving Hard *Jin*. This *Jin* can be done with the body, arms or legs. It acts like a speedy strong force thrusting through a door or gate. Often, it moves fast, like a gust of wind which surprises your opponent. Before you apply this *Jin*, you are acting at normal fighting speed, but when the time is right and the opportunity allows, suddenly apply the Thrusting *Jin* into the technique for an attack. Naturally, in order to reach this goal, you must train constantly, so that you develop extraordinary speed. Usually you will want to master this *Jin* along with one other to create a unique, devastating combination which is most effective for you.

13. Twisting Jin (*Zhuan Jin*, 轉勁) (*Nien Jin*, 搟勁)

Twisting *Jin* can be Hard or Soft-Hard. Twisting *Jin* is commonly used in *Qin Na*. The key words of effective *Qin Na* control are twisting and bending. That means once you have grabbed the opponent's joint, through twisting and bending, you can tear off his tendons or ligaments (Figure 8-68). Moreover often Twisting *Jin* is used to twist the joint out of its socket.

Twisting *Jin* is commonly practiced by twisting tree branches. In order to generate strong Twisting *Jin*, the joints of your wrists, elbows and shoulders must be strong since you are using strength against your opponent's strength. Therefore, if you intend to break a joint such as the elbow, you need Soft-Hard *Jin* to jerk the joint out of its socket (Figure 8-69).

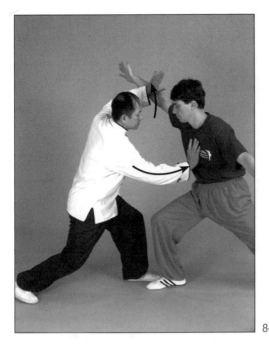
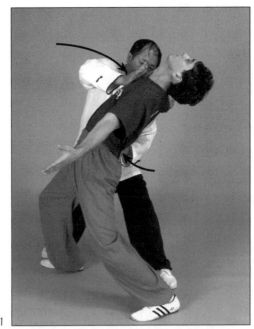

8–70   8–71

14. Pushing and Pressing Jin

(*Tui An Jin,* 推按勁)

Pushing can act like a palm strike (Figure 8-70). In this case, the *Jin* emitted is a Soft or Soft-Hard *Jin*. When pushing is used to push the opponent off balance, then the *Jin* is hard and firm (Figure 8-71). When the direction for pushing is downward, it is called Pressing *Jin*. Pressing *Jin* is often used to push the opponent's body or arms to limit his mobility (Figure 8-72). Pressing *Jin* is a steady growing Hard *Jin*, yet is neither stiff nor violent.

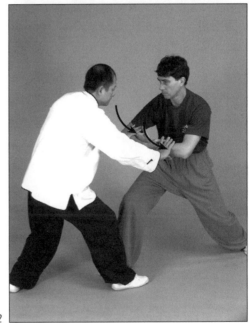

8–72

The trick to this *Jin* is normally obtained from wrestling and pushing hands training. You may use a punching bag as a target for the training.

15. Splitting Jin (*Chai Jin,* 拆勁) (*Lie Jin,* 捌勁)

Splitting *Jin* can be either a Soft-Hard or Hard *Jin*. From the name, you can see that this is an action of splitting. When this *Jin* is applied, your two arms generate two opposite forces into the opponent's body to split it apart. For example, using Splitting *Jin*, you may take your opponent

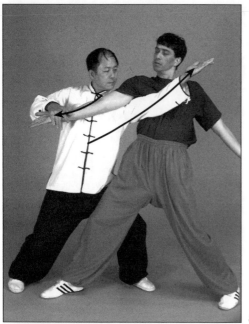

8–73

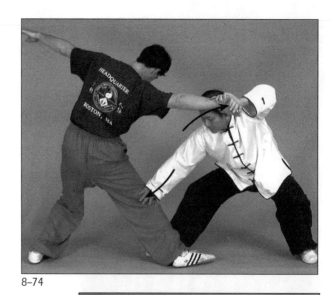

8–74

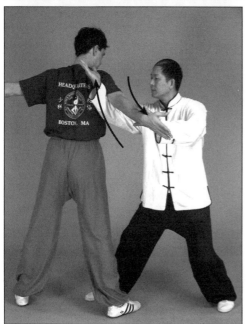

8–75

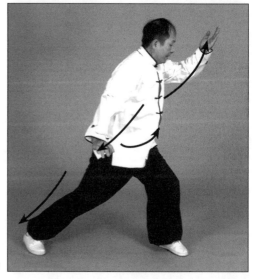

8–76

down (Figures 8-73 and 8-74). This *Jin* can also be used to lock your opponent's arm (Figure 8-75) or even used to break the elbow (Figure 8-76).

When you practice this *Jin*, you must generate the splitting force from your legs or waist. From the torso's twisting force, the hands separate in opposite directions (Figure 8-77). The key to this *Jin* can also be obtained from pushing hands practice.

8–77

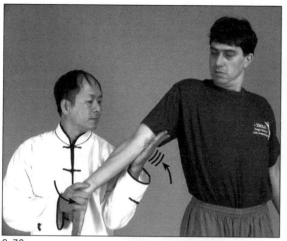

8–78

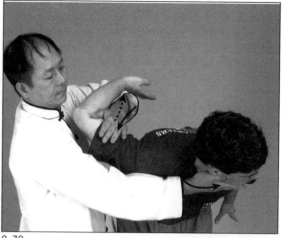

8–79

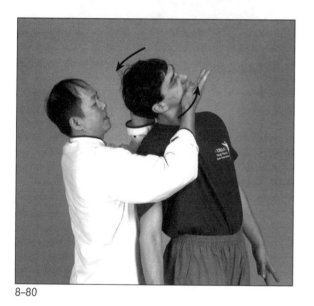

8–80

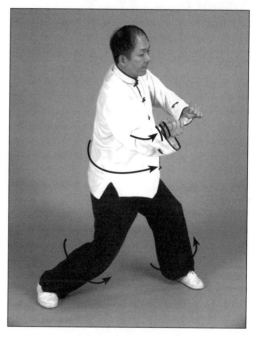

8–81

16. Breaking Jin (*Duan Jin,* 斷勁)

Breaking *Jin* is a Soft-Hard *Jin*. According to the name, you can see that this *Jin* is used to break the joints or to pop them out. The most common places for breaking are elbows (Figure 8-78), shoulders (Figure 8-79) and the neck (Figure 8-80). In the manifestation of this *Jin*, first lock the opponent's joints securely and then suddenly use a quick jerking power to break. When you do this, your mind must be concentrating on the deep joint areas and the angle of emission must be accurate. Moreover, the leverage of the forces is an essential key to the breaking.

Therefore, before you can apply this *Jin*, you must first find an opportunity which allows you to grab your opponent's arms or neck and twist it to an angle at which it can be broken easily. When this happens, his ligaments should always be taut. If you can apply the correct jerking, breaking power, his joints can be broken or easily popped out of their sockets.

To practice, learn how to generate quick, sharp and strong jerking power from the feet or the waist. With good coordination of the chest and the torso, the jerking power can be very strong (Figure 8-81).

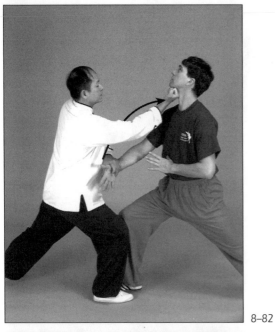
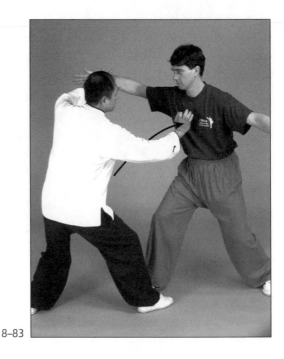

8–82   8–83

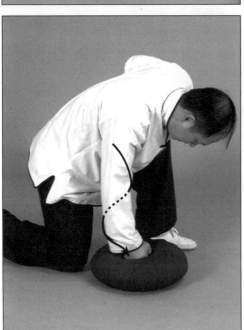

8–84

17. Drilling Jin (*Zuan Jin,* 鑽勁)

Drilling *Jin* can be used as either Hard or Soft-Hard. The idea of this *Jin* is to apply the drilling action in attacks such as a punch (Figure 8-82) or palm strike (Figure 8-83). When Drilling *Jin* is applied to these attacks, the power emitted will be more penetrating.

This *Jin* can be practiced by placing pads or cloths on a table (horizontal) or on the wall (vertical), then use your fist to press and drill them (Figure 8-84).

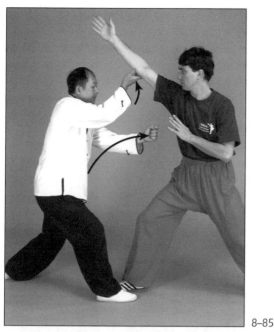
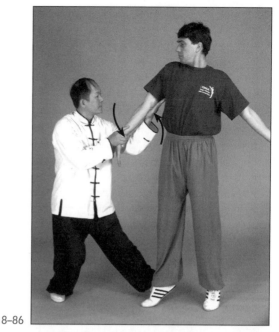

8–85   8–86

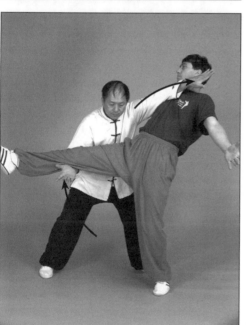
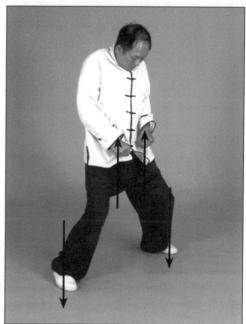

8–87   8–88

18. Lifting Jin (*Ti Jin*, 提勁)

Lifting *Jin* is a stationary moving Hard *Jin*. This *Jin* is commonly used to lift the opponent's elbows to expose the area under the armpit to attack (Figure 8-85). This *Jin* can also be used to lift an elbow for *Qin Na* control (Figure 8-86). Sometimes, Lifting *Jin* is used to lift up part of the opponent's body and destroy his root (Figure 8-87).

When you practice Lifting *Jin*, you should understand that the power for lifting is from the legs' downward pushing. That means your mind should go downward first in order to have upward lifting power. The first practice is imagining that both of your hands are grabbing a heavy object in your hands and then lifting it up (Figure 8-88).

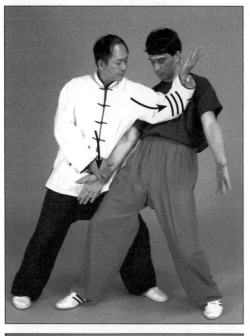

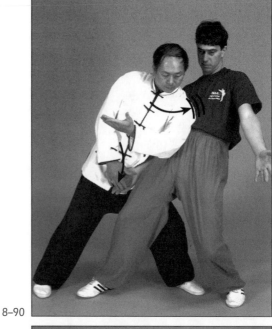

8–89   8–90

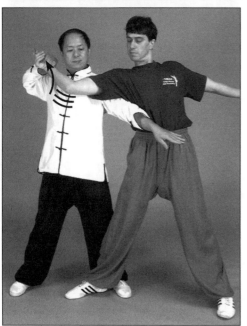

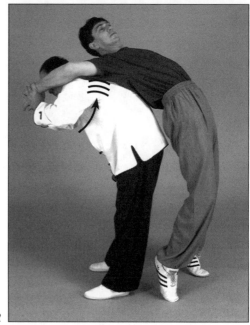

8–91   8–92

19. Bumping Jin (*Kao Jin,* 靠勁)

Bumping *Jin* is a Hard *Jin* which is used to bump your opponent off balance. The places used for bumping can be the elbows (Figure 8-89), shoulders (Figure 8-90), chest (Figure 8-91), back (Figure 8-92) and hips (Figure 8-93). This *Jin* is commonly used in wrestling to destroy the opponent's balance.

When you train Bumping *Jin*, first your legs must be firm and rooted. Otherwise, the power will bounce back to you when you apply this *Jin*. You may practice with a partner, a punching bag, or simply use a wall or post to practice your bumping (Figure 8-94).

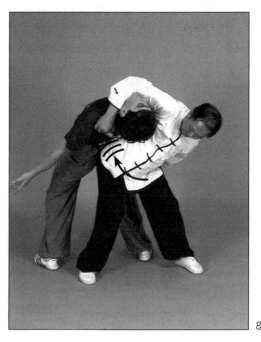 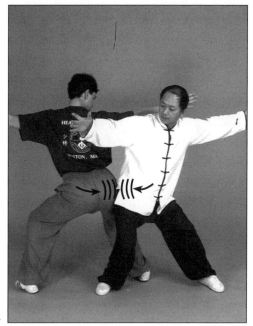

8-93   8-94

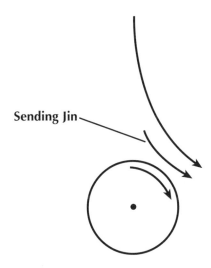

Figure 8–95. Sending Jin

20. Sending Jin (*Song Jin,* 送勁)

Sending *Jin* is a smooth and continuous Soft or Hard *Jin*. This *Jin* is used right after the opponent's incoming power is led to the sides and neutralized. When this happens, you follow his movement and add just a little more energy to send him away (Figure 8-95). This will enhance the unbalanced condition of the opponent.

To apply Sending *Jin* accurately, the timing has to be accurate and the force applied must follow the direction which caused your opponent lose his balance. Sending *Jin* is commonly used against stiff hard aggressive *Jin*. In order to make the technique work, you must be first soft, so you can neutralize the incoming strong offensive power before applying either Soft or Hard Sending *Jin*. The trick to this *Jin* can be obtained from pushing hands and wrestling practice.

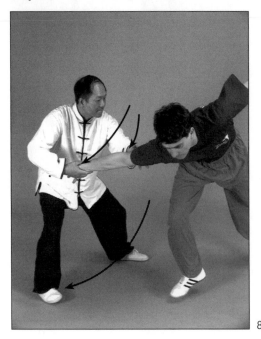
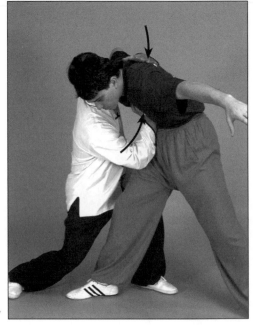

8-96   8-97

21. Pulling Jin (*La Jin*, 拉勁)

Pulling *Jin* is a steady and continuous Hard *Jin*. It is a steady strong force to pull part of your opponent's body. The main purpose is to pull him off balance or put him into a disadvantageous situation. For example, you may catch the opponent's right wrist with your right hand, then pull his wrist downward to your right to make him fall to your right (Figure 8-96). When this happens, you have created an opportunity for further attack since your opponent's mind is on regaining balance.

To train pulling, you must first recognize that the power is generated either from the legs or waist instead of your arms. If it is from the arm, the power will be weak and without a firm root. Generally, the training of this *Jin* can be done in wrestling, pushing hands or bridge hands training.

22. Pressing Upward Jin (*Ding Jin*, 頂勁)

Pressing Upward *Jin* can be a Soft-Hard or a steady and continuous Hard *Jin*. When it is applied to press a cavity, the *Jin* is Soft-Hard. For example, this *Jin* can be used to press the solar plexus upward to seal the opponent's breath (Figure 8-97). When it plays a role in controlling, then this *Jin* is a Hard *Jin*. For example, once you have controlled your opponent's wrist and elbow, you may press his wrist upward to cause pain and lock his arm (Figure 8-98).

When executing this *Jin*, you must have a good body structure for pressing. If you press simply with your arm, the power will be weak. In a good Pressing *Jin*, the entire body is involved (Figure 8-99). This *Jin* can be trained in Qin Na practice. This *Jin* is also commonly used together with Squeezing *Jin*.

B. JIN MANIFESTED ON LEG (*Tui Jin*) 腿勁

Generally speaking, it is harder to manifest leg *Jin* than arm *Jin*. The reason for this is that it is harder to use the waist to direct the jerking power to the legs. However, relatively speaking, the leg *Jin* manifested for low kicks is much easier than that of the higher kicks.

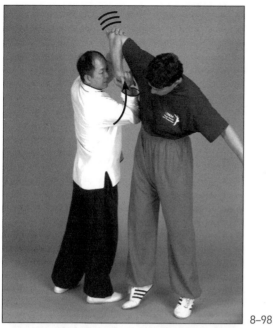

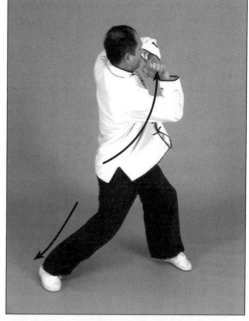

8-98   8-99

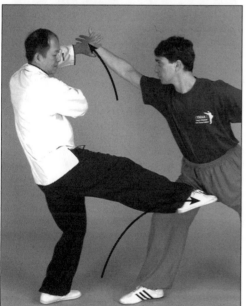

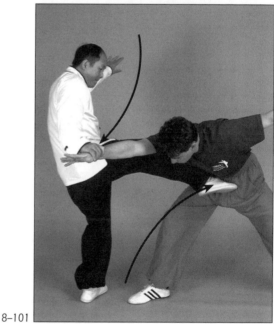

8-100   8-101

White Crane is a southern style. Consequently, most of the leg *Jin* emphasizes lower kicks. It is said in the southern styles that: "feet do not (pass) over the knees" (足不過膝). This implies that the kicks are low. As a matter of fact, when you are at short range fighting distance, high kicks are harder and not practical. Lower kicks are fast and powerful.

With many of the *Jin* manifested at the leg, the leg acts like a spring which expands the power out. Because of this, springing kicking training is also called "springing leg" (*Tan Tui*, 彈腿) in Chinese martial arts.

1. Toe Kicking Jin (*Ti Jin*, 踢勁)

Toe Kicking is a Soft-Hard Springing *Jin*. This kick uses the top of the toe area to kick the opponent's vital areas, such as the groin (Figure 8-100) or lower abdomen (Figure 8-101).

Toe kicking training is basic, since it is easy to catch the feeling of the leg springing. When training this *Jin*, first a beginner will learn how to make his leg like a spring to get the power out. In order to have a spring-like *Jin*, first the knee must be raised. After the knee is raised, the leg springs out (Figure 8-102). After you have developed a proficient *Jin* level, you should learn how to use the waist or hip area to generate more springing power.

In traditional Chinese martial arts training, when you kick, your other leg should be firmly rooted. When the kick is initiated, there is no twisting of the foot as in other oriental martial styles. The reason for this is simply that wrestling specializes against kicks. If you do not have a firm root when you initiate your kick, your opponent can take you down easily with wrestling techniques.

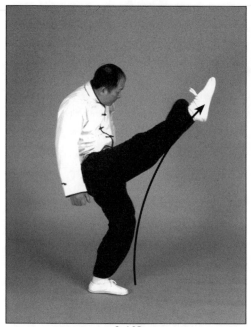

8–102

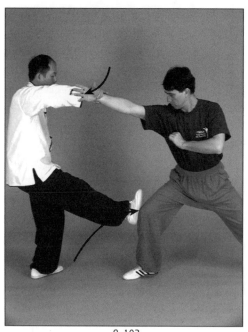

8–103

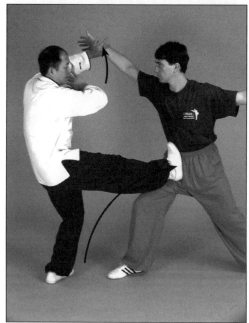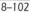

8–104

2. Heel Kicking Jin (*Deng Jin*, 蹬勁)

Heel Kicking *Jin* is a Soft-Hard Spring *Jin*. In many ways, this *Jin* is very similar to that of Toe Kicking *Jin*. The difference with this kick is that the heel is used to kick instead of the top area of toes. The general targets for this *Jin* are the knees (Figure 8-103), groin (Figure 8-104) and abdominal area (Figure 8-105).

For training, it is the same as with the toe kick explained earlier. While one of the legs is rooted firmly, the other leg kicks out under the control of the waist (Figure 8-106). You must practice until you feel your kicking is like a expanding spring. Normally, when you practice, you want to

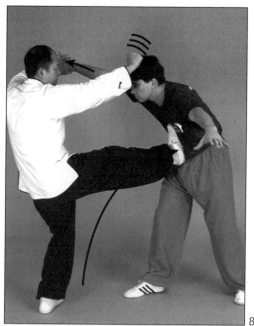
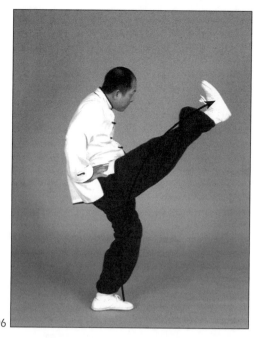

8-105   8-106

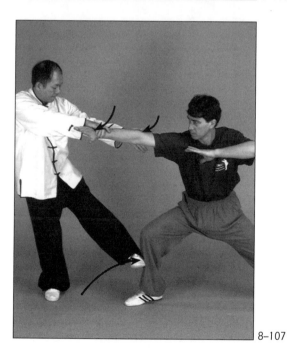
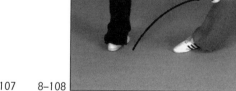

8-107   8-108

kick as high as possible. As mentioned earlier, it is harder to use your waist to direct the power for high kicks. However, if you are able to do so, then when you kick low, the speed will be much faster than that of a high kick. Naturally, the power will also be stronger.

3. Side Cut Jin (*Qie Jin*, 切勁)

Side Cut *Jin* is again a Soft-Hard *Jin*. The action of this *Jin* is a mixture of springing and pressing. The target of this kicking *Jin* is the shin (Figure 8-107) and knees (Figure 8-108) in southern styles.

When you initiate this kick, first raise up your kicking leg and then spring and press forward to the target (Figure 8-109). Again, you should practice with your leg's power first with a high kick. Later, when you become more proficient, learn how to use the waist to generate and direct the power. Naturally, you should pay attention to the standing leg. There is no twisting of the foot in traditional Chinese martial arts.

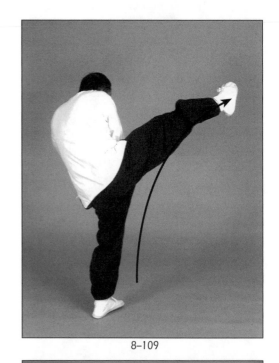

8-109

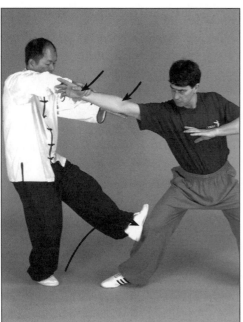 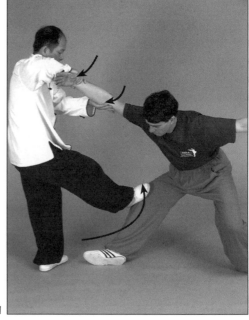

8-110   8-111

4. **Stepping On Jin** (*Cai Jin*, 踩勁)

Stepping On *Jin* is a Hard *Jin*. As the name says, you use the bottom of your foot to step on your opponent's knees to break them. You may step with your foot forward (Figure 8-110) or sideways (Figure 8-111).

When you train this *Jin*, you may first place a pad on a tree trunk the size of a leg, and learn how to step your power out. When the power is stronger and your leg is strong and more durable, gradually make the pad thinner until it is no longer necessary. In order to make the stepping more powerful, normally you have to control your opponent's arm. When his arm is pulled down, you

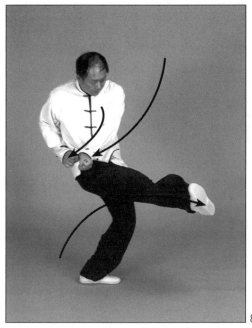

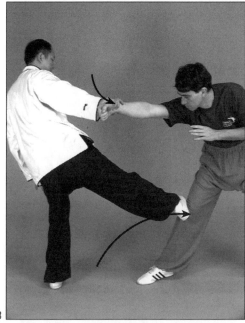

8-112   8-113

use the leverage of pulling to initiate your kicking. Therefore, this action is a common type of self-practice for this *Jin* (Figure 8-112).

5. Stamping Jin (*Duo Jin*, 跺勁) (*Chuai Jin*, 踹勁)

Stamping *Jin* is a Hard *Jin* which is classified as a kind of Stepping On *Jin*. The difference is that in Stepping On *Jin*, the kicking toes are facing upward while in Stamping *Jin* the toes are facing sideways. Again, Stamping *Jin* is commonly used to break the knee. You may stamp your foot forward (Figure 8-113) or sideways (Figure 8-114).

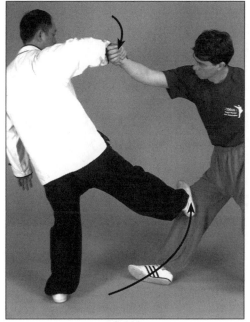

8-114

The training method is the same as that of Stepping On *Jin*. Please refer to the last *Jin* for information.

6. Sole Pressing Jin (*Ding Jin*, 頂勁)

This is a steady and continuous pressing Hard *Jin* executed by the front side of the sole. The general targets of pressing are the abdomen or solar plexus. Normally, in southern styles, the opponent's arms are grabbed and you use your foot to press his abdomen (Figure 8-115). Often, when the pressing has reached a maximum, a sudden jerking power can inflict injury.

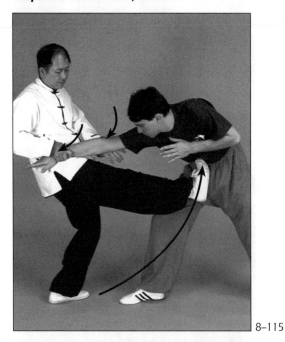
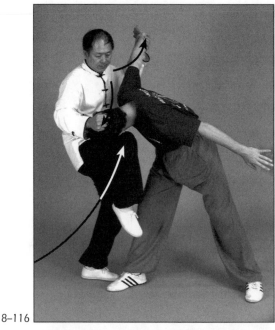

8-115   8-116

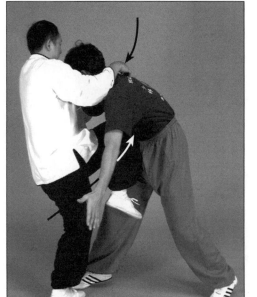
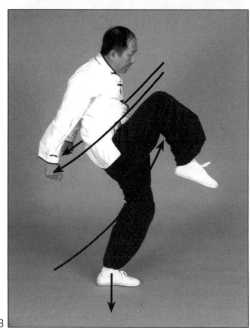

8-117   8-118

7. Knee Pressing Jin (*Xi Ding Jin,* 膝頂勁)

This is a Hard *Jin.* The targets of Knee Pressing *Jin* are usually the chin (Figure 8-116) and the abdominal area (Figure 8-117). This *Jin* is commonly used in Thai boxing because it is very useful for short range fighting situations.

When you practice this *Jin* without a partner, the downward power from the standing leg and both arms is very important. It is from this downward pulling that the leverage of the upward power is generated (Figure 8-118). Commonly, you can practice this *Jin* with a kicking bag.

8. Bumping Jin (*Kao Jin,* 靠勁)

The Leg Bumping *Jin* is a Soft-Hard *Jin,* although occasionally it is also used as a steady push-

– 298 –

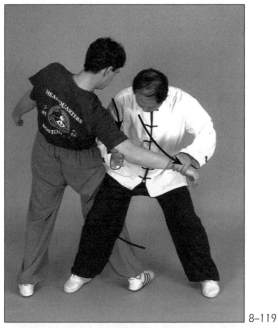
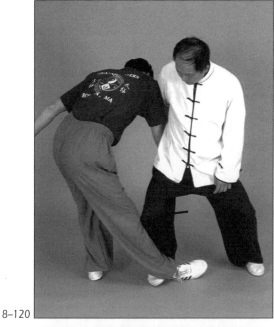

8-119   8-120

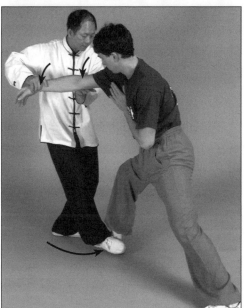
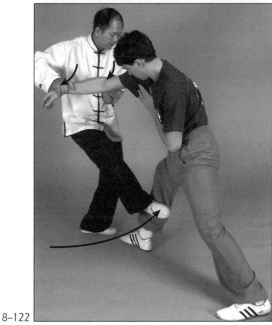

8-121   8-122

ing Hard *Jin*. The common places used to bump with your leg are the thighs and knees. The targets for bumping are also on the opponent's thighs (Figure 8-119) or knees (Figure 8-120). The purpose of leg bumping is to bump the opponent off balance by destroying his root.

When you practice Leg Bumping *Jin*, you may use a tree trunk for training. Naturally, in order to generate great bumping power, your root is extremely important. It is your opponent who should be bumped away instead of you.

9. Sweeping Jin (*Sao Jin,* 掃勁)

This *Jin* can be a Soft-Hard *Jin* or a steady strong Hard *Jin*. This *Jin* is commonly used to destroy the opponent's root in wrestling. When it is executed as a Soft-Hard *Jin*, the bottom of the foot is used to sweep the inner side of the opponent's foot (Figure 8-121), shin (Figure 8-122) or

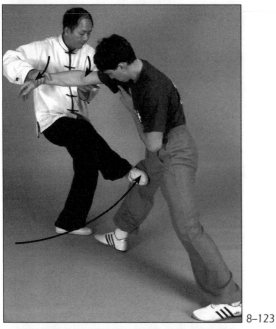
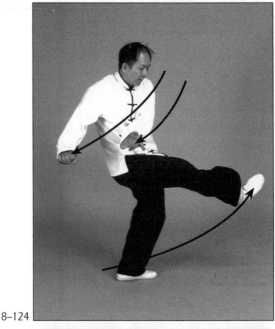

8–123   8–124

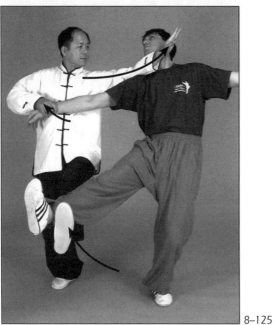
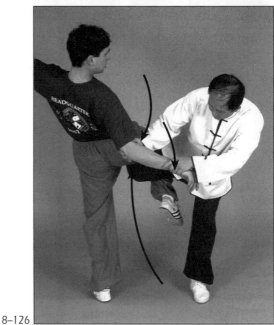

8–125   8–126

knee (Figure 8-123).

When you practice this sweeping, first place a pad on a tree trunk and sweep it. After you have become more proficient, remove the pad. Naturally, the rooting of the other foot is extremely important in this kicking. In order to generate good leverage for sweeping, commonly you control your opponent's arm and pull. This pulling action will offer you significant sweeping power (Figure 8-124).

10. Hooking Jin (Gou Jin, 勾勁) (Qiao Jin, 翹勁)

This *Jin* can be manifested as a Soft-Hard or steady strong Hard *Jin*. This *Jin* can be used to hook the opponent's front leg to make him fall (Figures 8-125 and 8-126). As you do this, the *Jin*

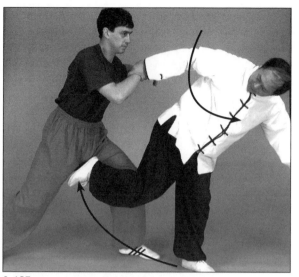

8-127

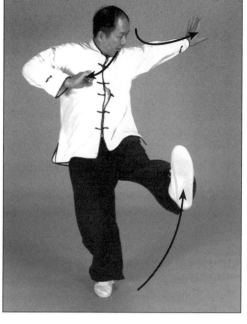

8-128

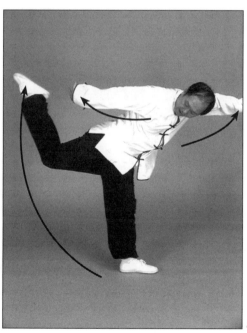

8-129

can be manifested as either Soft-Hard or Hard. Hooking *Jin* can also be used to hook upward as a kick to the rear at the opponent's groin (Figure 8-127). In this application, the *Jin* will be Soft Hard *Jin*.

As usual, you may place a pad on a tree trunk and learn how to hook it. For the back hooking kick, you may use a kicking bag. You may also practice this kicking technique by hooking against an imaginary opponent (Figures 8-128 and 8-129).

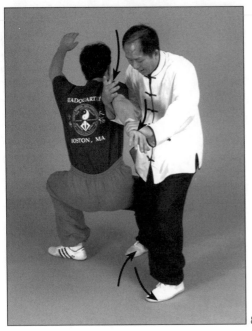

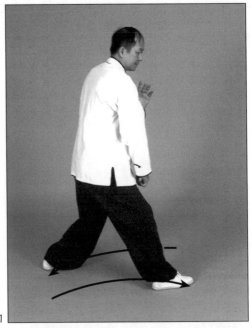

8–130   8–131

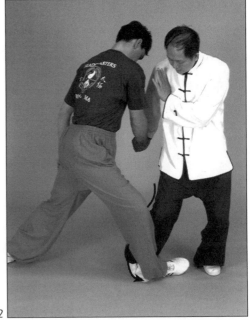

8–132

11. Splitting Leg Jin (*Tui Zhan Jin,* 腿展勁)

This *Jin* is commonly executed as a Hard *Jin*, though if the situation and timing allows, it can also be used as a Soft-Hard *Jin*. This *Jin* is done by splitting both of your legs, one forward and one backward. For example, if your right leg is on the right hand side of your opponent's right leg, you split both of your legs and use your right leg's backward splitting to sweep your opponent's right leg to make him fall (Figure 8-130).

When you practice this *Jin*, place some weight on your calf near the ankle areas, and then keep splitting one leg forward and one backward (Figure 8-131).

12. Coiling Jin (*Chan Jin,* 纏勁)

Coiling *Jin* is a Soft-Hard *Jin* which is used to coil the leg around an opponent's leg. Normally, it is used for leg *Qin Na*. In leg *Qin Na,* your front leg is coiling your opponent's front leg, and Hard *Jin* is used to press the leg to make your opponent fall (Figure 8-132).

To train Leg Coiling *Jin*, practice coiling your leg around a trunk or a post. Once you have coiled your leg around it, immediately apply Pressing *Jin* into it.

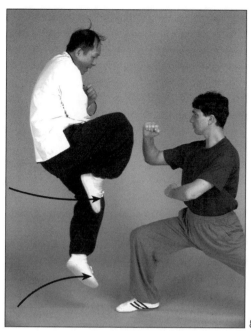
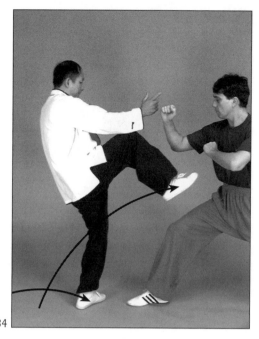

8-133   8-134

13. Jumping Jin (*Tiao Jin*, 跳勁)

Jumping *Jin* is a Soft-Hard *Jin* from which the body's posture is set up softly at first to store the jumping power. Once the posture is stored, then the Jumping *Jin* is manifested. Like a cat before it jumps, you first must position yourself in the best posture for the most efficient leap. In actual application, Jumping *Jin* is used to jump forward to shorten the fighting range, or to kick (Figure 8-133).

The best way of training Jumping *Jin* is to place some weight on the calf near the ankle area and run to build the strength of the torso and legs. Later, keep increasing the weight and jump over a high bar.

14. Hopping Jin (*Yao Jin*, 躍勁)

Hopping *Jin* is very similar to Jumping *Jin*. Again, you must store your hopping power into a correct posture and then use the leg to hop. This *Jin* is used to shorten the fighting range or to kick (Figure 8-134).

You may refer to Jumping *Jin* for the training methods.

III. DEFENSIVE JIN (*Yin Jin*) 守勁 (陰勁)

Defensive *Jins* are generally used to intercept or escape from the opponent's attack. Compared to offensive *Jins*, these *Jins* are more passive. Again, we will discuss these *Jins* by dividing them into those *Jins* manifested from the arms or body and those which are manifested from the legs.

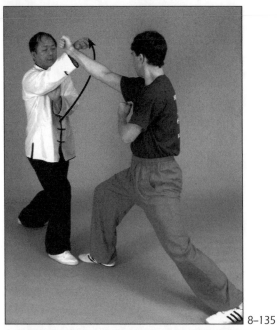
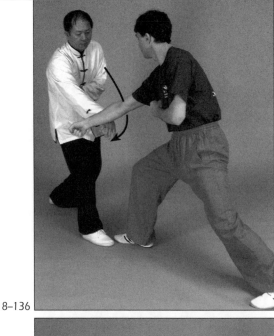

8-135   8-136

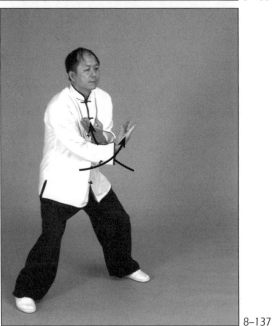
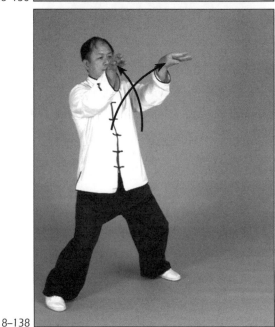

8-137   8-138

A. Jin MANIFESTED ON ARMS OR BODY 手勁與身勁

1. Repelling Jin (*Bo Jin,* 撥勁)

Repelling *Jin* is a steady Hard *Jin* which is commonly used to repel an incoming attack to the side. This *Jin* can be applied against both upper body attack (Figure 8-135) and lower body attack (Figure 8-136). When this *Jin* is used to repel incoming strong force, it must be firm, strong and fast.

The best way to train reaction for this *Jin* is to have someone punch you and you learn to intercept and repel the punch. Often, a tree branch or a specially designed dummy is used to train repelling power. To train the *Jin* itself, you can practice by yourself. Again, the repelling action is rooted in the feet and directed by the waist. First, cross both of your arms in front of your chest and then repel them upward and sideways (Figures 8-137 and 8-138). Then, cross your

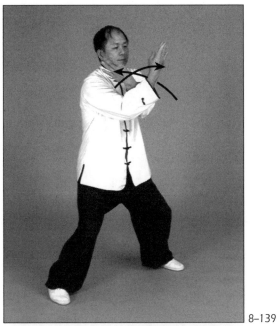
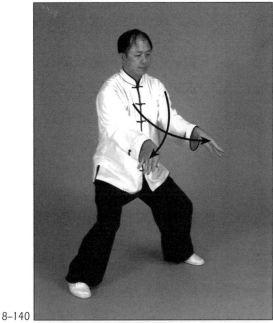

8-139   8-140

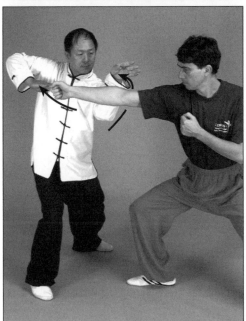
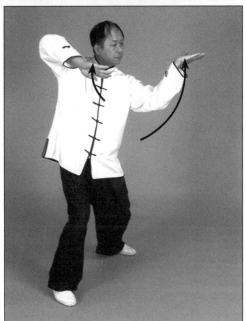

8-141   8-142

arms again and repel downward and sideways (Figure 8-139 and 8-140). You may also practice with a single hand.

2. Covering Jin (*Gai Jin*, 蓋勁)

Covering *Jin* is also a steady Hard *Jin* which is used to cover the incoming upper body attack downward (Figure 8-141). Again, the best way of training this *Jin* is to practice with a partner. You may also train with a tree branch. However, since the tree does not attack, when you train with a tree, you lose the feeling and the training of intercepting.

When you practice by yourself, you may first twist your body to your right and use your left forearm to intercept the incoming imaginary opponent's attack, palm facing upward (Figure 8-142). Next, cover your left hand down like the wing of a crane (Figure 8-143).

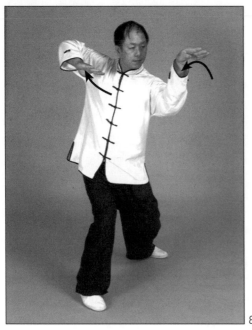

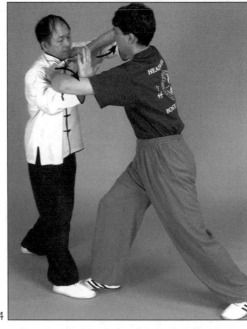

8–143   8–144

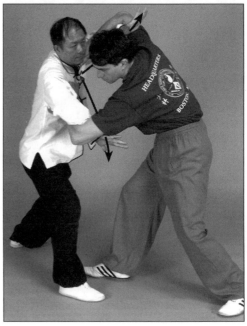

3. Developing or Expanding Jin

(*Zhan Jin*, 展勁)

Developing *Jin* is a steady and firm Hard *Jin* which is normally used against grabbing to the chest area. For example, if your opponent grabs your upper chest with both of his hands, expand both of your arms to split both of his arms apart (Figure 8-144). Naturally, this *Jin* can also be used to split the grab with one arm up and one down (Figure 8-145).

This *Jin* is normally trained in wrestling practice. In fact, this *Jin* can be called an extension of the Arcing *Jin* (or Wardoff *Jin*) from the chest to the arms.

8–145

4. Winding Jin (*Pan Jin*, 盤勁)

Winding *Jin* is an extremely Soft *Jin* which is used to prevent being picked up and then thrown down. This *Jin* is used mostly against wrestling. When this *Jin* is applied, your mind is sunk, which creates the feeling that the center of gravity is sunk. As you do this, you also twist your body sideways to wind the body down to the ground (Figure 8-146). This can effectively prevent you from being picked up.

This *Jin* is normally trained in wrestling practice. The mind and a soft body are the keys to manifesting this *Jin*.

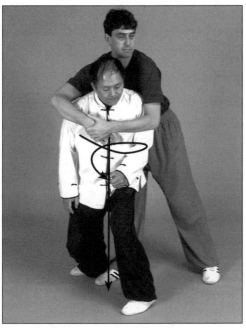

8–146

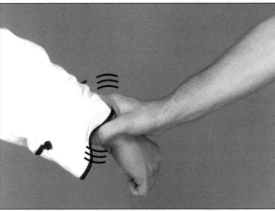

Figure 8–147

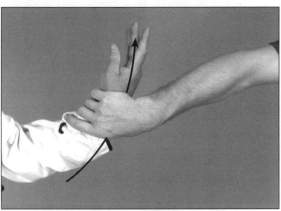

Figure 8–148

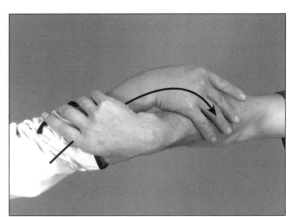

Figure 8–149

5. **Coiling Jin** (*Chan Jin,* 纏勁) (*Juan Jin,* 捲勁)

Coiling *Jin* is a steady coiling Hard *Jin* which is commonly used against grabbing in *Qin Na*. For example, if your wrist is grabbed (Figure 8-147), simply coil your arm out (Figures 8-148 and 8-149).

Coiling *Jin* can be trained in *Qin Na* and wrestling practice. In order to make the coiling effective, the coiling motion must be steady and firm. You should always remember that all *Jin* actions are initiated either from the legs or waist.

6. **Arcing Jin** (*Gong Jin,* 拱勁)

Arcing *Jin* is a steady Hard *Jin*. When this *Jin* is used, the chest is withdrawn, the back is arced backward and the arms are roundly expanded forward. The arms and the upper body form a ball. This *Jin* is used to arc the opponent away if you are embraced (Figure 8-150).

This *Jin* is generally practiced in wrestling.

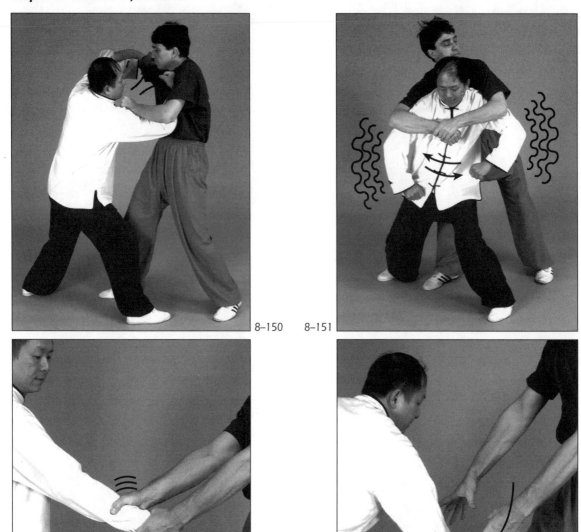

8-150   8-151

8-152   8-153

7. Trembling Jin (*Zhan Jin,* 顫勁)

Trembling *Jin* is a quick shaking Hard *Jin*. This *Jin* is commonly used to shake off the opponent's controlling. For example, when you are just being embraced, you may use Trembling *Jin* to prevent being embraced, or even to loosen the embrace if it has already been done (Figure 8-151). You may also use this *Jin* to shake off wrist or arm grabs executed by your opponent (Figures 8-152 and 8-153).

This *Jin* is commonly practiced in *Qin Na* and wrestling. To make this *Jin* strong and powerful, the trembling power must be generated from the legs or waist.

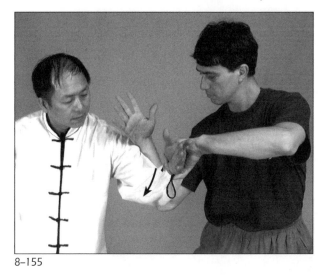

8–155

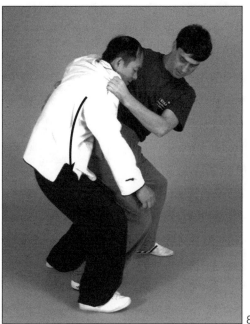

8–154

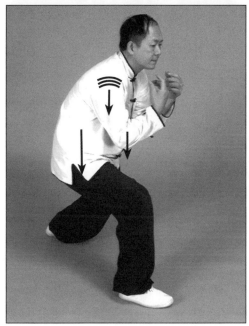

8–156

8. Sinking or Dropping Jin (*Chen Jin,* 沈勁) (*Zhui Jin,* 墜勁)

Sinking *Jin* is a steady and firm downward *Jin*. When this *Jin* is applied to the body, you can prevent being lifted and thrown in wrestling (Figure 8-154). When this *Jin* is used at the elbow, you can prevent your arm from being locked in a *Qin Na* application (Figure 8-155). When the shoulders are sunk, the arms will be firm and rooted. The shoulders are the foundation of the arms (Figure 8-156).

This *Jin* can be practiced in *Qin Na,* wrestling or pushing hands training.

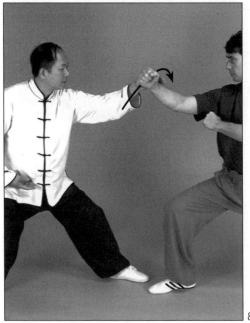 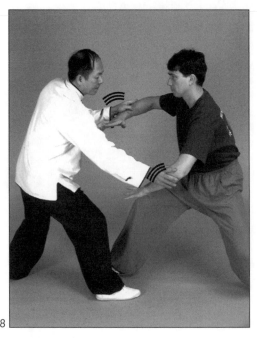

8-157   8-158

9. Sticking and Adhering Jin (*Zhan Nian Jin,* 沾黏勁)

Sticking is a Soft *Jin* and is an action of intercepting. It implies stickiness like wet paper stuck to a wall. When your opponent is attacking, use sticking to intercept his incoming arms (Figure 8-157).

Adhering *Jin* is the action of "listening" (i.e., feeling) and "following," which allows your hands to continue touching your opponent's body (Figure 8-158). It acts like fly paper adhering to his hands or arms. These two *Jin* are usually practiced together.

Sticking *Jin* must be practiced with a partner. Simply ask your partner to continue to touch your upper chest and you learn how to adjust your body and use your hands to stick to the incoming attack. Adhering *Jin* can be trained in pushing hands practice.

10. Hooking Jin (*Diao Jin,* 刁勁)

Hooking *Jin* is a firm hooking or grabbing Hard *Jin* which is used to immobilize the opponent's further action. For example, when your opponent punches you, you can use Hooking *Jin* to bring his arm down (Figure 8-159) and immediately follow with Grabbing or Controlling *Jin* to control his wrist's mobility (Figure 8-160). Grabbing *Jin* is an attacking *Jin*.

Hooking *Jin* can be practiced in bridging hands, *Qin Na,* or pushing hands training. In order to have strong hooking power, normally finger strength and endurance is important.

11. Twisting Jin (*Zhuan Jin,* 轉勁) (*Nien Jin,* 撏勁)

In defense, Twisting *Jin* is commonly use to twist the arms and get free from being grabbed. For example, if your arm is grabbed, twist your arm to loosen the grip (Figure 8-161). Twisting *Jin* can also be applied to your body and used to twist your body free when it is embraced (Figure 8-162).

Defensive Twisting *Jin* can be practiced in wrestling and *Qin Na.*

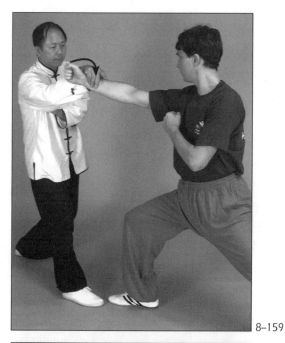
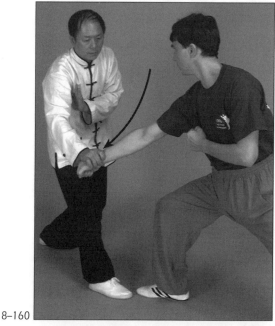

8–159   8–160

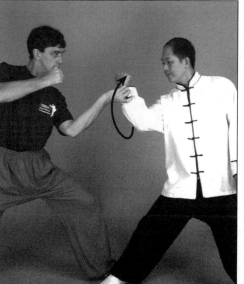
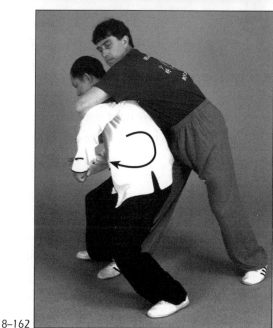

8–161   8–162

12. Controlling Jin (*Na Jin,* 拿勁)

Defensive Controlling *Jin* is not a grabbing *Jin* but a soft covering adhering contact *Jin* on the opponent's joints such as the wrists, elbows and shoulders. When this *Jin* is on top of these joints, you have put your opponent into a disadvantageous defensive situation for your attack to his upper body (Figure 8-163).

This *Jin* is very hard to train. To make this *Jin* effective, you must first master Listening, Following, Yielding, Leading and Neutralizing *Jin*. Without these foundations, controlling *Jin* will not be effective.

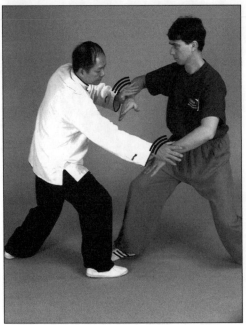

8-163

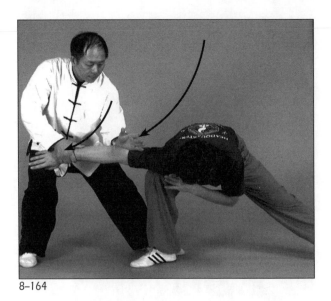

8-164

13. Rolling Back Neutralizing Jin (*Lu Hua Jin,* 擺化勁)

This *Jin* can be a Soft *Jin* or a Soft-Hard *Jin*. The main purpose of this *Jin* is to yield, lead and then neutralize incoming power to the side and backward (Figure 8-164). Theoretically, in order to neutralize the opponent's incoming force, you must first know how to listen (i.e., skin feeling), yield and then lead. Without mastering these three *Jins*, the neutralization will not be effective.

This *Jin* can be practiced from *Qin Na,* bridging hands and pushing hands training.

14. Splitting Jin (*Chai Jin,* 拆勁) (*Lie Jin,* 挒勁)

Splitting *Jin* is a steady Hard *Jin* in which two repelling *Jins* are applied. For example, when your opponent attacks you with both of his arms, use your left forearm to repel his right hand upward and to your left, while repelling his left attack to your right (Figure 8-165).

This *Jin* can be practiced in bridging hands training.

15. Carrying Jin (*Dai Jin,* 帶勁)

Carrying *Jin* is also called Following-Carrying *Jin* (*Shun Dai Jin,* 順帶勁). The reason for its name is that, when you are executing this *Jin*, you first listen and follow your opponent's incoming *Jin* and then lead or carry this *Jin* into emptiness (Figure 8-166). Normally, this *Jin* is used to neutralize the opponent's attack.

Carrying *Jin* can be practiced in wrestling or pushing hands. Normally, in order to lead and carry the opponent's power into emptiness, your waist and torso must be soft and the stepping must be properly and accurately executed.

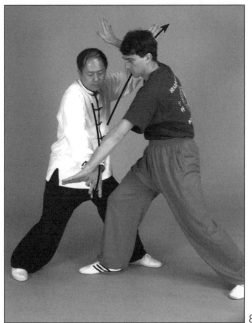
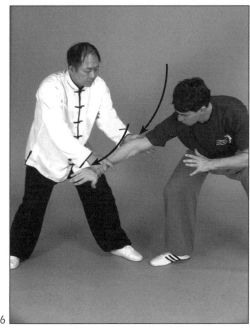

8–165   8–166

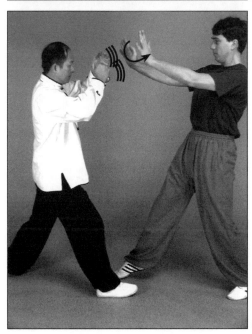

8–167

16. Borrowing Jin (*Jie Jin*, 借勁)

Borrowing *Jin* is executed when your opponent has generated an idea of attack (i.e., *Jin*'s emitting) and has just started to initiate power. At this moment, if you can sense this incoming *Jin* and generate a force against it, the opponent's mind will be interrupted suddenly and his *Jin* will be bounced back (Figure 8-167). It is like when you are about to step through a door and it is suddenly shut on you.

The timing of Borrowing *Jin* is a critical key to success. The best way of training is from continuous practice. Borrowing *Jin* is well known as one of the most difficult *Jin* manifestations. However, if you know how to do it naturally, you will often put your opponent into a defensive situation. This *Jin* again can be trained in wrestling and pushing hands practice.

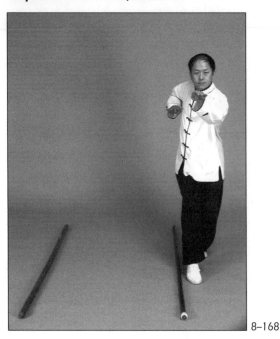

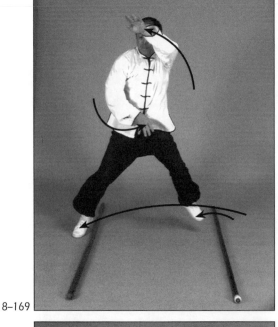

8-168 8-169

B. JIN MANIFESTED ON LEG

(Tui Jin) 腿勁

1. Dodging Jin *(Shan Jin,* 閃勁)

This is also called *Shan Duo Jin* (閃躲勁), meaning "Dodging to Shun *Jin.*" This *Jin* is purely defensive against an attack, though it is also used to set up a strategy for counter attack. This *Jin* trains the speed of dodging by hopping sideways. The hopping should be like a monkey, agile and light. In order to reach this goal, the legs must be strong, especially the ankles, knees and the hips. The legs should be like springs which bounce you up, down and sideways easily. To obtain agile hopping, not only must your legs be strong and speedy, but your body must also be agile.

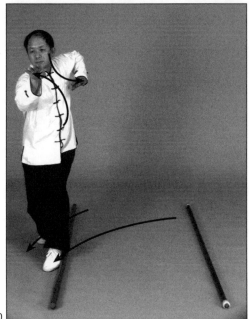

8-170

To practice this *Jin*, simply place two staffs or draw two lines about four feet apart. Next, hop from one side of the staff to the other side thirty times (Figures 8-168 to 8-170). You should measure the time of the hopping and then gradually improve your speed by shortening the time. If you can complete thirty hops in twenty seconds, you are pretty good.

Next, increase the distance between the staffs or lines to five feet, and repeat the same training. Later increase to six feet. If you can hop a six foot divide thirty times in twenty seconds, your speed has reached a very good level.

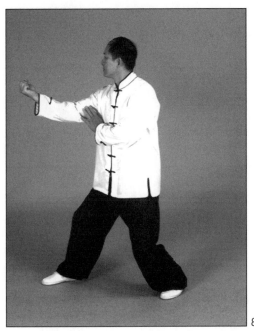 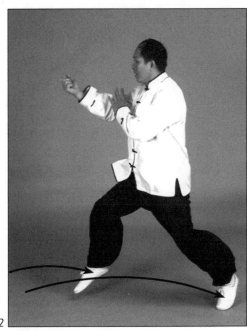

8-171   8-172

If this does not satisfy you, apply weight to your ankles and repeat the entire training process. When this time comes, you will realize that you must coordinate your breathing correctly and really concentrate on your hopping. This means you are changing from external into internal.

How deep you can reach depends on the individual. You are the one who makes the progress and therefore make the decisions. The art of training is alive and its potential is unlimited. The hardest part of training is actually the process of conquering your emotional, lazy mind. Remember, learning *Gongfu* is a process of self emotional regulation, i.e., self conquering. Through this training process, you can understand the meaning and the spirit of life.

2. Hopping Jin (*Yao Jin*, 躍勁)

As explained earlier, Hopping *Jin* can be divided into attacking hopping and defensive hopping. When you hop sideways, it is a Dodging *Jin*. When you hop forward to approach your opponent for an attack, it is an attacking Hopping *Jin*. Here, the hopping is for retreating, and the hopping power of the front leg must be strong. Naturally, speed and agility are two major concerns.

When you practice, use the same training theory as before. Draw lines about four feet apart. Then hop backward from line to line and time yourself (Figures 8-171 and 8-172). Train to make the time shorter and to make the distance between the lines longer and longer. You may also put some weight on your ankles and repeat the training process. Again, gradually you should change from external action to internal action through the coordination of the breathing and the mind. Often, hopping forward and backward are practiced together. Hop forward to attack and hop backward to retreat.

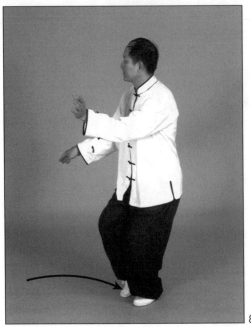 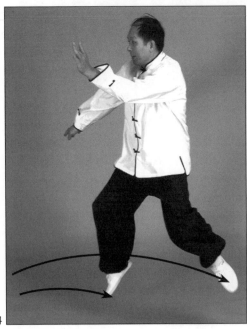

8-173   8-174

3. Jumping Jin (*Teng Jin,* 騰勁)

As explained previously, Jumping *Jin* can be distinguished into Offensive Jumping *Jin* and Defensive Jumping *Jin*. In Defensive Jumping *Jin* training, you jump backward for retreating. Jumping is different from the hopping discussed in the last two *Jins*. First, the hopping distance is shorter than that of jumping. Second, hopping is used for a temporary short retreat and to prepare for the next attack, while jumping is used for a complete retreat which increases the distance between you and your opponent from short or middle range to long range or beyond. When you use hopping for retreating, you are still in danger, since the distance between you and your opponent is still critical and in attacking range. However, if you use jumping to retreat, you are relatively safe unless your opponent also jumps forward to keep the distance between you short. Therefore, sometimes more than two hops or jumps are necessary to keep yourself at a safe distance.

In Jumping *Jin* training, you place obstacles in a line about three to five feet apart. Then, jump backward over the obstacles by first drawing your front leg back, next to your rear leg (Figure 8-173). Next, use the withdrawn leg to bounce the body upward and backward over the obstacle (Figure 8-174). Again, you should time yourself and make it as short as possible. In addition, you should increase the distance between the obstacles, and also make the obstacle higher and higher. After you have practiced for a long time, you may apply weight to your ankles and repeat the training.

4. Flying Jin (*Fei Jin,* 飛勁)

Flying *Jin* is a sideways jumping, imitating a White Crane's flying. This *Jin* is used to dodge sideways a greater distance from the opponent. This *Jin* is needed when your opponent is using a long distance high jump kick or a long weapon to attack you. This Jumping *Jin* is also commonly used to circle around your opponent before an attack.

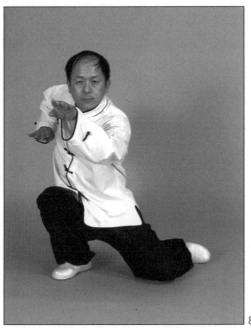
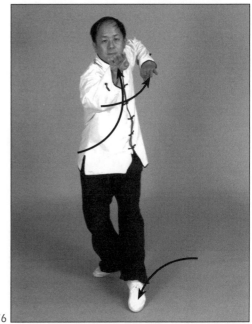

8-175   8-176

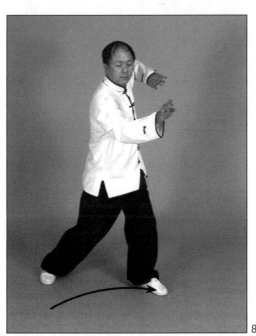
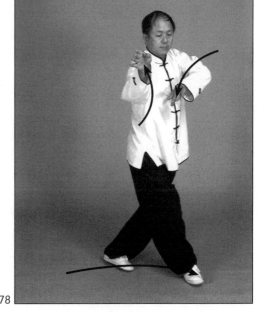

8-177   8-178

When you practice this *Jin*, first squat down in Crane Squatting Stance (Figure 8-175). Next, raise your body and change your stance into Crane False Stance (Figure 8-176). Step to your left with your left leg (Figure 8-177) and then follow with your right leg (Figure 8-178). Immediately after the right leg touches down, use it to bounce yourself upward and fly to the left (Figures 8-179 and 8-180). Finally, land on the ground and enter Crane Squatting Stance again (Figure 8-181). You may repeat your flying jump to the other side. Again, to make it more challenging, you should place obstacles on the path for you to jump over. After you have practiced for a while, you should increase the height of the obstacles and try to jump as far as possible. Later, apply weight to the ankles and repeat the training.

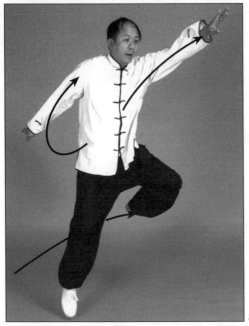

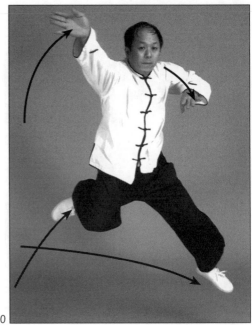

8–179　　8–180

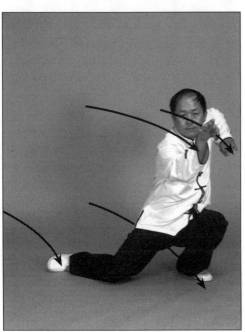

8–181

Reference

1. 太極拳論：有上即有下，有前即有後，有左即有右。如意要向上，
即寓下意。

Chapter 9

Conclusion

結論

Although this book has explained some of the most important basic concepts in Chinese martial arts - Martial Arts *Qigong* and *Jin* - you should remain humble, keep your eyes and mind open and practice intelligently. Study, ponder and practice are three key words which can lead your understanding and martial capability to a profound and proficient level.

Here, I would like to summarize some important points. First, Chinese martial arts includes external and internal styles. Generally speaking, the external styles emphasize the manifestation of *Jin* through the muscles and tendons, while internal styles focus on the tendons and ligaments. Consequently, the *Jin* manifested in the external styles is harder, and the *Jin* manifested is classified as "Hard *Jin*," while the *Jin* manifested in the internal styles is relatively softer, and is categorized as "Soft *Jin*." In order to make the manifested *Jin* efficient and powerful, *Qigong* training is important in both external and internal styles. Although the fundamental training theory and principles are the same, the methods of training are different. In order to manifest Hard *Jin*, Hard *Qigong* training is the root of the muscular *Jin* manifestation. Similarly, in order to manifest Soft *Jin* most effectively, Soft *Qigong*, which emphasizes relaxed and soft whipping motions, is the key to practice.

Second, Chinese martial arts can be divided into northern and southern styles. Generally speaking, northern styles emphasize long range fighting, consequently techniques using the legs are more developed, while southern styles prefer short and middle range fighting, and therefore the hand techniques are more perfected. From different styles, different types of *Jin* training were designed to suit the special characteristics of each style.

Third, it does not matter what style, there are always four fighting categories: kicking, punching, wrestling and *Qin Na* (seizing and controlling). All the *Qigong* and *Jin* are developed according to the uses of these four categories. If you wish to become a proficient Chinese martial artist, you must learn and study all of these categories.

Fourth, White Crane style is only one of the many southern styles which exist today. Moreover, there are more than four different Southern White Crane styles known in Chinese martial arts. Though the Martial Arts *Qigong* and *Jin* theory and principles explained in this book are universal, the training methods for both *Qigong* and *Jin* are developed from only one of the Southern White Crane styles, and also from my personal understanding. That means this book is not an authority, but should be considered only one of the sources which can offer you study and understanding. To make the entire art complete, we still need other qualified traditional masters to contribute from an open mind. Only then will Chinese martial arts be preserved and continue to be developed.

Finally, as explained in this book, White Crane is a Soft-Hard Style. Therefore, it emphasizes both Hard and Soft *Qigong*. As a consequence, both Hard and Soft *Jin* are trained. At the beginning, the training for a beginner is harder physically and more external. Later, the training will gradually become softer and more internal. Although this book offers you the concepts of only the Southern White Crane *Qigong* and *Jin* practice, since the basic foundation and *Dao* remain the same, its theory and training methods can be applied into all other Hard and Soft Styles.

Appendix A
Translation and Glossary of Chinese Terms

Ai 哀 Sorrow.

Ai 愛 Love.

Ba Duan Jin 八段錦 Eight Pieces of Brocade. A Wai Dan Qigong practice which is said to have been created by Marshal Yue Fei during the Southern Song Dynasty (1127-1279 A.D.).

Ba Mai 八脈 Referred to as the eight extraordinary vessels. These eight vessels are considered to be Qi reservoirs, which regulate the Qi status in the primary Qi channels.

Ba Kua Chang (Baguazhang) 八卦掌 Means "Eight Trigram Palms." The name of one of the Chinese internal martial styles.

Bagua 八卦 Literally, "Eight Divinations." Also called the Eight Trigrams. In Chinese philosophy, the eight basic variations; shown in the Yi Jing as groups of single and broken lines.

Baguazhang (Ba Kua Zhang) 八卦掌 Means "Eight Trigram Palms." The name of one of the Chinese internal martial styles.

Bai He 白鶴 Means "White Crane." One of the Chinese southern martial styles.

Bai, Yu-Feng 白玉峰 A well known Chinese martial artist during the Song Dynasty (Northern and Southern, 960-1278 A.D.). Later, he and his son joined the Shaolin Temple. His monk's name was Qiu Yue Chan Shi.

Baihui (Gv-20) 百會 Literally, "hundred meetings." An important acupuncture cavity located on the top of the head. The Baihui cavity belongs to the Governing Vessel.

Bao 豹 Panther. A Chinese martial style. This style is one of the Five Animal Patterns. The other four are Tiger, Crane, Snake and Dragon.

Batuo 跋陀 An Indian Buddhist monk who came to China to preach Buddhism in 464 A.D.

Bei 撐 Expelling. A hand technique or Jin pattern in White Crane style.

Bi 閉 Means "close" or "seal."

Bi Qi 閉氣 Qi here means "air." It refers to the oxygen we inhale. Therefore Bi Qi means to "seal the oxygen supply" or "seal the breath."

Bruce Lee 李小龍 A well known Chinese martial artist and movie star during the 1960's.

Cai 採 Plucking.

Canton (Guangdong) 廣東 A province in southern China.

Chai (Sai) 釵 A kind of hairpin for ancient Chinese women. Later, it was developed into a southern Chinese weapon.

Chan 纏 To wrap or to coil. A common Chinese martial arts technique.

Chan (Ren) 禪 A Chinese school of Mahayana Buddhism which asserts that enlightenment can be attained through meditation, self-contemplation and intuition, rather than through study of scripture. Chan is called Ren in Japan.

Chan Jin 纏勁 The martial power of wrapping or coiling.

Chang Chuan (Changquan) 長拳 Means "Long Range Fist." Chang Chuan includes all northern Chinese long range martial styles.

Chang Jiang 長江 Literally, long river. Refers to the Yangtze river in southern China.

Chang 長 Long.

Chang, San-Feng 張三丰 Chang, San-Feng is credited as the creator of Taijiquan during the Song Dynasty in China (960-1127 A.D.).

Chang, Xiang-San 張詳三 A well known Chinese martial artist in Taiwan.

Changquan (Chang Chuan) 長拳 Means "Long Range Fist." Changquan includes all northern Chinese long range martial styles.

Cheng, Gin-Gsao 曾金灶 Dr. Yang, Jwing-Ming's White Crane master.

Cheng, Man-Ching 鄭曼清 A well known Chinese Taijiquan master in America during the 1960's.

Chi (Qi) 氣 The energy pervading the universe, including the energy circulating in the human body.

Chi Kung (Qigong) 氣功 The Gongfu of Qi, which means the study of Qi.

Chiang, Kai-Shek 蔣介石 A well known president in China.

Chin Na (Qin Na) 擒拿 Literally means "grab control." A component of Chinese martial arts which emphasizes grabbing techniques, to control your opponent's joints, in conjunction with attacking certain acupuncture cavities.

Chong Mai 衝脈 Thrusting Vessel. One of the eight extraordinary Qi vessels.

Chu Qiao 出竅 Means "to exit the gate." It is believed that our spirit is able to exit our body through the Baihui cavity or from our third eye.

Chui Shou 捶手 Means "hammer hand." One of the hand forms used in southern Chinese martial styles.

Confucius 孔子 A Chinese scholar, during the period of 551-479 B.C., whose philosophy has significantly influenced Chinese culture.

Da 打 To strike. Normally, to attack with the palms, fists or arms.

Da Mo 達摩 The Indian Buddhist monk who is credited with creating the Yi Jin Jing and Xi Sui Jing while at the Shaolin monastery. His last name was Sardili and he was also known as Bodhidarma. He was once the prince of a small tribe in southern India.

Dabao (Sp-21) 大包 An acupuncture cavity belonging to the Spleen Channel.

Dan Tian 丹田 "Elixir field." Located in the lower abdomen. It is considered the place which can store Qi energy.

Dan Tian Qi 丹田氣 Usually, the Qi which is converted from Original Essence and is stored in the Lower Dan Tian. This Qi is considered "water Qi" and is able to calm down the body. Also called Xian Tian Qi (Pre-Heaven Qi).

Da Zhi 大智和尚 A Japanese Buddhist monk who lived in the Yuan Dynasty, in the year 1312 A.D. After he studied Shaolin martial arts (barehands and staff) for nearly 13 years (1324 A.D.), he returned to Japan and spread Shaolin Gongfu to Japanese martial arts society.

Da Zhou Tian 大周天 Literally, "Grand Cycle Heaven." Usually translated Grand Circulation. After a Nei Dan Qigong practitioner completes Small Circulation, he will circulate his Qi through the entire body or exchange the Qi with nature.

Dao 道 The "way," by implication the "natural way."

Dao De Jing 道德經 Morality Classic. Written by Lao Zi.

Dao Jia 道家 The Dao family. Daoism. Created by Lao Zi during the Zhou Dynasty (1122-934 B.C.). In the Han Dynasty (c. 58 A.D.), it was mixed with the Buddhism to become the Daoist religion (Dao Jiao).

Deng Feng Xian Zhi 登封縣志 Deng Feng County Recording. A formal historical recording in Deng Feng County, Henan, where the Shaolin Temple is located.

Di 地 The Earth. Earth, Heaven (Tian) and Man (Ren) are the "Three Natural Powers" (San Cai).

Di Li Shi 地理師 Di Li means "geomancy" and Shi means "teacher." Therefore Di Li Shi is a teacher or master who analyzes geographic locations according to the formulas in the Yi Jing (Book of Change) and the energy distributions in the Earth. Also called Feng Shui Shi.

Dian 點 "To point" or "to press."

Dian Mai (Dim Mak) 點脈 Mai means "the blood vessel" (Xue Mai) or "the Qi channel" (Qi Mai). Dian Mai means "to press the blood vessel or Qi channel."

Dian Qi 電氣 Dian means "electricity" and so Dian Qi means "electrical energy" (electricity). In China, a word is often placed before "Qi" to identify the different kinds of energy.

Dian Xue 點穴 Dian means "to point and exert pressure" and Xue means "the cavities." Dian Xue refers to those Qin Na techniques which specialize in attacking acupuncture cavities to immobilize or kill an opponent.

Dian Xue massage 點穴按摩 A school of Chinese massage in which the acupuncture cavities are stimulated through pressing. Dian Xue massage is also called acupressure and is the root of Japanese Shiatsu.

Diao 刁 Hooking.

Dim Mak (Dian Mai) 點脈 Cantonese of "Dian Mai."

Ding 定 "To stabilize" or "to firm."

Ding Gong 定功 Stationary Gongfu; implies that the legs are not moving. In some martial arts training, it also means the Gongfu of stability. This is a Gongfu training which stabilizes your body and mind.

Ding Shen 定神 To stabilize the spirit. To keep the spirit at one place (usually the Shang Dan Tian located at the third eye). One of the exercises for regulating the Shen (spirit) in Qigong.

Dong Jin 懂勁 "Understanding Jin." One of the Jins which uses the feeling of the skin to sense the opponent's energy.

Dong Gong 動功 Moving Gongfu.

Dou 抖 Shaking. One of the White Crane Jin manifestations.

Du Mai 督脈 Usually translated "Governing Vessel." One of the eight extraordinary vessels.

Duan 斷 "To break" or "to seal."

Emei 峨嵋 Name of a mountain in Sichuan Province, China.

Er Lu Mai Fu 二路埋伏 Second way of ambush. The name of a Shaolin Long Fist sequence.

Fa Jin 發勁 "Emitting Jin." Jin is martial power, in which muscular power is manifested to its maximum from mental concentration and Qi circulation.

Fan Hu Xi 反呼吸 Reverse breathing. Also commonly called "Daoist Breathing."

Fan Tong Hu Xi 返童呼吸 Back to childhood breathing. A breathing training in Nei Dan Qigong through which the practitioner tries to regain control of the muscles in the lower abdomen. Also called "abdominal breathing."

Fang, Zhen-Dong 方振東 A well known martial artist during the Chinese Qing Dynasty (1644-1912 A.D.). Also called Fang, Zhang-Guang.

Fei Gong Fei Shou Jin 非攻非守勁 The Jins which are not used to attack or defend.

Fei He Gong 飛鶴功 Literally, Flying Crane Gong. A soft, Moving Qigong training in White Crane martial styles.

Fei He Quan 飛鶴拳 One of the four known White Crane martial styles.

Feng 封 "To seal" or "to cover."

Feng Shui Shi 風水師 Literally, "wind water teacher." Teacher or master of geomancy. Geomancy is the art or science of analyzing the natural energy relationships in a location, especially the interrelationships between "wind" and "water," hence the name. Also called Di Li Shi.

Feng Yan Shou 鳳眼手 Literally, "phoenix eye hand." A hand form commonly used in southern Chinese martial styles.

Fu Shi Hu Xi 腹式呼吸 Literally, "abdominal way of breathing." As you breathe, you use the muscles in the lower abdominal area to control the diaphragm. It is also called "back to (the) childhood breathing."

Fujian Province 福建 A province located in southeast China.

Futu (LI-18) 伏兔 Name of an acupuncture cavity which belongs to the Large Intestine Primary Qi Channel.

Ge 戈 Spear, lance or javelin; implies general weapons in this book.

Gong Jin 攻勁 Attacking or offensive Jin.

Gong Zi Shou 弓字手 Literally, "Gong word hand." A hand form commonly used in southern Chinese martial styles.

Gong (Kung) 功 Energy or hard work.

Gongfu (Kung Fu) 功夫 Means "energy-time." Anything which will take time and energy to learn or to accomplish is called Gongfu.

Gu Qi Feng mountain 古奇峰 Name of a mountain located in Xinzhu, Taiwan.

Gu Shen 谷神 Valley Spirit. The Baihui cavity on the top of the head, believed to be the place or gate where the body's Qi communicates with the Heaven Qi.

Guan Jie Hu Xi 關節呼吸 Literally, "joints breathing." A Qigong practice in which the mind is used to lead the Qi in and out at the joint areas.

Gui Qi 鬼氣 The Qi residue of a dead person. It is believed by the Chinese Buddhists and Daoists that this Qi residue is a so called ghost.

Gung Li Chuan 功力拳 The name of a barehand sequence in Chinese Long Fist martial arts.

Guohuen 國魂 Country soul or spirit.

Guoshu 國術 Abbreviation of "Zhongguo Wushu," which means "Chinese Martial Techniques."

Ha 哈 A Qigong sound which is commonly used to lead an over abundance of Qi from inside the body out and therefore reduce over-accumulated Qi.

Han 漢 A Dynasty in Chinese history (206 B.C.-221 A.D.).

Han race 漢族 The major race in China.

Han, Ching-Tang 韓慶堂 A well known Chinese martial artist, especially in Taiwan in the last forty years. Master Han is also Dr. Yang, Jwing-Ming's Long Fist Grand Master.

He Chi 鶴翅 Crane wings.

He Ma Bu 鶴馬步 A horse stance used in Southern White Crane style.

He 呵 A Qigong sound related to the heart. This sound is also commonly used in Chinese martial arts fighting.

He 和 Harmony or peace.

He 合 Means "to close."

He 鶴 Crane.

Hei 嘿 A sound commonly used in Chinese martial arts fighting.

Hen 恨 Hate.

Hen 哏 A Yin Qigong sound which is the opposite of the Ha Yang sound.

Henan 河南省 The province in China where the Shaolin Temple is located.

Heng Xin 恆心 Literally, persistent heart. This implies patience, endurance and perseverance.

Hong Quan 洪拳 A Tiger Fist style created by Hong Xi-Guang.

Hou Tian Fa 後天法 Means "Post-Heaven Techniques." An internal Qigong style dating from 550 A.D.

Hou Tian Qi 後天氣 Post-Birth Qi. This Qi is converted from the Essence of food and air and is classified as "fire Qi" since it can make your body too Yang.

Hsing Yi Chuan (Xingyiquan) 形意拳 A style of internal Chinese martial arts.

Hu 呼 A Qigong sound used to regulate the Qi status of the spleen.

Hu 虎 Tiger. A martial arts style in southern China. One of the Five Animal Patterns in the Shaolin Temple.

Hu Zhua 虎爪 Tiger Claw. A southern Chinese martial style.

Hua 化 "To neutralize."

Hua Jin 化勁 The Jin (martial power) used to neutralize anopponent's attack.

Huan Jing Bu Nao 還精補腦 Literally, "to return the Essence to nourish the brain." A Daoist Qigong training process wherein Qi which is converted from Essence is led to the brain to nourish it.

Huan 緩 Slow.

Huo Qi 活氣
Huo means "alive." Huo Qi is the Qi of a living person or animal.

Ji 擠 Means "to squeeze" or "to press."

Jia Dan Tian 假丹田 False Dan Tian. Daoists believe that the Lower Dan Tian located on the front side of the abdomen is not the real Dan Tian. The real Dan Tian corresponds to the physical center of gravity. The False Dan Tian is called Qihai (Qi ocean) in Chinese medicine.

Jiache (S-6) 頰車 Name of an acupuncture cavity. It belongs to the Stomach Channel.

Jiaji 夾脊 Literally, squeeze spine. A cavity name used by Qigong practitioners. The acupuncture name for the same cavity is Lingtai. This cavity is on the Governing Vessel.

Jianneiling (M-UE-48) 肩內陵
Name of an acupuncture cavity. A special point.

Jiexi (S-41) 解溪
An acupuncture cavity belonging to the Stomach Primary Qi Channel.

Jin 筋 Means "tendons."

Jin (Jing) 勁 Chinese martial power. A combination of "Li" (muscular power) and "Qi."

Jin Di 勁敵 A strong and powerful enemy.

Jin Feng 勁風 A strong and powerful gust of the wind.

Jin Gong 勁弓 A strong and powerful bow.

Jin Gong 勁功 Gongfu which specializes in the training of Jin manifestation.

Jin Qiang Shuo Hou 金槍鎖喉 Literally, "metal spear to thread the throat." A Hard Qigong training in which a spear head is pressed against the throat.

Jin Zhong Zhao 金鐘罩 Literally, "golden bell cover." A higher level of Iron Shirt training.

Jin, Shao-Feng 金紹峰 Dr. Yang, Jwing-Ming's White Crane Grand Master.

Jing (Jin) 勁 Chinese martial power. A combination of "Li" (muscular power) and "Qi."

Jing 精 Essence. The most refined part of anything.

Jing 靜 Calm.

Jing 經 Channels. Sometimes translated "meridian." Refers to the twelve organ-related "rivers" which circulate Qi throughout the body.

Jing Zi 精子 Literally, "essence son." The most refined part of human essence. The sperm.

Judo 柔道 A style of Japanese martial arts which originated from Chinese wrestling.

Jue Jin 覺勁 Sensing Jin. The Jin of feeling.

Jueyuan 覺遠 The monk name of a Shaolin priest during the Chinese Song Dynasty (960-1278 A.D.).

Jujitsu 柔術道 A style of Japanese martial arts which uses theories similar to Chinese Taijiquan and Qin Na.

Jun Qing 君倩 A Daoist and Chinese doctor during the Chinese Jin Dynasty (265-420 A.D.). Jun Qing is credited as the creator of the Five Animal Sports Qigong practice.

Kan 坎 One of the Eight Trigrams.

Kao Tao 高濤 Dr.Yang, Jwing-Ming's first Taijiquan master.

Karate 空手道 Literally, "barehand." Karate Do is "the barehand way." A Japanese martial art rooted in Chinese Southern White Crane.

Kong Qi 空氣 Air.

Kun 坤 One of the Eight Trigrams.

Kung Fu (Gongfu) 功夫 Means "energy-time." Anything which will take time and energy to learn or to accomplish is called Kung Fu.

Kung (Gong) 功 Means energy or hard work.

La Ma 喇嘛 A Tibetan monk. Also used for Tibetan White Crane style.

Lan Zhou 蘭州 Name of a county in ancient times. Exact location unknown to the author.

Lao Zi 老子 The creator of Daoism, also called Li Er.

Laogong (P-8) 勞宮 Cavity name. On the Pericardium Channel in the center of the palm.

Le 樂 Joy or happiness.

Li 力 The power which is generated from muscular strength.

Li 離 One of the Eight Trigrams.

Li Sou 李叟 A well known Chinese martial artist during the Chinese Song Dynasty (960-1278 A.D.).

Li, Mao-Ching 李茂清 Dr. Yang, Jwing-Ming's Long Fist master.

Li-Qi 力氣　When you use Li (muscular power) you also need Qi to support it. However, when this Qi is led by a concentrated mind, the Qi is able to manifest the muscular power to a higher level and is therefore called Jin. Li-Qi (or Qi-Li) is a general definition of Jin and commonly implies manifested power.

Lian Jing Hua Qi 練精化氣　To refine the Essence and convert it into Qi. One of the Qigong training processes through which you convert Essence into Qi.

Lian Qi Hua Shen 練氣化神　To refine the Qi to nourish the spirit. Part of the Qigong training process in which you learn how to lead Qi to the head to nourish the brain and Shen (spirit).

Lian Qi 練氣　Lian means "to train, to strengthen and to refine." A Daoist training process through which your Qi grows stronger and more abundant.

Lian Shen 練神　To train the spirit. To refine and strengthen the Shen and make it more focused.

Lian Shen Liao Xing 練神了性　To refine the spirit and end human nature. This is the final stage of spiritual Qigong training for enlightenment. In this process you learn to keep your emotions neutral and try to be undisturbed by human nature.

Liang 梁　A Dynasty in Chinese history (502-557 A.D.)

Liang, Shou-Yu 梁守渝　A well-known Chinese martial arts and Qigong master. Currently resides in Vancouver, Canada.

Liang Wu 梁武　An emperor of the Chinese Liang Dynasty.

Lien Bu Chuan 連步拳　One of the basic Long Fist barehand sequences.

Lingtai (Gv-10) 靈台　An acupuncture cavity belonging to the Governing Vessel.

Liu He Ba Fa 六合八法　Literally, "six combinations eight methods." One of the Chinese internal martial arts, its techniques are combined from Taijiquan, Xingyi and Baguazhang. It is reported that his internal martial art was created by Chen Bo during the Song Dynasty (960-1279 A.D.).

Long 龍　Dragon. One of the original Five Animal Patterns martial arts developed in the Shaolin Temple.

Lu, Si-Niang 呂四娘　A well-known female martial artist in China during the Qing Dynasty(1644-1912 A.D.). Later, Lu, Si-Niang retired and became a Buddhist nun. Her nun name was Wumei. She was the creator of the Wumei martial style.

Luo 絡　The small Qi channels which branch out from the primary Qi channels and are connected to the skin and to the bone marrow.

Ma Bu 馬步　Horse Stance. One of the basic stances in Chinese martial arts.

Mai 脈　Means "vessel" or "Qi channel."

Mencius (372-289 B.C.) 孟子　A well-known scholar who followed the philosophy of Confucius during the Chinese Zhou Dynasty (909-255 B.C.).

Mian 綿　Soft.

Ming He Quan 鳴鶴拳　Shouting Crane Fist. One of the four major Southern White Crane styles.

Mo 摩　Rub. A major technique of Chinese Qigong massage.

Na 拿　Means "to hold" or "to grab."

Nanking Central Guoshu Institute 南京中央國術館　A national martial arts institute organized by the Chinese government in 1928.

Nei Dan 內丹　Literally, internal elixir. A form of Qigong in which Qi (the elixir) is built up in the body and spread out to the limbs.

Nei Jin 內勁　Internal power. The Jin power in which the Qi from the Lower Dan Tian is used to support the muscles. When the muscles predominate and local Qi is used to support them, it is called Wai Jin (external Jin).

Nei Shi Gongfu 內視功夫 Nei Shi means "to look internally," so Nei Shi Gongfu refers to the art of looking inside yourself to read the state of your health and the condition of your Qi.

Nei Wai He Yi 內外合一 Literally, "internal and external unified as one." Means the unification of the external action and the internal Qi.

Neiguan (P-6) 內關 An acupuncture cavity belonging to the Pericardium Primary Qi Channel.

Ni Wan Gong 泥丸宮 The place where the Mud Pill resides. The brain.

Ni Wan 泥丸 Mud Pill. Pituitary gland.

Ning Shen 凝神 To condense or focus on the spirit. In Qigong training, after you are able to keep your spirit in one place, you learn how to condense it into a tiny spot and make it stronger.

Nu 怒 Anger.

Ping 平 Peace and harmony.

Putian 浦田 Name of a county in China's Fujian Province.

Qi (Chi) 氣 Chinese term for universal energy. A current popular model is that the Qi circulating in the human body is bioelectric in nature.

Qi Jing Ba Mai 奇經八脈 Literally, "strange (odd) channels eight vessels." Usually referred to as the eight extraordinary vessels or simply as the vessels. Called odd or strange because they are not well understood and some of them do not exist in pairs.

Qi Hua Lun 氣化論 Qi variation thesis. An ancient treatise which discusses the variations of Qi in the universe.

Qi Huo 起火 To start the fire. In Qigong practice, when you start to build up Qi at the Lower Dan Tian.

Qi Qing Liu Yu 七情六慾 Seven emotions and six desires. The seven emotions are happiness, anger, sorrow, joy, love, hate and desire. The six desires are the six sensory pleasures associated with the eyes, nose, ears, tongue, body and mind.

Qi Shi 氣勢 Shi means the way something looks or feels. Therefore, the feeling of Qi as it expresses itself.

Qi-Li 氣力 When you use Li (muscular power) you also need Qi to support it. However, when this Qi is led by a concentrated mind, the Qi is able to manifest the muscular power to a higher level and is therefore called Jin. Li-Qi or Qi-Li is a general definition of Jin and commonly implies manifested power.

Qi-Xue 氣血 Literally, "Qi blood." According to Chinese medicine, Qi and blood cannot be separated in our body and so the two words are commonly used together.

Qian Xu 謙虛 Humility.

Qigong (Chi Kung) 氣功 The Gongfu of Qi, which means the study of Qi.

Qihai (Co-6) 氣海 An acupuncture cavity belonging to the Conception Vessel.

Qimen (Li-14) 期門 An acupuncture cavity belonging to the Liver Channel.

Qin (Chin) 擒 Means 'to catch" or "to seize."

Qin Na (Chin Na) 擒拿 Literally means "grab control." A component of Chinese martial arts which emphasizes grabbing techniques to control your opponent's joints, in conjunction with attacking certain acupuncture cavities.

Qing Dynasty 清朝 A Dynasty in Chinese history; The last Chinese Dynasty (1644-1912 A.D.).

Qiu Yue Chan Shi 秋月禪師 A Shaolin monk during the Chinese Song Dynasty (960-1278 A.D.). His layman name was Bai, Yu-Feng.

Quchi (LI-11) 曲池 Name of an acupuncture cavity. It belongs to the Large Intestine Channel.

Re Qi 熱氣 Re means warmth or heat. Generally, Re Qi is used to represent heat. It is used sometimes to imply that a person or animal is still alive since the body is warm.

Ren 人 Man or mankind.

Ren 仁 Humanity, kindness or benevolence.

Ren Mai 任脈 Conception Vessel. One of the Eight Extraordinary Vessels.

Ren Nai 忍耐 Endurance.

Ren Qi 人氣 Human Qi.

Ren Shi 人事 Literally, human relations. Human events, activities and relationships.

Rou Jin 柔勁 Soft Jin. The Jin manifested as softly as a whip.

Ru Jia 儒家 Literally, "Confucian family." Scholars following Confucian thoughts; Confucianists.

Ruan-Ying Jin 軟硬勁 Soft-Hard Jin. The Jin in which the body is soft at the beginning of manifestation and right before arriving on target, turns hard.

Sa 煞 A sound used in Chinese martial arts fighting.

Sai (Chai) 釵 A kind of hairpin for ancient Chinese women. Later, it was developed into a southern Chinese weapon.

San Bao 三寶 Three treasures. Essence (Jing), energy (Qi) and spirit (Shen). Also called San Yuan (three origins).

San Cai 三才 Three powers. Heaven, Earth and Man.

San Gong 散功 Literally, "energy dispersion." A state of premature degeneration of the muscles where the Qi cannot effectively energize them. It can be caused by earlier overtraining.

San Guan 三關 Three gates. In Small Circulation training, the three cavities on the Governing Vessel which are usually obstructed and must be opened.

San Shou 散手 Literally, "random hands." Implies techniques executed randomly. This means free sparring.

San Yuan 三元 Three origins. Also called "San Bao" (three treasures). Human Essence (Jing), energy (Qi) and spirit (Shen).

Sardili 沙地利 The last name of Da Mo. Also known as Bodhidarma.

Seng Bing 僧兵 Monk soldiers. The monks who also trained martial arts to protect the property of the temple.

Shang Dan Tian 上丹田 Upper Dan Tian. Located at the third eye, it is the residence of the Shen (spirit).

Shao Yuan 邵元和尚 A Japanese Buddhist monk who went to Shaolin Temple in 1335 A.D. During this stay, he mastered calligraphy, painting, Chan theory (i.e., Ren) and Shaolin Gongfu. He returned to Japan in 1347 A.D. and was considered a "Country Spirit" (Guohuen) by the Japanese people. This confirms that Shaolin martial techniques were imported into Japan for at least seven hundred years.

Shaohai (H-3) 少海 Name of an acupuncture cavity. It belongs to the Heart Channel.

Shaolin 少林 "Young woods." Name of the Shaolin Temple.

Shaolin Temple 少林寺 A monastery located in Henan Province, China. The Shaolin Temple is well known because of its martial arts training.

She 蛇 Snake. One of the original Five Animal Martial Patterns developed in the Shaolin Temple. The other four are tiger, crane, dragon and panther.

Shen Gu 神谷 Spirit valley. Formed by the two lobes of the brain, with the Upper Dan Tian at the exit.

Shen Hu Xi 深呼吸 Deep breathing. Means to breathe from the lower abdomen area.

Shen 神 Spirit. According to Chinese Qigong, the Shen resides at the Upper Dan Tian (the third eye).

Shen 深 Deep.

Shen Tai 神胎 Spiritual embryo. It is also called "Ling Tai."

Sheng Tai 聖胎 Holy embryo. Another name for the spiritual embryo (Shen Tai).

Shi Er Jing 十二經 The Twelve Primary Qi Channels in Chinese medicine.

Shi He Quan 食鶴拳 Eating Crane Fist. One of the four major Southern White Crane martial styles. Also called Zhao He Quan.

Shi Zi Tang 十字趟 Word Ten Sequence. A middle level Northern Long Fist sequence.

Shi, You-San 石友三 A military Warlord during the Chinese civil war in the 1920's. He was known as the one who burned the Shaolin Temple in 1928.

Shou Jin 守勁 Defensive Jin. Those Jins which are mainly used for defensive purposes.

Shou Shen 守神 To keep the mind at the spirit. A Qigong meditation training.

Shuai 摔 Means "to throw." An abbreviation of "Shuai Jiao" (wrestling).

Shuai Jiao 摔交 Chinese wrestling. Part of Chinese martial arts.

Shuxi (N-CA-6) 鼠蹊 An acupuncture cavity belonging to miscellaneous cavities.

Si Qi 死氣 Dead Qi. The Qi remaining in a dead body. Sometimes called "ghost Qi" (Gui Qi).

Si Xin Hu Xi 四心呼吸 A Qigong Nei Dan practice in which a practitioner uses his mind with the coordination of the breathing to lead the Qi to the centers of the palms and feet.

Song 宋 A Dynasty in Chinese history (960-1278 A.D.).

Southern Song Dynasty 南宋 After the Song was conquered by the Jin race from Mongolia, the Song people moved to the south and established another country, called Southern Song (1127-1278 A.D.).

Su He Quan 宿鶴拳 One of the major styles of Southern White Crane Chinese martial arts. This style is also called Zhan He Quan (Trembling Crane), Zong He Quan (Ancestral), Zong He Quan (Jumping Crane).

Suan Ming Shi 算命師 Literally, "calculate life teacher." A fortune teller who is able to calculate your future and destiny.

Sui Dynasty 隋 A dynasty in China during the period of 589-618 A.D.

Sui Xi 髓息 Sui means the marrow or brain. Therefore, Sui Xi means the Qigong breathing technique which is able to lead the Qi to the bone marrow and brain.

Sun, Yat-Sen 孫中山 Father of China.

Tai Chi Chuan (Taijiquan) 太極拳 A Chinese internal martial style which based on the theory of Taiji (grand ultimate).

Tai Xi 胎息 Embryo Breathing. One of the final goals in regulating the breath, Embryo Breathing enables you to generate a "baby Shen" at the Huang Ting (yellow yard).

Taiji 太極 Means "grand ultimate." It is this force which generates two poles, Yin and Yang.

Taiji Qigong 太極氣功 A Qigong training specially designed for Taijiquan practice.

Taijiquan (Tai Chi Chuan) 太極拳 A Chinese internal martial style which is based on the theory of Taiji (grand ultimate).

Taipei 台北 The capital city of Taiwan located in the north.

Taiwan 台灣 An island to the south-east of mainland China. Also known as "Formosa."

Taiwan University 台灣大學 A well known university located in northern Taiwan.

Taiyang (M-HN-9) 太陽 Name of an acupuncture cavity. A special point.

Taizuquan 太祖拳 A style of Chinese external martial arts.

Tamkang 淡江 Name of a University in Taiwan.

Tamkang College Guoshu Club 淡江國術社 A Chinese martial arts club founded by Dr. Yang when he was studying in Tamkang College.

Tan Tui 彈腿 Springing leg. The training which enables you to kick your leg as a spring.

Tan 彈 Rebounding or springing.

Tang Dynasty 唐 A dynasty in Chinese history during the period 713-907 A.D.

Ti 踢 Means "to kick."

Ti 提 Means "to lift."

Ti Sui Xi 體髓息 Skin Marrow Breathing.

Ti Xi 體息 Body breathing or skin breathing. In Qigong, the exchanging of Qi with the surrounding environment through the skin.

Tian Mountain 天山 Literally, "sky mountain." The name of a mountain located in Xinjiang Province, China.

Tian 天 Heaven or sky. In ancient China, people believed that Heaven was the most powerful natural energy in this universe.

Tian Qi 天氣 Heaven Qi. It is now commonly used to mean the weather, since weather is governed by Heaven Qi.

Tian Ren He Yi 天人合一 Literally, "Heaven and man unified as one." A high level of Qigong practice in which a Qigong practitioner, through meditation, is able to communicate his Qi with heaven's Qi.

Tian Shi 天時 Heavenly timing. The repeated natural cycles generated by the heavens such as: seasons, months, days and hours.

Tianron (SI-17) 天容 An acupuncture cavity belonging to the Small Intestine Primary Qi Channel.

Tiao Qi 調氣 To regulate the Qi.

Tiao Shen 調身 To regulate the body.

Tiao Shen 調神 To regulate the spirit.

Tiao Xi 調息 To regulate the breathing.

Tiao Xin 調心 To regulate the emotional mind.

Tie Ban Qiao 鐵板橋 Literally, "Iron Board Bridge." A special martial arts strength and endurance training for the torso.

Tie Bu Shan 鐵布衫 Iron shirt. Gongfu training which toughens the body externally and internally.

Tie Sha Zhang 鐵砂掌 Literally, "iron sand palm." A special martial arts conditioning for the palms.

Tie Tou Gong 鐵頭功 Literally, "iron head Gong." A special martial arts conditioning to make the head strong enough for attacking.

Ting Jin 聽勁 Listening Jin. A special training which uses the skin to feel the opponent's energy and from this feeling to further understand his intention.

Tui Na 推拿 Means "to push and grab." A category of Chinese massages for healing and injury treatment.

Tui 推 Push. A major technique in Chinese Tui Na Qigong massage.

Tuo 托 Lifting, raising or holding upward.

Wai Dan Chi Kung (Wai Dan Qigong) 外丹氣功 External Elixir Qigong. In Wai Dan Qigong, a practitioner will generate Qi to the limbs and then allow the Qi to flow inward to nourish the internal organs.

Wai Dan 外丹 External elixir. External Qigong exercises in which a practitioner will build up the Qi in his limbs and then lead it into the center of the body for nourishment.

Wai Jia 外家 External family. Those martial schools which practice the external styles of Chinese martial arts.

Wai Jin 外勁 External power. The type of Jin where the muscles predominate and only local Qi is used to support the muscles.

Wei Qi 衛氣 Protective Qi or Guardian Qi. The Qi at the surface of the body which generates a shield to protect the body from negative external influences such as colds.

Weilu 尾閭 Tail bone. The same place is called Changqiang (Gv-1) in Chinese medicine.

Wen Huo 文火 Scholar fire. One of the soft types of breathing used in Chinese Qigong practice.

Wilson Chen 陳威伸 Dr. Yang, Jwing-Ming's friend.

Wingchun (Wing Chun) 詠春拳 (永春拳) Also called Yongchun Quan. A southern Chinese martial style derived from Southern White Crane during the Qing Qian Long period (1736-1796 A.D.). There is a saying that Yongchun Quan was started by the lady Yan, Yong-Chun who learned Southern White Crane techniques from the Buddhist nun Wumei in the mountains of Yunnan Province.

Wu 武 Means "martial."

Wu Huo 武火 Martial fire. One of the hard and fast types of breathing used in Chinese Qigong practice.

Wu Qin Shi 五禽戲 Five Animal Sports. A set of medical Qigong practices created by Jun Qing during Chinese Jin Dynasty (265-420 A.D.).

Wu Xin 五心 Five centers. The face, the Laogong cavities in both palms and the Yongquan cavities on the bottoms of both feet.

Wu Xin Hu Xi 五心呼吸 One of the Qigong Nei Dan practices in which a practitioner uses his mind in coordination with breathing to lead the Qi to the center of the palms, feet and head.

Wudang Mountain 武當山 Located in Fubei Province in China.

Wude 武德 Martial morality.

Wuji Qigong 無極氣功 A style of Taiji Qigong practice.

Wuji 無極 Means "no extremity."

Wumei 五枚 A well-known female martial artist in China during Qing Dynasty(1644-1912 A.D.). Her layman name is Lu, Si-Niang. Later, she retired and became a Buddhist nun. Her nun name was Wumei. She was the creator of the Wumei martial style.

Wushu 武術 Literally, "martial techniques."

Wuxing Quan 五形拳 Five Shape Fists or Five Animal Patterns. The martial art styles developed in the Chinese Shaolin Temple. The five animals include: Tiger, Crane, Dragon, Snake and Panther.

Wuyi 武藝 Literally, "martial arts."

Xi 細 Slender.

Xi 喜 Joy, delight and happiness.

Xi Sui Gong 洗髓功 Gongfu for marrow and brain washing Qigong practice.

Xi Sui Jing 洗髓經 Literally, Washing Marrow/Brain Classic, usually translated Marrow/Brain Washing Classic. A Qigong training which specializes in leading Qi to the marrow to cleanse it or to the brain to nourish the spirit for enlightenment. It is believed that Xi Sui Jing training is the key to longevity and achieving spiritual enlightenment.

Xia Dan Tian 下丹田 Lower Dan Tian. Located in the lower abdomen, it is believed to be the residence of water Qi (Original Qi).

Xian Jin 顯勁 The Jins which are manifested externally and can be seen.

Xian Tian Qi 先天氣 Pre-Birth Qi or Pre-Heaven Qi. Also called Dan Tian Qi. The Qi which is converted from Original Essence and is stored in the Lower Dan Tian. Considered to be "water Qi," it is able to calm the body.

Xiao Jiu Tian 小九天 Small Nine Heaven. A Qigong style created around 550 A.D.

Xiao Zhou Tian 小周天 Literally, small heavenly cycle. Also called Small Circulation. In Qigong, when you can use your mind to lead Qi through the Conception and Governing Vessels, you have completed "Xiao Zhou Tian."

Xiao 孝 Filial Piety.

Xin Yong 信用 Trust.

Xin Yuan Yi Ma 心猿意馬 Literally, "heart monkey Yi horse." Xin (heart) is used to represent the emotional mind which is acting as a monkey, unsteady and disturbing. Yi is the mind which is generated from calm and clear thinking and judgment (i.e. wisdom mind). The Yi is like a horse, calm and powerful.

Xin 心 Means "heart." Xin means the mind generated from emotional disturbance.

Xin 信 Trust.

Xinglong 星龍 A Shaolin monk who was sent to Tibet for Buddhism research. It is said that he brought White Crane martial arts to Tibet, which became Northern Tibetan White Crane style, La Ma.

Xingyi 形意 An abbreviation of Xingyiquan.

Xingyiquan (Hsing Yi Chuan) 形意拳 One of the best known Chinese internal martial styles created by Marshal Yue Fei during the Chinese Song Dynasty (1103-1142 A.D.).

Xinzhu Xian 新竹縣 Birthplace of Dr. Yang, Jwing-Ming in Taiwan.

Xiong Er mountain 熊耳山 Literally, "bear ear mountain." Name of a mountain located near the Shaolin Temple.

Xiong Shang Shui Shi 胸上碎石 To break a cement block on the chest. A hard martial Qigong training.

Xiu Qi 修氣 Cultivate the Qi. Cultivate implies to protect, maintain and refine. A Buddhist Qigong training.

Yan 言 Talking or speaking.

Yan, San-Niang 嚴三娘 Another name of Yan, Yong-Chun.

Yan, Yong-Chun 嚴永春 A female Chinese martial artist who is credited as the creator of the Wingchun (Wing Chun) martial style (also known as Yongchun Quan) during the Qing Qian Long period (1736-1796 A.D.).

Yang 陽 Too sufficient. One of the two poles. The other is Yin.

Yang Jin 陽勁 The Jins which are aggressive and mainly used for offense.

Yang, Jwing-Ming 楊俊敏 Author of this book.

Yang, You-Ji 養由基 A famous archer during the Chinese Spring and Autumn period (722-481 B.C.).

Yi 意 Wisdom mind. The mind generated from wise judgment.

Yi 義 Justice or righteousness.

Yi Jin Jing 易筋經 Literally, Changing Muscle/Tendon Classic, usually called The Muscle/Tendon Changing Classic. Credited to Da Mo around 550 A.D., this book discusses Wai Dan Qigong training for strengthening the physical body.

Yi Jing 易經 Book of Changes. A book of divination written during the Zhou Dynasty (1122-255 B.C.).

Yi Li 毅力 Perseverance.

Yi Lu Mai Fa 一路埋伏 A Long Fist middle level sequence.

Yi Shou Dan Tian 意守丹田 Keep your Yi on your Lower Dan Tian. In Qigong training, you keep your mind at the Lower Dan Tian in order to build up Qi. When you are circulating your Qi, you always lead your Qi back to your Lower Dan Tian before you stop.

Yi Yi Yin Qi 以意引氣 Use your Yi (wisdom mind) to lead your Qi. A Qigong technique. Yi cannot be pushed, but it can be led. The is best done with the Yi.

Yi Zhi 意志 Will.

Yifeng (TB-17) 翳風 An acupuncture cavity belonging to the Triple Burner Primary Qi Channel.

Yin 陰 Deficient. One of the two poles. The other is Yang.

Yin Jin 引勁 The Jin (martial power) of leading.

Ying Gong 硬功 Hard Gongfu. Any Chinese martial training which emphasizes physical strength and power.

Ying Jin 硬勁 Hard Jin. The Jin which is manifested mainly with muscles.

Ying Qigong 硬氣功 Hard Qigong. A Qigong training which emphasizes muscular strength and endurance. Hard Qigong is the foundation of Hard Jin.

Yong Gan 勇敢 Bravery.

Yongchun Quan (Wingchun) 詠春拳 (永春拳) A southern Chinese martial style derived from Southern White Crane during the Qing Qian Long period (1736-1796 A.D.). There is a saying that Yongchun Quan was started by the Lady Yan, Yong-Chun, who learned Southern White Crane techniques from the Buddhist nun Wumei in the mountains of Yunnan Province.

Yongquan (K-1) 湧泉 Bubbling Well. Name of an acupuncture cavity belonging to the Kidney Primary Qi Channel.

You 悠 Long, far, meditative, continuous, slow and soft.

Yu 慾 Desire.

Yuan Dynasty 元代 A Chinese Dynasty during the period of 1206-1368 A.D.

Yuan Jing 元精 Original Essence. The fundamental, original substance inherited from your parents, it is converted into Original Qi.

Yuan Qi 元氣 Original Qi. The Qi created from the Original Essence inherited from your parents.

Yue Fei 岳飛 A Chinese hero in the Southern Song Dynasty (1127-1279 A.D.). Said to have created Ba Duan Jin, Xingyiquan and Yue's Ying Zhua.

Yun 勻 Uniform or even.

Yun 雲 Cloud. When it is used in martial arts, it means a smooth horizontal circular movement.

Yunnan Province 雲南 A province in southern China.

Yuzhen 玉枕 Jade pillow. One of the three gates of Small Circulation Qigong training.

Zhan He Quan 顫鶴拳 Means Trembling or Shaking Crane. One of the four main Southern White Crane styles. This style is sometimes called: Zong He Quan (Ancestral Crane), Zong He Quan, (Jumping Crane), Su He Quan (Sleeping Crane).

Zhan Jin 顫勁 Trembling Jin.

Zhang Dao-Ling 張道陵 A Daoist who combined scholarly Daoism with Buddhist philosophies and created Religious Daoism (Dao Jiao) during the Chinese Eastern Han Dynasty (25-221 A.D.).

Zhao 趙 One of the kingdoms during the period of the Warring States (475-222 B.C.).

Zhao He Quan 朝鶴拳 One of four major Southern White Crane styles. It is also called Shi He Quan (Eating Crane Fist).

Zhen Dan Tian 眞丹田 The Real Dan Tian, which is located at the physical center of gravity.

Zheng Hu Xi 正呼吸 Formal Breathing. More commonly called Buddhist Breathing.

Zheng Qi 正氣 Righteous Qi. When a person is righteous, it is said that he has righteous Qi which evil Qi cannot overcome.

Zheng Yi 正義 Righteousness.

Zhi 止 Stop.

Zhong 忠 Loyalty.

Zhong Cheng 忠誠 Literally, loyalty sincerity. Loyalty to someone or something from the deep heart.

Zhong Dan Tian 中丹田 Middle Dan Tian. Located in the area of the solar plexus, it is the residence of fire Qi.

Zhong Guo Wushu 中國武術 Chinese Wushu.

Zhong Guo 中國 Literally, "central country." This name was given by the neighboring countries of China. China was considered the cultural and spiritual center from the point of view of the Asian countries in ancient times.

Zhou 周 Roundness or completeness.

Zhuan 轉 Means "to turn around" or " to twist."

Zhuang Zhou 莊周 A contemporary of Mencius who advocated Daoism.

Zhuang Zi 莊子 Zhuang Zhou. A contemporary of Mencius who advocated Daoism. Zhuang Zi also means the works of Zhuang Zhou.

Zhuang 撞 Bumping.

Zong He Quan 宗鶴拳 Ancestral Crane Fist. One of the main Southern White Crane styles. It is also called: Zhan He Quan (Trembling Crane Fist), Zong He Quan (Jumping Crane Fist) or Su He Quan (Sleeping Crane Fist).

Z'ong He Quan 蹤鶴拳 Jumping Crane Fist. One of the main Southern White Crane styles. It is also called: Zong He Quan (Ancestral Crane Fist), Zhan He Quan (Trembling Crane Fist) or Su He Quan (Sleeping Crane Fist).

Zong Jin 宗勁 Ancestral Jin; trembling or shaking Jin.

Zun Jing 尊敬 Respect.

SELECTED BOOKS FROM YMAA

more products available from...

YMAA Publication Center, Inc. 楊氏東方文化出版中心
4354 Washington Street Roslindale, MA 02131
1-800-669-8892 • ymaa@aol.com • www.ymaa.com